New Frontiers in Hepatology

New Frontiers in Hepatology

Edited by Amy McMahon

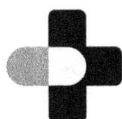

AMERICAN
MEDICAL PUBLISHERS
www.americanmedicalpublishers.com

American Medical Publishers,
41 Flatbush Avenue,
1st Floor, New York,
NY 11217, USA

Visit us on the World Wide Web at:
www.americanmedicalpublishers.com

ISBN: 978-1-63927-196-2

Cataloging-in-Publication Data

New frontiers in hepatology / edited by Amy McMahon.
    p. cm.
Includes bibliographical references and index.
ISBN 978-1-63927-196-2
1. Hepatology. 2. Gastroenterology. 3. Liver--Diseases. I. McMahon, Amy.
RC801 .N49 2022
616.33--dc23

Table of Contents

Preface

This book aims to highlight the current researches and provides a platform to further the scope of innovations in this area. This book is a product of the combined efforts of many researchers and scientists, after going through thorough studies and analysis from different parts of the world. The objective of this book is to provide the readers with the latest information of the field.

Hepatology is a field of medicine which studies the pathologies of the liver, including their management and diagnosis. Hepatic disease or liver disease causes damage to the liver. They are majorly caused by viral or parasitic infections, alcohol overconsumption, obesity and metabolic syndrome, genetics and genetic disorders, etc. Certain signs of liver disease are jaundice, coagulopathy and thrombocytopenia, confusion and altered consciousness, ascites and bleeding symptoms. The assessment of the liver is possible through a variety of liver function tests. Imaging allows the examination of liver tissue and bile ducts. Ultrasound, transient elastography and magnetic resonance imaging are used to assess the condition. Liver biopsy is another definitive diagnostic test for liver disease. The treatment of each liver disease requires a unique therapeutic modality. Antiviral medications are generally prescribed for the treatment of hepatitis B. Steroid-based drugs are useful in autoimmune hepatitis, while venesection is a routine procedure in hemochromatosis. This book discusses the fundamentals as well as modern approaches of hepatology. It unfolds the innovative aspects of hepatology which will be crucial for the progress in the understanding and management of liver diseases. The extensive content of this book provides the readers with a thorough understanding of the subject.

I would like to express my sincere thanks to the authors for their dedicated efforts in the completion of this book. I acknowledge the efforts of the publisher for providing constant support. Lastly, I would like to thank my family for their support in all academic endeavors.

Editor

Development of a transgenic mouse model of hepatocellular carcinoma with a liver fibrosis background

Sook In Chung[1,2†], Hyuk Moon[1,2†], Dae Yeong Kim[1], Kyung Joo Cho[1], Hye-Lim Ju[1], Do Young Kim[3], Sang Hoon Ahn[3], Kwang-Hyub Han[3*] and Simon Weonsang Ro[1,4*]

Abstract

Background: Liver fibrosis and its end-stage disease, cirrhosis, are major risk factors for hepatocellular carcinoma (HCC) and present in 80 to 90 % of patients with HCC. Current genetically engineered mouse models for HCC, however, generally do not feature liver fibrosis, which is a critical discrepancy between human HCC and murine models thereof. In this study, we developed a simple transgenic mouse model of HCC within the context of a fibrotic liver.

Methods: Employing hydrodynamic transfection (HT), coupled with the *Sleeping Beauty* (SB) transposon system, liver was stably transfected with transposons expressing cMyc and a short hairpin RNA down-regulating p53 (shp53). A chronic liver injury model, induced by hepatotoxic carbon tetrachloride (CCl_4), was applied to the transgenic mice, allowing cells expressing cMyc plus shp53 to become malignant in the background of liver fibrosis.

Results: Livers harvested about 3 months after HT had excessive collagen deposition and activated hepatic stellate cells surrounding the tumors. Hepatocarcinogenesis was significantly accelerated in the fibrotic livers compared to those of the control, significantly decreasing the life span of the mice. The tumor incidence and average number of tumors per mouse were significantly higher in the group treated with CCl_4 compared to the vehicle-treated control mice, following HT ($p < 0.01$).

Conclusions: Considering the simplicity and efficiency in generating HCC for fibrotic livers, the transgenic HCC model has the potential to be effectively used in preclinical testing of HCC anticancer therapy and in studies of hepatocarcinogenesis in fibrotic livers.

Keywords: Transgenic mouse, Hepatocellular carcinoma, Fibrosis, Hydrodynamic transfection, Liver injury

Background

Hepatocellular carcinoma (HCC) is one of the most prevalent and lethal cancers worldwide, ranking third among all cancer-related mortalities and accounting for 500,000 deaths annually [1, 2]. Most patients with HCC have a long history of chronic liver disease caused by diverse factors including hepatitis B and C viral infection, alcohol abuse, diabetes, and obesity [3–6]. Persistent injury to the liver from such factors leads to fibrotic scars in the tissue, characterized by an excessive accumulation of collagen fibers in the space of Disse [7, 8]. Liver fibrosis and its end-stage disease, cirrhosis, are highly associated with HCC. Fibrosis and cirrhosis are present in 80 to 90 % of patients with hepatocellular carcinoma and the 5-year cumulative risk for the development of HCC in patients with cirrhosis is between 5 and 30 % [2, 9].

Genetically engineered mouse (GEM) models for HCC have been generated for activated oncogenic signaling pathways or inactivated tumor-suppressing pathways, making significant contributions to our understanding of the genetic mechanism underlying the pathogenesis [10, 11]. Development of a GEM model usually involves expensive and time-consuming processes, such as genetic

* Correspondence: gihankhy@yuhs.ac; simonr@yuhs.ac
†Equal contributors
3Department of Internal Medicine, Yonsei University College of Medicine, Seoul 120-752, South Korea
1Institute of Gastroenterology, Yonsei University College of Medicine, Seoul 120-752, South Korea
Full list of author information is available at the end of the article

manipulation of target cells, subsequent implantation, and breeding of the animal. Furthermore, current GEM models for HCC generally do not feature liver fibrosis, calling into question whether the models can reliably recapitulate human HCC [10, 12]. Given the high association of chronic liver injury and fibrosis with the development of human HCC, a novel animal model is needed in which HCC is induced within the microenvironment of hepatic injury and fibrosis.

A very elegant and simple method was recently developed for liver-specific transgenesis in which the hydrodynamics-based transfection (HT) method was coupled with the *Sleeping Beauty* (SB) transposase system [13]. This simple liver-specific transgenic approach allowed generation of various HCC transgenic models with reduced time and resources [14]. In this study we developed a transgenic model for HCC via HT of transposons expressing cMyc and short hairpin RNA down-regulating $p53$ (shp53). To induce HCC within the context of hepatic injury and fibrosis, mice transfected with cMyc plus shp53 were repeatedly treated with carbon tetrachloride (CCl_4), a hepatotoxic chemical that induces chronic liver damage [15, 16]. Using the mouse model, the effect of CCl_4 treatment and liver fibrosis on hepatocarcinogenesis was investigated.

Methods
Animals
All experiments involving live mice were performed according to the Guidelines and Regulations for the Care and Use of Laboratory Animals in AAALAC-accredited facilities, and were approved by the Animal Policy and Welfare Committee of the Yonsei University College of Medicine (Permit number: 2014–0261). The mice were 5–to 6-week-old C57BL/6 males purchased from the Orientbio (Seongnam, Korea).

Plasmids and hydrodynamic transfection
The plasmid pT2/GFP harboring a transposon encoding the enhanced green fluorescent protein (GFP) was described previously [17]. The cDNA encoding murine cMyc was PCR amplified from pCX-cMyc, a gift from Dr. Shinya Yamanaka (Addgene plasmid # 19772). The amplified cDNA replaced the GFP cDNA in pT2/GFP, generating pT2/cMyc. The pPGK-SB13 plasmid, encoding SB transposase under the control of the phosphoglycerate kinase (PGK) promoter, was a gift from Dr. John Ohlfest. The transposon plasmid, pT2/shp53/GFP4, which encodes a short hairpin RNA against the tumor suppressor p53, with GFP as a reporter, was a gift from Dr. John Ohlfest and is referred to as pT2/shp53 [18]. For hydrodynamic injection, 14 µg of pT2/cMyc and 14 µg of pT2/shp53 (or pT2/GFP as a control) were mixed with 9 µg of pPGK-SB13 and then suspended in 2 ml of Lactated

Ringer solution. The DNA solution was injected into the lateral tail veins of 6-week-old mice (0.1 ml/g body weight) in less than 7 s.

Carbon tetrachloride (CCl_4) treatment
CCl_4 was administered to mice twice weekly at a dose of 1 ml/kg body weight [16]. Mice were monitored regularly following administration of the CCl_4, and treated and sacrificed according to institutional guidelines.

Liver harvest and tissue processing
Mice were deeply anesthetized by intraperitoneal injection of zoletil (30 mg/kg) and xylazine (10 mg/kg). Livers were harvested after a midline laparotomy incision and then carefully inspected for tumor nodules. Extracted livers were then immersed in 10 % neutral-buffered formalin. Fixed liver specimens were embedded in paraffin blocks.

H&E staining and histopathological examination
Liver specimens embedded in paraffin blocks were sectioned into 4-µm slices, which were stained with hematoxylin and eosin (H&E) and picro-sirius red following standard protocols. Liver lesions were assessed as described by Frith et al. [19]. Slides were analyzed and photographed using a microscope (Eclipse Ti; Nikon, Tokyo, Japan) equipped with a digital camera.

Western blotting
Liver tissues were homogenized and digested in 1× RIPA buffer containing phosphatase inhibitor cocktail solution (GenDEPOT, Barker, TX, USA). Western blot experiments were performed following the standard protocol. The following primary antibodies were used: anti-c-Myc (ab32072; Abcam, Cambridge, UK), anti-p53 (sc-6243; Santa Cruz Biotechnology, Santa Cruz, CA, USA), and anti-GAPDH (#2118; Cell Signaling Technology, Danvers, MA, USA). Anti-rabbit IgG–HRP (Sigma-Aldrich, St. Louis, MO, USA) was used as the secondary antibody. Bands were detected using the enhanced chemiluminescence (ECL) Western blot detection system (Amersham Pharmacia Biotech, Piscataway, NJ, USA).

Immunohistochemistry
Paraffin sections were deparaffinized in xylene and rehydrated through a gradual decrease in concentration of ethanol. The antigen epitopes were then unmasked using sodium citrate buffer (pH 6.0). Subsequently, the sections were incubated overnight at 4 °C with the following primary antibodies: anti-α-smooth muscle actin (ab5694; Abcam), anti-c-Myc (ab32072; Abcam) and anti-GFP (#2555; Cell Signaling Technology). After primary incubation, sections were incubated with the appropriate biotinylated secondary antibodies, followed by

treatment with freshly prepared DAB substrates (Vector Laboratories, Burlingame, CA, USA). Sections were lightly counter-stained with hematoxylin and mounted.

Mouse survival and statistical analysis

Mice were monitored daily for illness symptoms. Kaplan–Meier survival data were analyzed using a log-rank test. Statistical analyses were conducted using an unpaired parametric Student's t-test or Fisher's exact test, as appropriate. A value of $p < 0.01$ was taken to indicate statistical significance.

Results

Mice expressing cMyc plus shp53 develop well-differentiated HCC

Transgenic mice were developed expressing cMyc and short hairpin RNA down-regulating p53 (shp53) in the liver via hydrodynamics-based transfection. Inactivation of P53 has been frequently observed across the diversity of etiologic factors in human HCC [20, 21]. In particular, allelic deletions or mutations in P53 have been frequently detected in hepatocellular carcinoma after HBV or HCV infection [22]. The Myc protein is a transcription factor that promotes cell proliferation and growth, and is overexpressed in up to 70 % of viral and alcohol-related HCC [23–25]. Thus, overexpression of cMyc and downregulation of p53 in the model are genetic characteristics relevant to human hepatocarcinogenesis.

Transposons encoding cMyc plus shp53 (or GFP, as a control) were mixed with plasmids expressing the SB transposase and then hydrodynamically delivered to the liver (Fig. 1a). Livers were harvested at 7 months post-hydrodynamic injection (PHI). About 43.5 % (10 of 23) of the mice developed liver tumors in the cMyc plus shp53 group, while no mice in the cMyc plus GFP group ($n = 10$) had hyperplastic nodules in their livers (Fig. 1b). Liver tumors of cMyc plus shp53 mice showed overexpression of cMyc and down-regulation of p53, indicating that they originated from cells transfected with the oncogene-encoding transposons (Fig. 1c). Overexpression of cMyc and shp53 in tumors was confirmed via IHC staining for cMyc and GFP, respectively (Fig. 1d). IHC staining in liver sections from the cMyc plus GFP mice revealed scattered GFP-positive and cMyc-positive clusters consisting of 1–3 hepatocytes (Fig. 1d), suggesting that overexpression of cMyc alone was insufficient to induce tumor in the liver. Consistent with previous reports, no nodules were found in livers of the 10 control mice expressing shp53 alone, when analyzed at 7 months PHI (data not shown) [17]. Thus, the data indicate that oncogenic collaboration between cMyc overexpression and p53 down-regulation is required to induce tumors in the liver. Histopathological examination revealed that the tumors from the

cMyc plus shp53 group exhibited typical features of highly differentiated hepatocellular carcinomas, with broadened trabeculae (Fig. 1b).

Combining the transgenic HCC model with a chronic liver injury model

To develop HCC in the background of liver fibrosis, we attempted to induce fibrosis in livers expressing cMyc plus shp53 via treatment with carbon tetrachloride (CCl_4), a hepatotoxic chemical that induces chronic liver damage [15, 16]. Mice were hydrodynamically injected with transposons encoding cMyc plus shp53, and assigned randomly to the CCl_4 and vehicle-treated groups ($n = 10$ for each group). Treatment was started at 15 d PHI and performed twice per week throughout the experiment (Fig. 2a). Cells transfected with cMyc and shp53 remained as single cells at 15 d PHI and no lesions were observed in the livers (Additional file 1). As a control (referred to as 'CT'), 10 mice were treated with CCl_4 without hydrodynamic injection.

A few mice treated with CCl_4 were severely ill and died within 1 month of treatment. A similar frequency of lethality followed treatment with CCl_4, regardless of hydrodynamic injection (40 % for mice without hydrodynamic injection vs. 30 % for mice with hydrodynamic injection), indicating that hydrodynamic injection does not affect lethality. The mice treated with the vehicle following hydrodynamic injection did not die. No tumors were detected in the livers of mice that died during this period. None of the mice that survived the first 30 d of CCl_4 treatment died during the remainder of the study period.

A few mice hydrodynamically transfected with cMyc plus shp53, and treated with CCl_4 (referred to as "MPC mice") showed signs of discomfort starting at about 14 weeks after hydrodynamic injection. Livers were harvested from mice of all groups at 102 d PHI, after 87 d of treatment (Fig. 2a). Gross examination revealed that the CT mice ($n = 6$) had no hyperplastic nodules in the liver, although the surface was somewhat rough (Fig. 2b). Two of the ten mice transfected with cMyc plus shp53, and then treated with the vehicle (referred to as "MP mice"), had a single liver tumor. All remaining MPC mice ($n = 7$) had multiple large tumors in the liver (Fig. 2b). Of note, livers of MPC mice had a roughened appearance as seen in those of CT mice.

Successful generation of a transgenic mouse model of HCC with concurrent hepatic fibrosis

Histopathological examination revealed that liver tumors from both MP and MPC had similarly well-differentiated HCCs (Fig. 2c) [19]. No microscopic nodules were observed in livers from the CT mice, while an increased

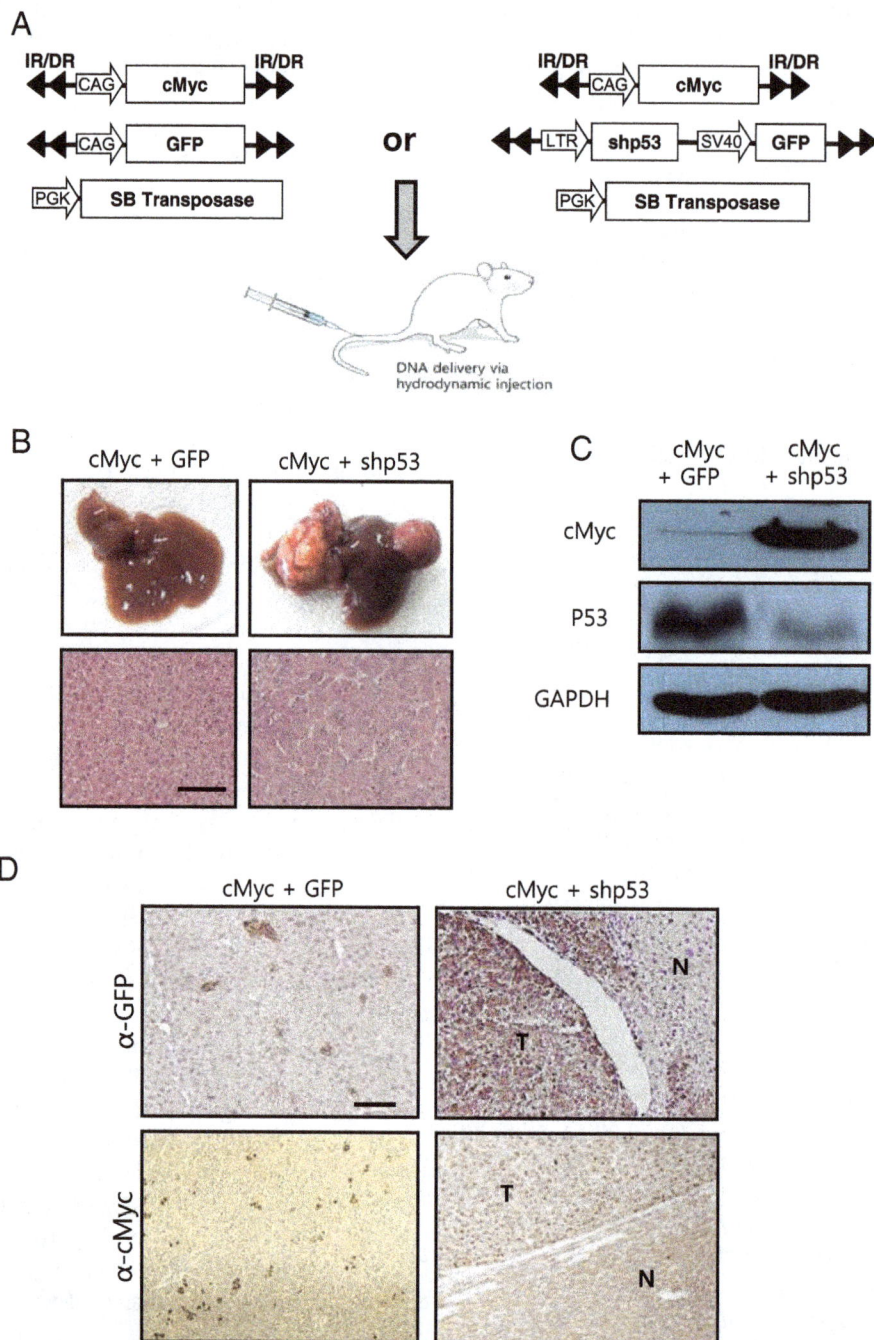

Fig. 1 Expression of cMyc plus shp53 in the liver induces well-differentiated HCC. **a** Schematic illustration of the experimental procedure to generate transgenic livers expressing cMyc plus GFP (control), and cMyc plus shp53. Hydrodynamic transfection was performed using a mixture of indicated plasmids. **b** Gross morphology (upper panels) of livers harvested from mice of each group at 7 months post hydrodynamic injection. Images of H&E staining in liver sections are shown below. Well-differentiated HCCs developed in cMyc plus shp53 mice, while the control mice did not develop tumors. Scale bar, 100 μm. **c** Protein expression levels of cMyc and p53 in liver of cMyc plus GFP mice (control) and liver tumor of cMyc plus shp53 mice. **d** Images of IHC staining for GFP and cMyc in liver sections of indicated groups. "T" denotes tumor and "N" denotes non-tumorous liver parenchyma tissue. Scale bar, 100 μm

number of inflammatory cells were observed in the tissue, likely due to liver injury induced by CCl₄ (Fig. 2c).

Picro-sirius red staining revealed that fibrosis was present throughout the tissues of CT mice (Fig. 2c).

Fibrosis was not observed in tumor-bearing livers of MP mice (Fig. 2c). In stark contrast to MP mice, MPC mice had fibrosis in non-tumorous liver parenchyma tissue surrounding the tumors (Fig. 2c). Liver tumors in both

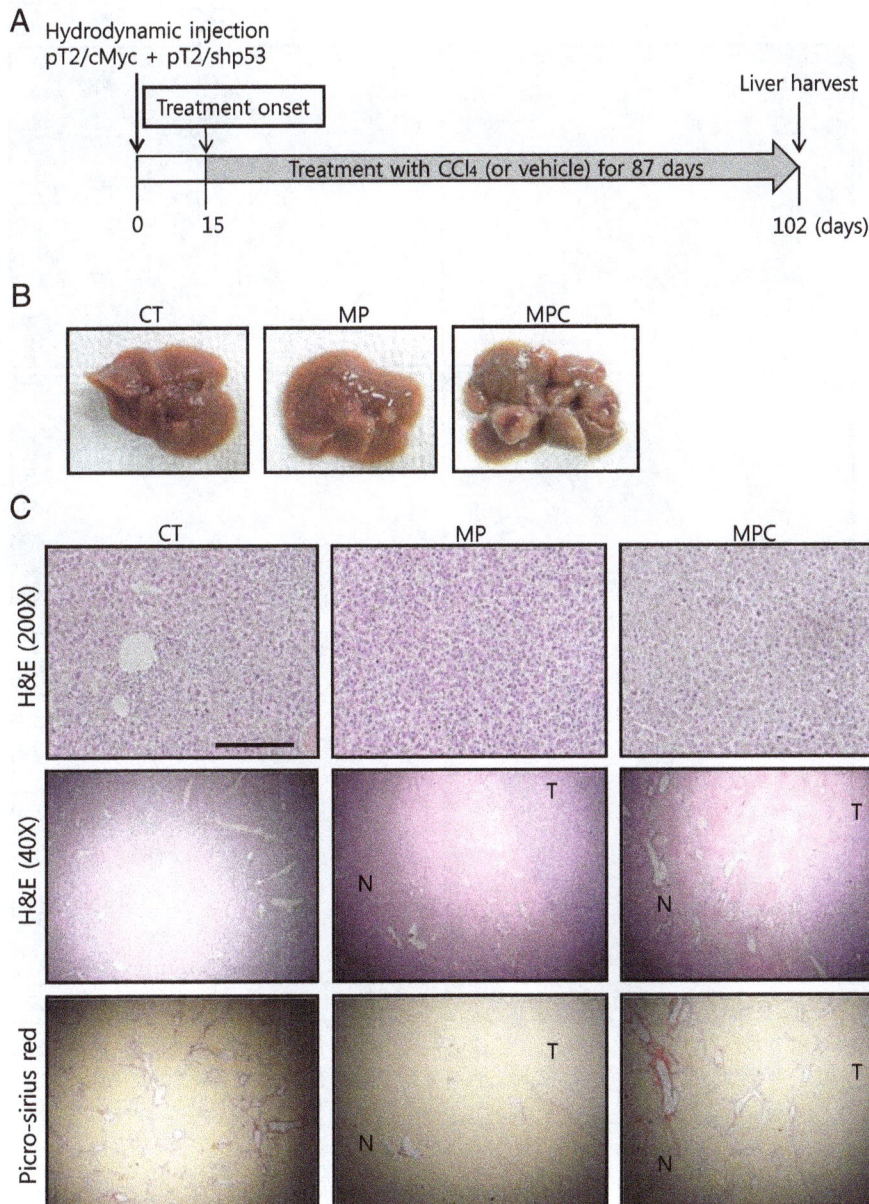

Fig. 2 Application of a chronic liver injury model to the cMyc plus shp53 mice induces HCC in a fibrotic liver background. **a** Diagram of experimental procedures. Starting at 15 d post hydrodynamic transfection, mice were treated with CCl₄ or the vehicle twice per week for about 12 weeks. **b** Gross images of representative livers of CT, MP, and MPC mice that were harvested at 102 d post hydrodynamic transfection. **c** H&E (200× and 40×) and picro-sirius red staining in liver sections of indicated groups. Tumors from both MP and MPC show similar well-differentiated HCC phenotypes (upper panels). Low-magnification images of the tumor seen in upper panels reveal boundaries between tumor (T) areas and areas of non-tumorous (N) liver parenchyma tissue (middle panels). Images of picro-sirius red staining from the same area seen in middle panels are presented in lower panels. Note the presence of accumulated collagen bands in the area surrounding the liver tumor in an MPC mouse. Scale bars, 200 μm for upper panels and 1 mm for middle and lower panels

MP and MPC mice were GFP and cMyc-positive, indicating that the tumors were induced by transfection with the oncogene-encoding transposons (Fig. 3).

Activation of hepatic stellate cells (HSCs) represents a critical event in fibrosis, mediating secretion of fibrillar collagens and accumulation of the extracellular matrix components [7, 8]. In fibrotic areas around tumors in MPC mice, activated hepatic stellate cells were observed based on immunohistochemistry (IHC) analysis with antibodies against α-SMA, a marker of activated HSC (Fig. 3) [26]. Thus, treatment with CCl₄ resulted in successful production of a transgenic mouse model for HCC, accompanied by liver fibrosis within less than 4 months at a 100 % incidence.

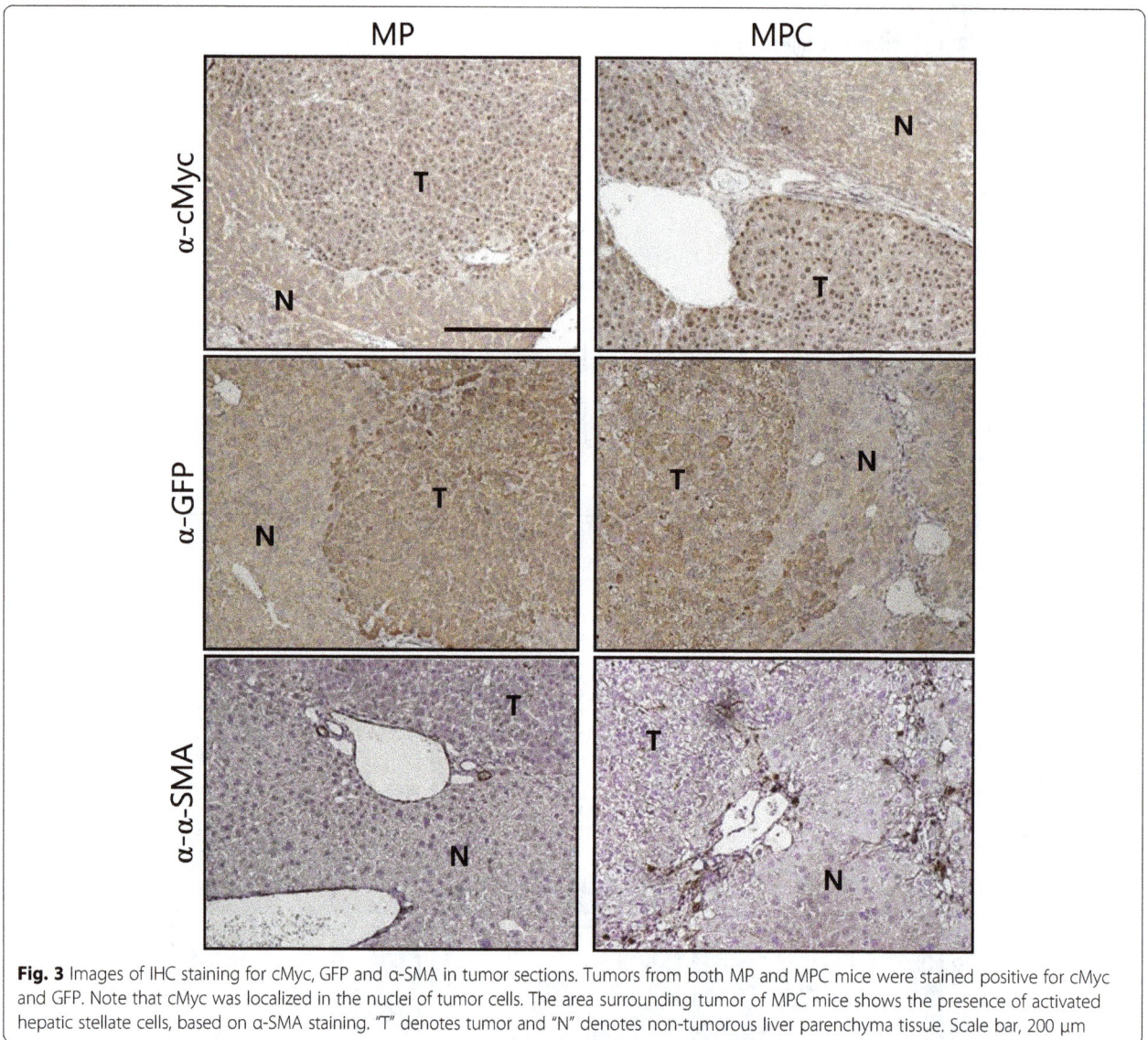

Fig. 3 Images of IHC staining for cMyc, GFP and α-SMA in tumor sections. Tumors from both MP and MPC mice were stained positive for cMyc and GFP. Note that cMyc was localized in the nuclei of tumor cells. The area surrounding tumor of MPC mice shows the presence of activated hepatic stellate cells, based on α-SMA staining. "T" denotes tumor and "N" denotes non-tumorous liver parenchyma tissue. Scale bar, 200 μm

Survival of MP and MPC mice

To perform a statistical comparison of the survival of MP and MPC mice, we replicated the experiment using an increased number of mice. MP mice ($n = 21$) and MPC mice ($n = 31$) were monitored for survival following HT. As control groups, mice hydrodynamically transfected with transposons encoding cMyc and GFP were used (Additional file 2). As in the previous experiment, treatment with CCl_4 or the vehicle was started at 15 d PHI and administered twice per week thereafter.

About 23 % of the mice died within the first 30 d of CCl_4 treatment in the MPC group (i.e., within 45 days post PHI), as observed in the previous experiment. Again, no tumors were observed in livers of MPC mice that died during the early period. The remaining MPC mice ($n = 24$) showed signs of discomfort, starting around 90 d PHI, and they died between 97 and 125 d

PHI. None of the MP mice died or developed illness during this period. The treatment part of the experiment was terminated at 150 d PHI and livers from all MP mice ($n = 21$) were harvested. The Kaplan-Meier survival analysis showed a significantly shorter life span of MPC mice compared to the MP mice (Fig. 4a). Even when mice that had died before 50 d PHI were excluded from the MPC group due to CCl_4-induced toxicity, a significant difference was observed in survival of the MPC and MP groups ($p < 10^{-4}$; Fig. 4b). Therefore, treatment with fibrosis-inducing CCl_4 significantly shortened the life span of mice expressing cMyc plus shp53. As observed in MPC mice, control mice expressing cMyc and GFP treated with CCl_4 displayed a similar percentage of lethality (~30 %) within the first 30 d of the treatment, however no death was observed in the group later on until the experiment end point (Additional file 2). Mice

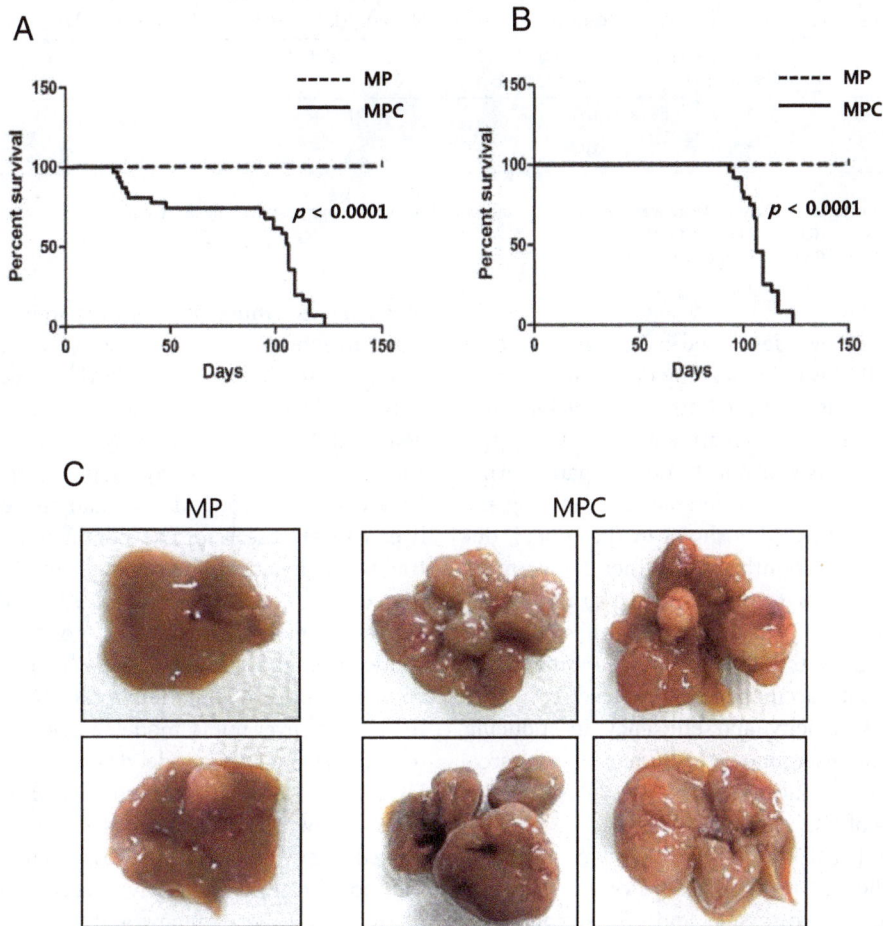

Fig. 4 Short life span of MPC mice and increased tumor burdens in their livers. **a, b** Kaplan–Meier survival curves of MP and MPC mice in the entire cohort (**a**) and with the exclusion of mice that died initially due to CCl$_4$-induced toxicity (**b**). Note that MPC mice had a significantly shorter life span compared to MP mice, even with the exclusion of the mice that died early in the MPC group ($p < 0.0001$). **c** Gross images of representative livers of MP and MPC mice. Livers were harvested following death for the MPC group and at the end of the experiment in the MP group

that were transfected with cMyc and GFP followed by the vehicle treatment showed no deaths throughout the experiment. The control mice expressing cMyc and GFP exhibited no tumors in their livers regardless of the treatment with CCl$_4$ when livers were investigated at 150 d PHI (data not shown).

Short life span of MPC mice is correlated with effects of liver tumors

To determine if the short life span of MPC mice was due to the liver tumors in the mice, livers were harvested from MPC mice following death. All of the 24 MPC mice that died between 97 and 125 d PHI had multiple large tumors in their livers (Fig. 4c). Livers were harvested from MP mice ($n = 21$) at 150 d PHI (the experiment end point) and inspected for the presence of tumors. Only 38 % of the MP mice (8 of 21 mice) had one or two small nodules in their livers (Fig. 4c). The incidence of HCC in MPC mice was significantly higher than in MP mice ($p < 10^{-4}$; Table 1).

Inclusion of seven MPC mice that died initially due to CCl$_4$-induced toxicity reduced the incidence to 77 % in that group (24 of 31 mice), but the incidence was still significantly higher compared to that for MP mice ($p < 0.01$).

The average tumor number of MPC group livers was about 15-fold that in the MP group ($p < 10^{-4}$; Table 1). The difference was larger when the seven MPC mice that died early in the study were excluded, as they did not have tumors.

The increased number of tumor nodules observed in MPC mice suggests that the fibrotic environment induced by CCl$_4$ treatment enhanced tumor initiation induced by cMyc overexpression and p53 down-regulation. Furthermore, the liver tumors in the MPC group appeared larger than those in the MP group (Fig. 4c), suggesting that the growth of tumors induced by cMyc plus shp53 was accelerated in fibrotic livers. Overall, the increased tumor burden in the liver of MPC mice likely led to a shortened life span.

Table 1 Summary of tumor incidence in cMyc + shp53 mice treated with vehicle (MP) vs. cMyc + shp53 mice treated with CCl₄ (MPC) from the survival study. Livers were harvested from MPC mice following death and from MP mice at the end of the experiment

	Total # of mice[a]	% of mice with liver tumors	Average # of tumors per mouse	Total # of mice[b]	% of mice with liver tumors	Average # of tumors per mouse
MP	21	38 % (8/21)[*]	0.6[†]	21	38 % (8/21)[‡]	0.6[§]
MPC	31	77 % (24/31)[*]	9[†]	24	100 % (24/24)[‡]	11.7[§]

[a]Entire cohort
[b]Mice that died initially due to CCl₄-induced toxicity were excluded (i.e., those died before 50 days post hydrodynamic transfection)
[*]$P < 0.01$, Fisher's exact test. [†]$P < 0.0001$, Student's t-test
[‡]$P < 0.0001$, Fisher's exact test. [§]$P < 0.0001$, Student's t-test

Discussion

In the present study, we developed a transgenic model system in which HCC was induced by oncogenic expression in the background of liver fibrosis, mimicking human hepatocarcinogenesis. Treatment with CCl₄ not only induced liver fibrosis in non-tumorous parenchyma surrounding HCC but also accelerated the carcinogenic process induced by cMyc plus shp53 in the model, developing HCC within 3 months of treatment. Treatment with CCl₄ alone, even for 6 months, failed to induce tumors in our experiment (data not shown), suggesting that the CCl₄ treatment could not induce tumor, but promoted the hepatocarcinogenesis induced by cMyc plus shp53. The simplicity and efficiency in inducing HCC, as well as the resemblance to human hepatocarcinogenesis, suggests the utility of this model system in preclinical studies of HCC [12].

Our data showed that CCl₄ induced background liver fibrosis and significantly enhanced hepatocarcinogenesis initiated by cMyc overexpression and p53 suppression. However, the molecular mechanism underlying the increased tumorigenesis remains unclear. As a hepatotoxic chemical inducing chronic liver injury, CCl₄ has been widely used to induce fibrosis in livers. A persistent injury to the liver leads to hepatocyte death, followed by compensatory regeneration, chronic inflammation, accumulation of extracellular matrix components, and subsequent changes in the tissue microenvironment [7, 26, 27]. A regenerative microenvironment promoting cellular proliferation might enhance tumor initiation in cells expressing cMyc plus shp53 [28]. Upregulation of inflammatory cytokines (e.g., IL-6 and TNF-α) in livers with chronic injury is known to support tumor-promoting microenvironments [29, 30]. Finally, the possibility cannot be ruled out that the treatment caused a genetic alteration directly or via upregulation of reactive oxygen species [15, 31], further enhancing tumor initiation induced by cMyc plus shp53. Ongoing studies are needed to investigate the molecular mechanism underlying the increased hepatocarcinogenesis of fibrotic livers in the model.

Several genetically engineered mouse (GEM) models for HCC have been developed, with alterations in candidate oncogenes or tumor suppressor genes, and significantly contributed to a better understanding of the genetic mechanisms underlying hepatocarcinogenesis [10, 11]. Circumventing procedures requiring excessive time and resources in developing a GEM model, a new methodology has been developed for simple generation of a transgenic HCC model, employing HT coupled with the SB transposon system [13, 14]. Many transgenic HCC models have been developed via HT and successfully applied to liver cancer research. The common problem with both traditional genetic models and HT models for HCC is that they do not consider background liver fibrosis. Considering that human HCC develops mostly in a fibrotic or cirrhotic liver, the lack of fibrosis in the background liver could be a critical limitation in the HCC models. Applying the chronic liver injury model, induced by CCl₄ treatment, to a transgenic HCC model developed by HT, a transgenic HCC model with background liver fibrosis was efficiently developed within a few months. Considering the simplicity and efficiency, as well as the resemblance to human HCC, the model can be effectively applied to preclinical testing of HCC anticancer therapy and studies of hepatocarcinogenesis in fibrotic livers.

Conclusions

A transgenic mouse model of hepatocellular carcinoma (HCC) with background liver fibrosis was developed, combining a chronic liver injury model with liver transgenesis via hydrodynamics-based transfection. Liver fibrosis significantly accelerated hepatocarcinogenesis induced by cMyc overexpression and p53 suppression.

Abbreviations
α-SMA: α-smooth muscle actin; CCl₄: carbon tetrachloride; CT: CCl₄-treated mouse; GEM: genetically engineered mouse; GFP: green fluorescent protein; HCC: hepatocellular carcinoma; H&E: hematoxylin & eosin; HSC, hepatic stellate cell; HT: hydrodynamic transfection; IHC: immunohistochemistry; MP: cMyc plus shp53; MPC: cMyc plus shp53 with CCl₄ treatment; PHI: post hydrodynamic injection; SB: Sleeping Beauty; shp53: short hairpin RNA down-regulating p53; WT: wild-type.

Competing interests
The authors declare that they have no competing interests.

Authors' contributions
SC and HM carried out molecular biology and histology experiments, and participated in study design, data analyses, and manuscript preparation. DaK, KC, and HJ were responsible for animal handling and the histopathological investigation. DoK, SH, KH participated in data analyses and manuscript preparation. SR conceived of the study, participated in study design, and wrote the manuscript. All authors read and approved the final manuscript.

Acknowledgements
This research was supported by the Basic Science Research Program through the National Research Foundation of Korea, which is funded by the Ministry of Education (NRF-2010-0025261 to DoK, 2010–0024939 to SA, and 2011–0021830 to SR).

Author details
[1]Institute of Gastroenterology, Yonsei University College of Medicine, Seoul 120-752, South Korea. [2]Brain Korea 21 Project for Medical Science College of Medicine, Yonsei University, Seoul 120-752, South Korea. [3]Department of Internal Medicine, Yonsei University College of Medicine, Seoul 120-752, South Korea. [4]Room 407, ABMRC, Severance Hospital, Yonsei University College of Medicine, Yonsei-ro 50-1, Seoul 120-752, South Korea.

References
1. Ince N, Wands JR. The increasing incidence of hepatocellular carcinoma. N Engl J Med. 1999;340:798–9.
2. El-Serag HB. Hepatocellular carcinoma. N Engl J Med. 2011;365:1118–27.
3. Hassan MM, Hwang LY, Hatten CJ, Swaim M, Li D, Abbruzzese JL, et al. Risk factors for hepatocellular carcinoma: synergism of alcohol with viral hepatitis and diabetes mellitus. Hepatology. 2002;36:1206–13.
4. El-Serag HB, Rudolph KL. Hepatocellular carcinoma: epidemiology and molecular carcinogenesis. Gastroenterology. 2007;132:2557–76.
5. Ascha MS, Hanouneh IA, Lopez R, Tamimi TA, Feldstein AF, Zein NN. The incidence and risk factors of hepatocellular carcinoma in patients with nonalcoholic steatohepatitis. Hepatology. 2010;51:1972–8.
6. Yang HI, Yuen MF, Chan HL, Han KH, Chen PJ, Kim DY, et al. Risk estimation for hepatocellular carcinoma in chronic hepatitis B (REACH-B): development and validation of a predictive score. Lancet Oncol. 2011;12:568–74.
7. Friedman SL. Mechanisms of hepatic fibrogenesis. Gastroenterology. 2008;134:1655–69.
8. Hernandez-Gea V, Friedman SL. Pathogenesis of liver fibrosis. Annu Rev Pathol. 2011;6:425–56.
9. Fattovich G, Stroffolini T, Zagni I, Donato F. Hepatocellular carcinoma in cirrhosis: incidence and risk factors. Gastroenterology. 2004;127:S35–50.
10. Newell P, Villanueva A, Friedman SL, Koike K, Llovet JM. Experimental models of hepatocellular carcinoma. J Hepatol. 2008;48:858–79.
11. Heindryckx F, Colle I, Van Vlierberghe H. Experimental mouse models for hepatocellular carcinoma research. Int J Exp Pathol. 2009;90:367–86.
12. Farazi PA, DePinho RA. Hepatocellular carcinoma pathogenesis: from genes to environment. Nat Rev Cancer. 2006;6:674–87.
13. Carlson CM, Frandsen JL, Kirchhof N, McIvor RS, Largaespada DA. Somatic integration of an oncogene-harboring Sleeping Beauty transposon models liver tumor development in the mouse. Proc Natl Acad Sci U S A. 2005;102:17059–64.
14. Chen X, Calvisi DF. Hydrodynamic transfection for generation of novel mousemodels for liver cancer research. Am J Pathol. 2014;184:912–23.
15. Weber LW, Boll M, Stampfl A. Hepatotoxicity and mechanism of action of haloalkanes: carbon tetrachloride as a toxicological model. Crit Rev Toxicol. 2003;33:105–36.
16. Sakaida I, Terai S, Yamamoto N, Aoyama K, Ishikawa T, Nishina H, et al. Transplantation of bone marrow cells reduces CCl4-induced liver fibrosis in mice. Hepatology. 2004;40:1304–11.
17. Ju HL, Ahn SH, Kim do Y, Baek S, Chung SI, Seong J, et al. Investigation of oncogenic cooperation in simple liver-specific transgenic mouse models using noninvasive in vivo imaging. PLoS One. 2013;8:e59869.
18. Wiesner SM, Decker SA, Larson JD, Ericson K, Forster C, Gallardo JL, et al. De novo induction of genetically engineered brain tumors in mice using plasmid DNA. Cancer Res. 2009;69:431–9.
19. Frith CH, Ward JM, Turusov VS. Tumours of the liver. IARC Sci Publ. 1994;111: 223–69.
20. Bressac B, Kew M, Wands J, Ozturk M. Selective G to T mutations of p53 gene in hepatocellular carcinoma from southern Africa. Nature. 1991;350:429–31.
21. Tannapfel A, Busse C, Weinans L, Benicke M, Katalinic A, Geissler F, et al. INK4a-ARF alterations and p53 mutations in hepatocellular carcinomas. Oncogene. 2001;20:7104–9.
22. Nose H, Imazeki F, Ohto M, Omata M. p53 gene mutations and 17p allelic deletions in hepatocellular carcinoma from Japan. Cancer. 1993;72:355–60.
23. Pelengaris S, Khan M, Evan G. c-MYC: more than just a matter of life and death. Nat Rev Cancer. 2002;2:764–76.
24. Schlaeger C, Longerich T, Schiller C, Bewerunge P, Mehrabi A, Toedt G, et al. Etiology-dependent molecular mechanisms in human hepatocarcinogenesis. Hepatology. 2008;47:511–20.
25. Dang CV. MYC on the path to cancer. Cell. 2012;149:22–35.
26. Pellicoro A, Ramachandran P, Iredale JP, Fallowfield JA. Liver fibrosis and repair: immune regulation of wound healing in a solid organ. Nat Rev Immunol. 2014;14:181–94.
27. Guicciardi ME, Gores GJ. Apoptosis: a mechanism of acute and chronic liver injury. Gut. 2005;54:1024–33.
28. Kuwata K, Shibutani M, Hayashi H, Shimamoto K, Hayashi SM, Suzuki K, et al. Concomitant apoptosis and regeneration of liver cells as a mechanism of liver-tumor promotion by beta-naphthoflavone involving TNFalpha-signaling due to oxidative cellular stress in rats. Toxicology. 2011;283:8–17.
29. Grivennikov SI, Karin M. Inflammatory cytokines in cancer: tumour necrosis factor and interleukin 6 take the stage. Ann Rheum Dis. 2011;70 Suppl 1:i104–8.
30. Kuraishy A, Karin M, Grivennikov SI. Tumor promotion via injury- and death-induced inflammation. Immunity. 2011;35:467–77.
31. Sipes IG, el Sisi AE, Sim WW, Mobley SA, Earnest DL. Reactive oxygen species in the progression of CCl4-induced liver injury. Adv Exp Med Biol. 1991;283:489–97.

2

Polymorphism in asparagine synthetase is associated with overall survival of hepatocellular carcinoma patients

Wei Li[1] and Chengwei Dong[2]* (iD)

Abstract

Background: Recently, it is reported that asparagine synthetase (ASNS) is an independent predictor of surgical survival in hepatocellular carcinoma (HCC) patients. It is also reported that activating transcription factor 6 (ATF6) expression is decreased in HCC patients. So in the present study, we explored the relationship between ASNS and ATF6, and whether ASNS expression was associated with HCC.

Methods: ATF6 was over expressed in 3 HCC cell lines (HepG2, HepG2.2.15 and SMMC-7721). We then examined the mRNA levels of ASNS and ATF6 in 90 HCC patients, 77 chronic hepatitis B patients and 70 controls. We also genotyped 2 functional polymorphisms in *ASNS* in a case–control study.

Results: The expression of ASNS was significantly elevated when ATF6 was over expressed. The expressions of these 2 genes were both decreased in HCC patients, and it was more significantly with ASNS. The mRNA levels of ASNS and ATF6 were positively correlated with each other. rs34050735 was associated with HCC in the case–control study ($P = 0.003$) and also an independent predictor of overall survival of HCC patients ($P = 0.001$).

Conclusions: Taken together, these findings indicated that rs34050735 in *ASNS* may associate with HCC and may be a promising biomarker of HCC.

Keywords: Hepatocellular carcinoma, ASNS, Realtime PCR, Association study, Survival analysis

Background

Hepatocellular carcinoma (HCC) is common cancer mortality worldwide. There are about 564,000 new cases of HCC each year throughout the world [1]. Recently, Zhang et al. reported that asparagine synthetase (ASNS) was an independent predictor of surgical survival and a potential therapeutic target in HCC [2]. Meanwhile, Wu et al. reported that HBsAg-negative healthy individuals and chronic hepatitis B (CHB) patients had higher ATF6 mRNA levels than HCC patients [3].

The *ASNS* gene encodes a protein involved in the synthesis of asparagine [4]. Asparagine is an essential amino acid for cell growth and survival. The transcription of *ASNS* is regulated by the nutritional status of the cell [5]. ASNS has been considered as a predictive biomarker in ovarian cancer [6], pancreatic cancer [7] and prostate cancer [8]. The *ATF6* gene encodes a transcription factor, acting as an unfolded protein response (UPR) transcriptional activator which regulates gene expression of endoplasmic reticulum (ER) chaperones, ER-associated proteins, and apoptotic genes [9, 10]. ATF6 works to alleviate ER stress by decreasing the amount of misfolded/unfolded proteins in the ER, or if this cannot be achieved, by initiating cell apoptosis [11]. As suggested by computational analysis (AliBaba 2 software), there is an ATF6 binding site in the promoter region of *ASNA* gene. So we speculated that ATF6 may regulate the expression of ASNS, and ASNA may also associated with HCC tumorigenesis. We carried out the present study to test this hypothesis.

* Correspondence: qzhdcw@163.com; lihuipumc@163.com
[2]Department of Hepatobiliary Surgery, Weifang People's Hospital, Weifang, Shandong 261041, China
Full list of author information is available at the end of the article

Methods

Subjects, ethics, consent and permissions

The subjects enrolled in this study were constituted of 2 independent groups of patients.

The first was constituted of 90 HCC patients, 77 CHB patients and 70 non-HBV controls which were enrolled from the Weifang People's Hospital from Jan 2011 to Nov 2014. The second was constituted of 337 HCC patients and 310 CHB patients enrolled from the same hospital from May 2005 to Jan 2010. Among the 337 HCC patients, clinical outcomes of 146 patients that had undergone surgical resection of a HCC tumor were recorded until October 2015, with a median follow-up time of 39.5 months (range 5.0–76.5 months).

HCC patients, CHB patients and non-HBV controls were defined as previously reported [3]. The main features of the subjects were summarized in Table 1. The study was carried out in accordance with the guidelines of the Helsinki Declaration after obtaining written informed consent from all the subjects and was approved by the ethics committee of the Weifang People's Hospital. All patients consented to participate this study.

Gene expression experiment

HepG2, HepG2. 2.15, and SMMC-7721 cells were were kindly gifts from professor Xiaopan Wu (National Laboratory of Medical Molecular Biology, Institute of Basic Medical Sciences, Chinese Academy of Medical Sciences, Beijing, China). The cells were propagated in MEM/NEAA or RPMI-1640 medium with 10% fetal calf serum. All cells were maintained with 5% CO_2 at 37 °C. We seeded 2×10^5 HepG2, HepG2. 2.15, or SMMC-7721 cells each well in 24-well plates. The ATF6 expression plasmid was constructed as previous reported [3]. Half Wells were transfected with ATF6 expression plasmid by Lipofectamine™ 2000 (Invitrogen, Carlsbad, CA). The rest half were non-transfected cells regarded as controls. All transfections were repeated 3 times. The primers used for qPCR and detailed qPCR methods were according to previously reported [2, 3]. Total RNA was extracted from the peripheral blood of 90 HCC patients, 77 CHB patients and 70 non-HBV controls and mRNA levels of ATF6 and ASNS were tested. The detailed qPCR methods were the same as above mentioned.

Plasmids and luciferase assay

We constructed a pGL3-Basic (Promega, Madison, WI) reporter plasmid encompassing –395 to +145 bp of ASNS promoter. The ATF6 eukaryotic expression plasmid and FLAG control plasmid were gifts from Dr. Wu (Institute of Basic Medical Sciences, Chinese Academy of Medical Sciences). The luciferase assay was performed as previously reported [3] in HepG2 cells.

Table 1 Clinical features of the subjects included in the study

A. Realtime PCR Study

	Non-HBV controls $n = 70$	CHB patients $n = 77$	HCC patients $n = 90$
Age, y mean ± SD	48.2 ± 7.5	49.1 ± 10.1	50.3 ± 9.5
Gender, n. (%)			
Male	39(55.7)	43(55.8)	50(55.6)
Famale	31(44.3)	34(44.2)	40(44.4)
Smoking, n. (%)			
Yes	30(42.9)	45(58.4)	55(61.1)
No	40(57.1)	32(41.6)	35(38.9)
Drinking, n. (%)			
Yes	33(47.1)	50(64.9)	73(81.1)
No	37(52.9)	27(35.1)	17(18.9)

B. Case–control Study

	HCC	CHB	P
Number	337	310	
Age, y mean ± SD	44.7 ± 11.0	44.3 ± 12.3	0.67
Gender (male/female)	298/39	254/56	0.02
Smoking (Yes/No)	141/192	128/182	0.79
Drinking (Yes/No)	98/239	92/218	0.87
Family history of HCC (Yes/No)	58/279	14/296	<0.001

HCC hepatocellular carcinoma, CHB chronic hepatitis B

SNP selection and genotyping

Genomic DNA were extracted from peripheral blood using the salting-out protocol. Using the NCBI dbSNP database (http://www.ncbi.nlm.nih.gov/snp/), potential functional SNPs (SNPs in promoter region and mRNA sequence) with minor allele frequency (MAF) greater than 0.05 for the Han Chinese Beijing population were selected. Only 2 SNPs were found, namely rs1049674 (nonsynonymous coding) and rs34050735 (5'UTR). These 2 SNPs were genotyped using TaqMan method (Applied Biosystems, Foster City, CA), according to the manufacture's protocols. All the samples were successfully genotyped.

Statistical analysis

ANOVA was used to examine the differences in mRNA expression levels between different groups. By using the $\chi 2$ test, we tested whether the genotype distributions of SNP were in the Hardy–Weinberg equilibrium (HWE). We used 2×2 or 2×3 contingency tables for comparing allele and genotype frequencies between different groups. We calculated the linkage disequilibrium values (r2, D') and the haplotype estimation using the SHEsis online software [12]. The associations between overall survival and demographic characteristics, and rs1049674 and rs34050735 were estimated using the Kaplan–Meier method. A survival curve was drawn with the Kaplan–Meier method for each genotype. $P < 10.05$ was the criterion for statistical significance. All statistical analyses were performed using the Statistical Package for the Social Sciences (SPSS), version 15.0 (SPSS Inc., Chicago, Illinois).

Results

ASNS was positively regulated by ATF6

We transiently transfected HepG2, HepG2.2.15, and SMMC-7721 cells with ATF6 expression plasmid, and then examined the mRNA expression of ASNS. Final abundance figures were adjusted to yield an arbitrary value of 1 for non-transfected cells. The result showed that when ATF6 was over expressed, the mRNA level of ASNS was elevated by 1.86-fold, 1.95-fold and 1.65-fold in HepG2, HepG2.2.15, and SMMC-7721 cells, respectively ($P < 0.001$) (Fig. 1).

We then examined levels of total ATF6 and ASNS mRNA using quantitative realtime PCR. The mRNA levels of ATF6 and ASNS were measured. As shown in Table 1, the 3 groups of subjects had similar age and sex distribution, but CHB and HCC groups had higher smoking and drinking ratio than non-HBV controls. Final abundance figures were adjusted to yield an arbitrary value of 1 for ATF6 expression level in HCC patients (Figs. 2 and 3). The result showed that non-HBV controls and CHB patients had 2.67-fold and 2.08-fold higher ATF6 mRNA levels than HCC patients ($P = 5.38E-79$), and 2.78-fold and 2.16-fold higher ASNS mRNA levels than HCC patients ($P = 9.05E-82$). We also found that ASNS expression level was positively correlated with ATF6 level (r2 = 0.98).

To further confirm whether ATF6 regulated *ASNS* promoter, we transiently transfected HepG2 cells with pGL3-ASNS promoter together with ATF6 expressing plasmid or FLAG control plasmid. The result showed that the ATF6 expressing plasmid group had 1.59-fold higher luciferase activity compared with FLAG control group ($P = 0.002$). This result indicated that ATF6 could indeed positively regulate the promoter region of *ASNS* gene.

Case–control study of SNPs in *ASNS* gene

We next conducted genotyping experiments for the 2 ASNS polymorphisms in the case–control samples. Genotype distributions of the studied SNPs were in HWE in both cases and controls. The genotype distributions and allelic frequencies of ASNS polymorphisms in

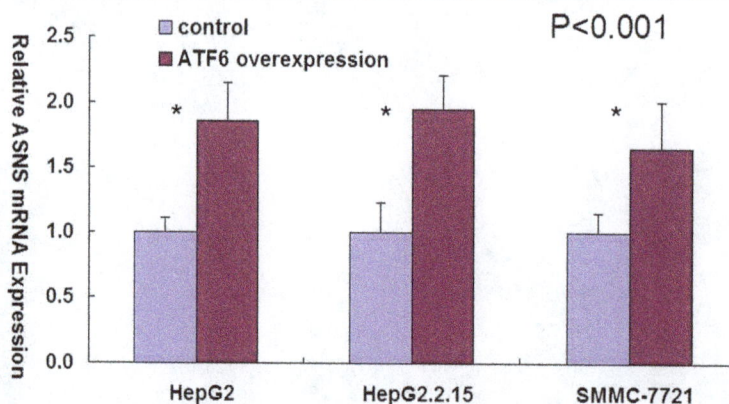

Fig. 1 Relative ASNS mRNA Expression in HepG2, HepG2. 2.15, and SMMC-7721 cells. Final abundance figures were adjusted to yield an arbitrary value of 1 for non-transfected cells. Data are means ± SD. *$P < 0.001$

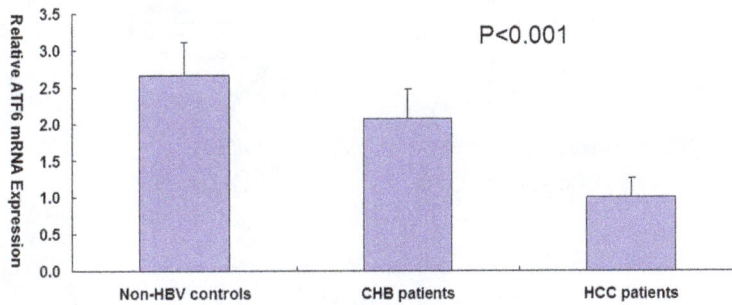

Fig. 2 Quantification of ATF6 mRNA expression by real-time PCR. GAPDH was used as an internal control gene. Final abundance figures were adjusted to yield an arbitrary value of 1 for HCC patients. Data are means ± SD

CHB and HCC patients were represented in Table 2. The frequency of T allele of rs34050735 was 16.5% in HCC patients vs. 10.8% in CHB patients ($P = 0.003$, OR = 1.63, 95%CI = 1.18–2.25). The Cochran-Armitage trend test (assuming an additive model for T allele) revealed an allele dose-dependent association of rs34050735 with HCC ($P = 0.005$), with decreased OR of 0.71 and 0.44 for GT and GG genotypes, respectively.

We then used binary logistic regression to adjust for confounding factors as age, gender, smoking drinking and family history under additive model, and the results showed that rs34050735 was still independently associated with HCC ($P = 0.005$, OR = 1.59, 95%CI = 1.15–2.20). While the other SNP rs1049674 was not associated with HCC under any model. We analyzed the degree of LD for these 2 SNPs, and found there was no apparent LD (D' ≤ 0.05, $r^2 ≤ 0.002$). Table 3 shows 4 haplotypes constructed by these 2 SNPs. The A-T haplotype was associated with HCC ($P = 0.02$).

Survival analysis

Finally, we asked the question whether these 2 SNPs influencing overall survival of HCC patients. Among the 146 HCC patients with clinical outcomes, 127 patients were died and were included in the final analysis. As shown in Table 4 and Fig. 4, SNP rs34050735 was

significantly associated with overall survival ($P = 0.001$). Patients who carried the TT genotype had a significantly shorter survival time compared to those with the GT or GG genotypes. We used Receiver Operating Characteristic (ROC) curve to establish the prognosis of HCC patients. According to the ROC curve, patients whose survival time more than or equal to 38 months were defined as the better group, survival time less than 38 months were defined as the poor group ($P = 0.025$).

Discussion

As an UPR-stimulating gene, ATF6 plays an important role in tumor genesis, and *ASNS* gene is important in tumor genesis due to its function of synthesis of asparagine, which is an essential amino acid for normal tissue or tumor growth. We found in this study that the mRNA levels of ASNS and ATF6 were positively correlated with each other, and the decrease of ASNS mRNA level in HCC patients was greater than ATF6. So as the disease progressed, the ASNA mRNA level was negatively correlated with the severity of HCC. This result may have potential application value as ASNA might be a useful diagnoses bio-marker of HCC.

Recent progresses have been made in determining the role of ATF6 and ASNS in varies tumors. ATF6 are reported to contribute to enhanced viability in glioblastoma [13], and important for survival of melanoma cells

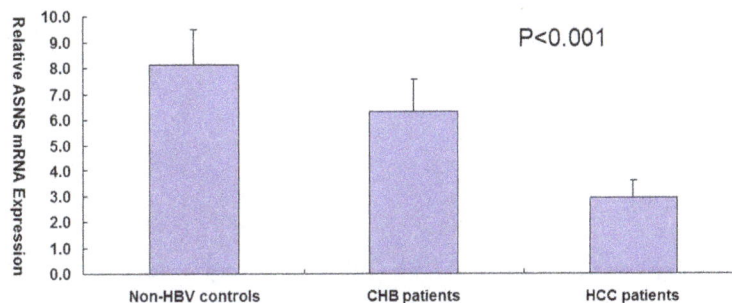

Fig. 3 Quantification of ASNS mRNA expression by real-time PCR. GAPDH was used as an internal control gene. Data are means ± SD

Table 2 Genotype distributions of 2 SNPs in ASNS gene

	Allele, n (ratio)				Genotype, n (ratio)			Cochran Armitage trend test	logistic regression[#]
	1/2	1	2	P/OR (95% CI)	11	12	22	P	P/OR (95% CI)
rs1049674	T/A								
HCC (n = 337)		57(0.085)	617(0.915)	0.72	2(0.006)	53(0.157)	282(0.837)	0.72	0.55
CHB (n = 310)		49(0.079)	571(0.921)	1.08(0.72–1.60)	3(0.010)	43(0.139)	264(0.852)		1.14(0.75–1.72)
rs34050735	T/G								
HCC (n = 337)		111(0.165)	563(0.835)	0.003	13(0.039)	85(0.252)	239(0.709)	0.005	0.005
CHB (n = 310)		67(0.108)	553(0.892)	1.63(1.18–2.25)	6(0.019)	55(0.177)	249(0.803)		1.59(1.15–2.20)

[#]P values were adjusted for age, gender, smoking drinking and family history of HCC by binary logistic regression under additive model

undergoing ER stress [14]. Knockdown of ASNS suppresses cell growth in human melanoma cells and epidermoid carcinoma cells [15]. Polymorphisms of asparaginase pathway genes are related with asparaginase-related complications in children with acute lymphoblastic leukemia [16], probably by affecting early response to treatment [17]. Down-regulation of ASNS induces cell cycle arrest and inhibits cell proliferation of breast cancer [18].

In the present study, we replicated Wu's work that ATF6 mRNA level decreased in turn from non-HBV controls to CHB patients and HCC patients [3]. However, Zhang's work revealed that the expression of ASNS was higher in HCC tumor tissues [2]. Our results showed that ASNS mRNA decreased in the peripheral blood of HCC patients, which was deviated to Zhang's. On the other hand, although Zhang's work showed ASNS was higher expressed in HCC tumor tissue, ASNS seemed to have antitumor effect, for patients with low ASNS expression levels had a poor prognosis and ASNS significantly inhibited the proliferation, migration and tumourigenicity of HCC cells. We speculated that the essential role of ASNS (synthesis of asparagine) made it a double-edge sword to HCC, whether it exercise good or bad effect on tumourigenicity depended on the complicated interaction between ASNS and other related genes. So further studies are needed to clarify the exact role of ASNS in tumourigenicity.

rs34050735 is in the 5'UTR region of ASNS gene. The 5'UTR region maybe the target of transcription factor. So further studies are needed to clarify the exact functional role of rs34050735.

Table 3 Common haplotypes constructed with SNPs rs1049674 and rs34050735 in ASNS gene

Haplotypes	HCC (n = 337)	CHB (n = 310)	P	OR (95%CI)
A-G	520.76(0.773)	508.74(0.821)	0.09	0.79(0.60–1.04)
A-T	96.24(0.143)	62.26(0.100)	0.02	1.52(1.08–2.13)
T-G	42.24(0.063)	44.26(0.071)	0.58	0.88(0.57–1.37)
T-T[a]	14.76(0.022)	4.74(0.008)		

[a]Haplotypes with frequency < 0.03 was ignored in analysis

Table 4 Clinical characteristics and their prediction of overall survival in 127 HCC patients

Characteristics	Number	Survival Time, m mean (95%CI)	P	OR (95%CI)
Gender			0.68	1.12(0.65–1.93)
male	107	39.1(35.1–43.2)		
female	20	41.8(31.0–52.6)		
Smoking			0.24	0.72(0.41–1.25)
No	86	40.8(36.1–45.4)		
Yes	41	37.0(30.7–43.4)		
Drinking			0.90	1.04(0.57–1.89)
No	97	40.3(36.0–44.6)		
Yes	30	37.1(29.3–45.0)		
Family history of HCC			0.16	0.65(0.36–1.19)
No	114	40.6(36.7–44.6)		
Yes	13	30.2(18.0–42.4)		
rs1049674			0.829	0.80(0.10–6.17)
TT	1	54.2		
TA	22	33.6(24.0–43.2)		
AA	104	40.7(36.6–44.8)		
rs34050735			0.001	7.21(2.30–22.6)
TT	4	15.2(−2.4–32.7)		
TG	35	34.4(27.7–41.1)		
GG	88	42.7(38.2–47.2)		
Vascular invasion			0.51	0.86(0.55–1.34)
No	78	39.2(34.4–44.1)		
Yes	49	40.1(34.1–46.0)		
Differentiation			0.28	1.27(0.82–1.97)
I + II	65	38.9(33.4–44.4)		
III + IV	62	40.3(35.1–45.4)		
TNM stage			0.53	0.88(0.60–1.30)
I + II	75	39.6(34.8–44.5)		
III + IV	52	39.4(33.4–45.5)		

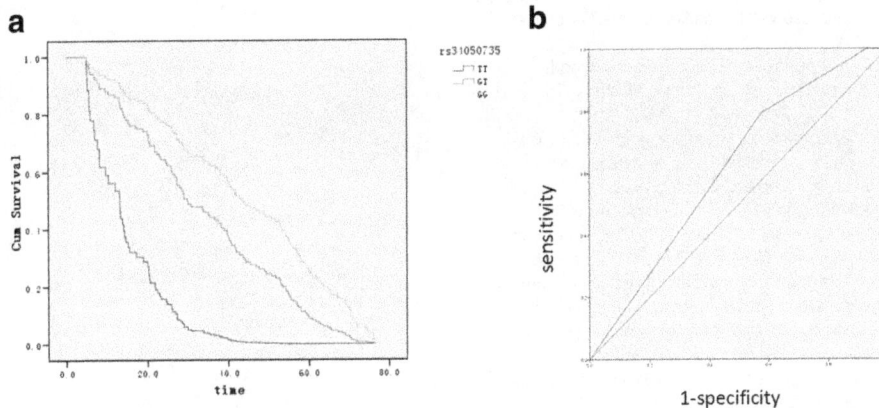

Fig. 4 rs34050735 genotype and HCC survival. **a** Kaplan–Meier survival curves of overall survival for HCC patients by rs34050735 genotype. **b** Using ROC curve to establish the prognosis of HCC patients

Several limitations of the present study need to be addressed. Further tests of ATF6 and ASNS mRNA levels in HCC tumor tissues and corresponding non tumor tissues should be done. The protein levels of ATF6 and ASNS should also be tested.

Conclusions

We found in the present study that ASNS and SNP in this gene may associate with HCC and be a promising bio-marker of HCC.

Abbreviations

ASNS: Asparagine synthetase; CHB: Chronic hepatitis B; ER: Endoplasmic reticulum; HCC: Hepatocellular carcinoma; MAF: Minor allele frequency; UPR: Unfolded protein response

Acknowledgements

We are thankful to all the subjects participated in the present study.

Funding

This work was supported by grants from Weifang Municipal Science and Technology Bureau (Grant No.20130225).

Authors' contributions

WL carried out the molecular genetic studies, participated in the sequence alignment and drafted the manuscript. CD participated in the design of the study and performed the statistical analysis and helped to draft the manuscript. Both authors read and approved the final manuscript.

Competing interests

The authors declare that they have no competing interests.

Consent for publication

Not applicable.

Author details

[1]Department of Interventional Radiology, the Affiliated Hospital of Qingdao University, Qingdao, Shandong 266003, China. [2]Department of Hepatobiliary Surgery, Weifang People's Hospital, Weifang, Shandong 261041, China.

References

1. Bosch FX, Ribes J, Cleries R, Diaz M. Epidemiology of hepatocellular carcinoma. Clin Liver Dis. 2005;9:191–211. v
2. Zhang B, Dong LW, Tan YX, et al. Asparagine synthetase is an independent predictor of surgical survival and a potential therapeutic target in hepatocellular carcinoma. Br J Cancer. 2013;109:14–23.
3. Wu X, Xin Z, Zhang W, et al. A missense polymorphism in ATF6 gene is associated with susceptibility to hepatocellular carcinoma probably by altering ATF6 level. Int J Cancer. 2014;135:61–8.
4. Richards NG, Schuster SM. Mechanistic issues in asparagine synthetase catalysis. Adv Enzymol Relat Areas Mol Biol. 1998;72:145–98.
5. Kilberg MS, Barbosa-Tessmann IP. Genomic sequences necessary for transcriptional activation by amino acid deprivation of mammalian cells. J Nutr. 2002;132:1801–4.
6. Lorenzi PL, Llamas J, Gunsior M, et al. Asparagine synthetase is a predictive biomarker of L-asparaginase activity in ovarian cancer cell lines. Mol Cancer Ther. 2008;7:3123–8.
7. Cui H, Darmanin S, Natsuisaka M, et al. Enhanced expression of asparagine synthetase under glucose-deprived conditions protects pancreatic cancer cells from apoptosis induced by glucose deprivation and cisplatin. Cancer Res. 2007;67:3345–55.
8. Sircar K, Huang H, Hu L, et al. Integrative molecular profiling reveals asparagine synthetase is a target in castration-resistant prostate cancer. Am J Pathol. 2012;180:895–903.
9. Namba T, Ishihara T, Tanaka K, Hoshino T, Mizushima T. Transcriptional activation of ATF6 by endoplasmic reticulum stressors. Biochem Biophys Res Commun. 2007;355:543–8.
10. Kaneko M, Nomura Y. ER signaling in unfolded protein response. Life Sci. 2003;74:199–205.
11. So AY, de la Fuente E, Walter P, Shuman M, Bernales S. The unfolded protein response during prostate cancer development. Cancer Metastasis Rev. 2009;28:219–23.
12. Shi YY, He L. SHEsis, a powerful software platform for analyses of linkage disequilibrium, haplotype construction, and genetic association at polymorphism loci. Cell Res. 2005;15:97–8.

13. Dadey DY, Kapoor V, Khudanyan A, et al. The ATF6 pathway of the ER stress response contributes to enhanced viability in glioblastoma. Oncotarget. 2015;7:2080–92.

14. Tay KH, Luan Q, Croft A, et al. Sustained IRE1 and ATF6 signaling is important for survival of melanoma cells undergoing ER stress. Cell Signal. 2014;26:287–94.

15. Li H, Zhou F, Du W, et al. Knockdown of asparagine synthetase by RNAi suppresses cell growth in human melanoma cells and epidermoid carcinoma cells. Biotechnol Appl Biochem. 2016;63:328–33.

16. Ben Tanfous M, Sharif-Askari B, Ceppi F, et al. Polymorphisms of asparaginase pathway and asparaginase-related complications in children with acute lymphoblastic leukemia. Clin Cancer Res. 2015;21:329–34.

17. Pastorczak A, Fendler W, Zalewska-Szewczyk B, et al. Asparagine synthetase (ASNS) gene polymorphism is associated with the outcome of childhood acute lymphoblastic leukemia by affecting early response to treatment. Leuk Res. 2014;38:180–3.

18. Yang H, He X, Zheng Y, et al. Down-regulation of asparagine synthetase induces cell cycle arrest and inhibits cell proliferation of breast cancer. Chem Biol Drug Des. 2015;84:578–84.

3

Survival benefit of transarterial chemoembolization in patients with metastatic hepatocellular carcinoma

Dominik Bettinger[1,2]* (iD), Renan Spode[1], Nicolas Glaser[1], Nico Buettner[1], Tobias Boettler[1], Christoph Neumann-Haefelin[1], Thomas Baptist Brunner[3], Eleni Gkika[3], Lars Maruschke[4], Robert Thimme[1] and Michael Schultheiss[1]

Abstract

Background: As prognosis of patients with metastatic hepatocellular carcinoma (HCC) is mainly determined by intrahepatic HCC progression, local treatment with TACE may result in improved OS, although it is not recommended. The purpose of this study was to analyze retrospectively the efficacy of TACE and its impact on OS in patients with metastatic hepatocellular carcinoma (HCC).

Methods: Two hundred and fifteen patients with metastatic HCC who were treated at our Liver Center between 2003 and 2014 were included in this retrospective analysis. Medical records, laboratory parameters and imaging studies were analyzed. Treatment of metastatic HCC and OS were assessed

Results: One hundred and two patients (47.4%) did not receive any HCC specific treatment while 48 patients (22.3%) were treated with sorafenib, 42 patients (19.5%) with TACE and 23 patients (10.7%) received treatment with TACE and sorafenib in combination. Survival analyses and Cox regression models revealed that TACE and a combination therapy of TACE and sorafenib were significant prognostic factors in metastatic HCC. However, further analyses revealed that there was no additional prognostic effect of adding sorafenib to TACE treatment in this patient cohort.

Conclusions: In metastatic HCC, treatment of intrahepatic tumor by TACE may be associated with improved survival. These results support the prognostic importance of treating intrahepatic HCC even in patients with metastatic disease. Therefore, we suggest evaluating the technical feasibility of TACE in all metastatic patients.

Keywords: Hepatocellular carcinoma, Metastases, Sorafenib, Transarterial chemoembolization, Prognosis

Background

Hepatocellular carcinoma (HCC) is the fifth most common cancer worldwide and its incidence is increasing due to the high incidence of non-alcoholic steatohepatitis (NASH) in the Western world [1–3]. Moreover, HCC is the third leading cause of cancer-related deaths worldwide [4]. Detection of HCC in surveillance programs has markedly improved, but patients with HCC are often diagnosed in advanced stages with the presence of vascular invasion or with extrahepatic tumor spread that is present in 15-42% of patients [5–10]. Prognosis in these patients is limited as there are no curative treatment options available.

Treatment of advanced HCC is determined according to the Barcelona Clinic Liver Cancer (BCLC) classification. Patients with advanced HCC, defined as presence of portal vein invasion or extrahepatic spread, are classified as BCLC stage C and if liver function or the performance status deteriorates, they are staged as BCLC D. In patients with BCLC stage C with and without metastases, sorafenib

* Correspondence: dominik.bettinger@uniklinik-freiburg.de
[1]Department of Medicine II, Medical Center University of Freiburg, Faculty of Medicine, University of Freiburg, Hugstetter Str. 55, D-79106 Freiburg, Germany
[2]Berta-Ottenstein-Programme, Faculty of Medicine, University of Freiburg, Freiburg, Germany
Full list of author information is available at the end of the article

is the treatment of choice although it only leads to a modest improvement of overall survival (OS) compared to treatment with best supportive care [11, 12]. Previous studies have shown that prognosis of patients with metastatic HCC is mainly determined by intrahepatic HCC, hepatic failure due to progression of intrahepatic tumor disease or progression of the underlying liver disease rather than by extrahepatic metastases [13, 14]. These results provide the rationale for treatment of intrahepatic HCC in order to preserve liver function and argue against systemic treatment. In the last years, several studies revealed that transarterial chemoembolization (TACE), the recommended treatment in patients with intermediate HCC, can also be safely and effectively performed in patients with advanced HCC defined by vascular invasion or extrahepatic spread [15]. As patients with advanced HCC are a very heterogeneous group with vascular invasion, extrahepatic metastases or both, it is not clear which subgroup will benefit most from an intrahepatic treatment approach using TACE [10, 16]. The aim of this retrospective study was to assess the efficacy of TACE and its impact on OS in patients with metastatic hepatocellular carcinoma (HCC).

Methods
Selection of patients
Between January 2003 and January 2013 1030 patients who presented with newly diagnosed HCC at our Liver Center were included in an HCC database. 215 of these patients (20.9%) presented with metastatic HCC and were included in these analyses. Patients with history of malignancies other than HCC within the last 5 years were excluded from the analyses to ensure that present metastases were linked to HCC. Further, patients who have been treated with systemic chemotherapy or with radiation therapy in clinical studies were not included in the analyses. Demographic data including etiology of liver disease, blood count, liver function test, the international normalized ratio (INR), alpha-fetoprotein (AFP) and tumor characteristics were collected from the electronical medical records and included in the database retrospectively.

Definitions and methods
HCC was diagnosed according to current guidelines by histopathology or computerized tomography (CT) scan or dynamic contrast-enhanced magnetic resonance imaging (MRI) showing the typical hallmark of HCC imaging (hypervascularity in the arterial phase with washout in the portal venous or delayed phases) [17, 18]. The number of focal hepatic lesions, the maximum tumor diameter and portal vein thrombosis and its extent were detected during contrast enhancement. The numbers of intrahepatic lesions are summarized in oligonodular (one or two intrahepatic lesions) and in multifocal HCC (three or more lesions or diffuse HCC growth pattern).

HCC was staged according to the Barcelona Clinic Liver Cancer (BCLC) classification.

The site of metastasis was determined by CT or MRI scan of the chest and abdomen. In the case that suspected bone metastases were not sufficiently classified in the mentioned imaging modalities, bone scintigraphy was performed for confirmation.

Liver function was assessed using the recently developed ALBI score [19]. The ALBI score was calculated using the following equation: linear predictor = ($\log_{10}$ bilirubin μmol/l × 0.66) + (albumin g/l × –0.085). Bilirubin was recorded in mg/dl and albumin in g/dl, but for the calculation of the linear predictor of the ALBI score, these parameters were transformed in the corresponding units (bilirubin in μmol/l and albumin in g/l). The linear predictor of the ALBI score was categorized in three prognostic groups as published by Johnson et al. [19]: grade 1 (less than –2.60), grade 2 (between –2.60 and –1.39) and grade 3 (above –1.39) with a higher ALBI score being associated with an impaired liver function.

TACE procedure
All HCC patients were discussed interdisciplinary in a review board with hepatologists, interventional radiologists, surgeons, nuclear medicine physicians and radiotherapists. As TACE is not recommended as the treatment of choice for patients with metastatic HCC, the decision to perform TACE was made on an individual basis in each patient. Clinical data, such as liver function and the ECOG performance score, as well as tumor characteristics including portal vein thrombosis and the hepatic vascular architecture were reviewed. If TACE was technically feasible and the patient presented in good performance status and preserved liver function, TACE was performed using a selective or super-selective approach. Intra-arterial infusion of the chemotherapeutic agent and lipiodol was performed after having localized the target lesion. Epirubicin or mitomycin (doses of max. 100 mg) were used as chemotherapeutic agents in our group. The chemotherapeutic agent was not defined in the study protocol. The lipiodol infusion was stopped when intra-arterial stasis was observed in the angiographic control. Further, gelatin sponge particles or PVA particles were used for embolization. The extent of embolization was selected individually. On the total number of 65 patients treated with any type of TACE, 11 cases received drug-eluting beads TACE (DEB-TACE; 16.9%) and 54 patients were treated with conventional TACE (cTACE; 83.1%). A mean number of 1.7 TACE sessions were performed on demand.

Sorafenib treatment
Decision for sorafenib treatment was also made in an interdisciplinary review board. In total, 71 patients were treated with sorafenib. The full dose of 800 mg sorafenib

per day was administered only in 16 of the 71 patients (22.5%) receiving sorafenib treatment. In the remaining 55 of the 71 patients (77.5%), sorafenib was started at a dose of 400 mg per day. Only in 58% of these patients, the dose of sorafenib could be increased to 800 mg per day due to side effects. The median time of sorafenib application was 59 (2 – 690) days.

Statistical analyses

The present study was a retrospective observational study. All patients were followed-up until death or last contact. At the end of the observation 194 of the 215 analyzed patients (90.2%) had died. The primary endpoints were the administered treatment modalities as well as OS stratified according to the individual therapy modalities. OS was calculated from the day of detection of metastases. The cut-off point for survival data was 25th of February 2017.

Continuous variables are expressed as median with the minimum and maximum whereas categorical variables are reported as frequencies and percentages unless stated otherwise.

For continuous variables, differences were determined using Wilcoxon-Mann-Whitney and Kruskal-Wallis tests as there was no Gaussian distribution of the data confirmed by the Kolmogorov-Smirnov test. χ^2 tests or Fisher's Exact tests were used for categorial variables. For sub-analyses of statistically significant tests, the Bonferroni correction was applied. P values <0.05 were considered being significant.

Overall survival was calculated using Kaplan Meier analyses with death being recorded as event. Differences in survival were assessed using logRank tests. To analyze prognostic factors univariate Cox regression models were performed. Age as a continuous variable, gender, ECOG performance score, intrahepatic tumor expansion (oligonodular vs. multifocal), BCLC (stage C vs. D), treatment modalities, the ALBI score, segmental portal vein thrombosis and etiology of liver disease (stratified in viral and non-viral liver disease), tumor size expressed as the large tumor diameter and AFP as a categorial variable with a cut-off of 400 ng/ml were included in the regression model. The ALBI score was used for the assessment of liver function as the Child score incoporates investigator-dependent variables such as hepatic encephalopathy and ascites which might be biased by the retrospective design of the study. Laboratory parameters representing liver function were not included in the models to avoid collinearity with regard to the ALBI score. After univariate analyses of possible predictive factors, multivariate Cox regression model was established using the forward selection method. A limit of $p < 0.05$ for candiate variables to enter the stepwise Cox model was used.

Subgroup analyses were performed in patients who were treated before and after introduction of sorafenib in daily clinical practice in 2007.

Statistical analyses were performed with SPSS (version 24.0, IBM, New York, USA) and GraphPad Prism (version 6, GraphPad Software, San Diego, CA, USA).

Results
Patient characteristics
Demographic and clinical characteristics of the 215 enrolled patients at the time of study inclusion are summarized in Table 1. The median age was 69 (33 – 87) years. 68.4% of the patients presented with non-viral liver disease while 31.6% of the patients had viral liver disease. 60.3% of these patients had chronic hepatitis B virus (HBV) infection and 39.7% were diagnosed with chronic hepatitis C virus (HCV) infection. In total, 35 patients of the included 215 patients (16.3%) had cyroptogenic liver cirrhosis. At the time of HCC diagnosis, the underlying etiology of the liver cirrhosis was not clearly assessable in these patients. Probably, some of them may have had previous non-alcoholic fatty liver disease and due to progression of liver cirrhosis they developed sarcopenia so that the typical features of non-alcoholic fatty liver disease were not present anymore. All patients had typical imaging features of liver cirrhosis in ultrasound examination or in CT or MRI imaging. Assessing liver function with the ALBI score, 24,7% were classified as ALBI 1, 56.7% as ALBI 2 and 18.6% as ALBI 3. In comparison 67.9% of the included patients were classified Child A, 26.5% Child B and 5.6% Child C.

All patients had advanced HCC as classified according to the BCLC classification. One hundred and eighty three patients (85.1%) were in BCLC C and 32 patients (14.9%) were in BCLC D. 73.4% of the patients had multifocal intrahepatic HCC and 30.7% displayed HCC larger than 7 cm. Intrahepatic segmental portal vein thrombosis was detected in 17.4%. None of the patients had extrahepatic portal vein thrombosis.

30.2% of the patients were diagnosed with pulmonary metastases and in 23.3% metastases at multiple sites (all with pulmonary metastases) were found. Lymph node metastases, bone, peritoneal and adrenal gland metastases were found in 19.5%, 11.2%, 5.6% and 1.9%, respectively.

Treatment of patients with metastatic HCC
In our cohort,102 patients (47.4%) with metastatic HCC did not receive any HCC specific therapy. Forty-eight patients (22.3%) were treated with sorafenib. In 42 patients (19.5%) TACE was performed as an individual treatment approach as outlined in the methods section. In 23 patients (10.7%), TACE was performed in combination with ongoing sorafenib treatment. In 17 patients (73.9%) sorafenib was started 5.5 ± 2.0 days after TACE

Table 1 Baseline characteristics of study patients

	All patients	No treatment	Sorafenib	TACE	TACE and sorafenib	p value[#]
Parameter	n = 215	n = 102	n = 48	n = 42	n = 23	
Epidemiology						
Gender, m/f (%)	185/30 (86.0/14.0)	85/17 (83.3/16.7)	42/6 (87.5/12.5)	36/6 (85.7/14.3)	22/1 (95.7/4.3)	0.480
Age, median (min.- max.)	69 (33 – 87)	70 (41 -87)	64 (33 – 85)	68 (46 – 85)	70 (50 -87)	0.150
ECOG						0.163
0	149 (69.3)	65 (63.7)	35 (72.9)	29 (69.1)	20 (87.0)	0.164
1	31 (14.4)	14 (13.7)	6 (12.5)	8 (19.0)	3 (13.0)	0.844
2	35 (16.3)	23 (22.6)	7 (14.6)	5 (11.9)	0	0.042
Etiology of liver disease						
Viral (%)	68 (31.6)	29 (28.4)	16 (33.3)	16 (38.1)	7 (30.4)	0.718
HBV (%)[l]	41 (60.3)	18 (62.1)	7 (43.8)	12 (75.0)	4 (57.1)	
HCV (%)[l]	27 (39.7)	11 (37.9)	9 (56.2)	4 (25.0)	3 (42.9)	
Non-viral (%)	147 (68.4)	73 (71.6)	32 (66.7)	26 (61.9)	16 (69.6)	0.658
Alcohol (%)[l]	82 (55.7)	42 (57.5)	18 (56.3)	14 (53.8)	8 (50.0)	
NAFLD (%)[l]	21 (14.4)	12 (16.4)	1 (3.1)	6 (23.1)	2 (12.4)	
cryptogenic (%)[l]	35 (23.8)	16 (21.9)	9 (28.1)	6 (23.1)	4 (25.0)	
hemochromatosis (%)[l]	8 (5.4)	3 (4.1)	4 (12.5)	-	1 (6.3)	
autoimmune (%)[l]	1 (0,7)	-	-	-	1 (6.3)	
Child Score						
Score, median	5 (5-14)	6 (5-14)	5 (5-9)	5 (5-9)	5 (5-9)	0.001
(min.-max.)					18 (78.3)	0.003
Child A	146 (67.9)	57 (55.8)	38 (79.2)	33 (78.6)	5 (21.7)	0.005
Child B	57 (26.5)	33 (32.4)	10 (20.8)	9 (21.4)	0	0.340
Child C	12 (5.6)	12 (11.8)	0	0		0.004
ALBI score[##]median (min.- max.)	−2.11 (−4.69 – −0.32)	−1.79 (− 3.25 – −0.32)	−2.36 (−3.36 – −0.85)	−2.19 (−4.69 – −0.76)	−2.23 (−3.32- - 1.13)	<0.001
ALBI grade[##](%)						<0.001
ALBI 1	53 (24.7)	16 (15.7)	17 (35.4)	11 (26.2)	9 (39.1)	0.018
ALBI 2	122 (56.7)	54 (52.9)	29 (60.4)	28 (66.7)	11 (47.9)	0.355
ALBI 3	40 (18.6)	32 (31.4)	2 (4.2)	3 (7.1)	3 (13.0)	<0.001
Tumor characteristics						
Intrahepatic HCC: oligonodular vs. multifocal (%)	51 / 149 (26.6/73.4)	22 /80 (21.6/78.4)	8 /40 (16.7/83.3)	17 / 25 (40.5/59.5)	7/16 (30.4/69.6)	0.071
Segmental portal vein thrombosis (%)	36 (17.4)	19 (18.6)	5 (10.4)	7 (16.7)	5 (21.7)	0.611
BCLC (%)						<0.001
C	183 (85.1)	74 (72.5)	44 (91.7)	42 (100)	23 (100)	
D	32 (14.9)	28 (27.5)	4 (8.3)	0	0	
Largest tumor diameter [cm], median (min.-max.)	5.2 (1 – 18)	5.8 (1 – 17	4.4 (1 – 17)	5.3 (1- 17)	7 (2- 18)	0.308
Largest tumor size >7 cm (%)	66 (30.7)	34 (33.3)	9 (18.8)	12 (28.6)	11 (47.8)	0.078
Location of metastases						0.006
Lung	65 (30.1)	38 (37.3)	11 (22.9)	9 (21.4)	7 (30.4)	0.012
Bone	24 (11.2)	11 (10.8)	5 (10.4)	3 (7.1)	5 (21.7)	0.012

Table 1 Baseline characteristics of study patients *(Continued)*

Lymph nodes	42 (19.5)	14 (13.7)	8 (16.7)	17 (40.5)	3 (13.1)	0.012
Peritoneum	12 (5.6)	5 (4.9)	3 (6.3)	3 (7.1)	1 (4.4)	0.718
Adrenal gland	4 (1.9)	3 (2.9)	0	1 (2.4)	0	0.425
Others	18 (8.4)	10 (9.8)	2 (4.2)	6 (14.3)	0	0.416
Multiple sites*	50 (23.3)	21 (20.6)	19 (39.5)	3 (7.2)	7 (30.4)	0.002
Laboratory analyses Median (min.-max.)						
White blood count [10^6/µl]	6. 7 (2.1 – 34.4)	6,4 (2.1 – 28.0)	6.8 (2.6 – 23.0)	6.6 (2.4 – 34.4)	6.8 (2.6 – 14.4)	0.689
Platelets [10^6/µl]	157 (9 -702)	150 (9 -702)	201 (29 – 363)	145 (56 – 480)	161 (51 -401)	0.400
Hemoglobin [g/dl]	12.3 (6.8 – 19.1)	11.9 (6.8 – 16.4)	12.9 (7.8 – 19.1)	13.1 (8.9 – 17.3)	12.6 (7.8 -14.9)	0.002
INR	1.13 (0.7 – 10.0)	1.17 (0.7 – 10.0)	1.12 (0.8 – 2.6)	1.10 (0.8 – 3.4)	1.01 (0.8 – 3.2)	0.078
Creatinine [mg/dl]	0.9 (0.4 – 7.4)	0.9 (0.4 – 5.5)	0.9 (0.5 – 7.4)	0.9 (0.4 – 2.1)	0.9 (0.6 – 1.3)	0.123
AST [U/l]	75 (12 – 674)	96 (18 – 674)	75 (25 – 450)	56 (12 – 252)	65 (20 -472)	0.002
ALT [U/l]	47 (8 - 640)	48 (13 -640)	49 (16 – 205)	45 (8 – 234)	46 (15 – 253)	0.555
Bilirubin [mg/dl]	1.0 (0.3 – 30.9)	1.5 (0.3 -30.9)	0.9 (0.3 – 6.8)	0.9 (0.4 – 14.9)	0.8 (0.4 – 2.5)	<0.001
Albumin [g/dl]	3.5 (2.0 – 6.4)	3.3 2.0 – 4.7)	3.7 (2.4 – 4.6)	3.5 (2.5 – 6.4)	3.7 (2.4 – 4.6)	<0.001
AFP [ng/ml]	222.0 (0.6 – 502,900.0**)	303.1 1.1 – 502,900.0)	174.6 (1.1 – 60,500.0**)	71.4 (0.6 – 60,500.0)	174.0 (1.5 – 60,500.0)	0.098
AFP > 400 ng/ml (%)	93 (43.3)	49 (48.0)	20 (41.7)	16 (38.1)	8 (34.8)	0.557

p values are referred to group comparisons between the different therapies
| relative frequencies are referred either to viral or non-viral etiology
a *higher* ALBI score is associated with *impaired* liver function. ALBI grade 1 represents good liver function while ALBI 3 shows worse liver function
*All patients with multiple metastases had pulmonary metastases
** 502,900 ng/ml and 60,500 ng/ml were the highest values which could have been measured with the AFP assay. As the assay has changed the highest measurable values has also changed

and in 6 patients (26.1%) sorafenib was ongoing when TACE was additionally performed.

Compared to patients who received sorafenib, TACE or a combination of both, patientswho did not receive any HCC specific therapy had impaired liver function as indicated by a higher ALBI score (Table 1, Fig. 1). The ALBI score did not differ significantly between patients who had been treated with TACE, sorafenib or a combination of both ($p = 0.579$).

Patients with multiple extrahepatic metastases were also treated less commonly compared to patients with solitary metastases ($p = 0.002$, Table 1). In this subgroup sorafenib was significantly more often used than TACE (39.6% vs. 7.1%, $p < 0.001$, Table 1). The site of the metastasis did not influence the treatment approach.

Patients with BCLC D did not receive any HCC specific treatmentexcept from four patients who were treated with sorafenib. The decision to treat these patients against current guideline recommendations was based on an interdisciplinary discussion.

The intrahepatic growth pattern (oligonodular vs. multifocal, $p = 0.071$) and the size of the largest tumor diameter ($p = 0.308$) did not differ between the treatment approaches.

We included patients who had been treated between 2003 and 2013. Before 2007 sorafenib had not been

introduced in daily clinical practice for treatment of HCC. Therefore, we divided the cohort in two subgroups (treatment before [$n = 83$] and after 2007 [$n = 132$]). Before 2007, 64 of 83 patients (77.1%) did not receive any HCC-specific treatment while 19 of 83

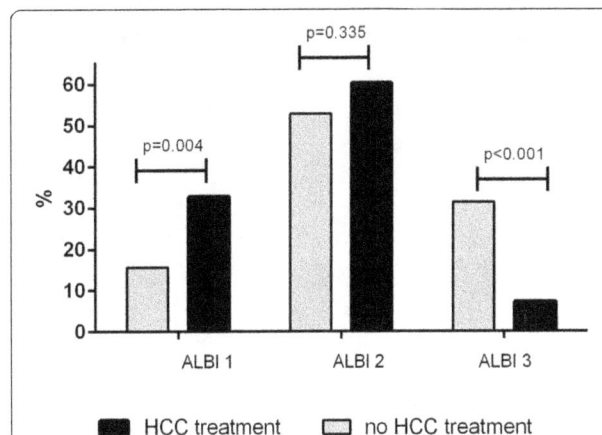

Fig. 1 Liver function assessed by the ALBI score in patients with no HCC specific treatment compared to patients with different treatment approaches. Patients who did not receive any HCC specific treatment had impaired liver function as shown by a higher ALBI grade. * The group "HCC treatment" includes all patients who received either sorafenib, TACE or a combination of both

patients (22.9%) were treated with TACE. After sorafenib had been introduced in daily clinical practice, 48 of 132 patients (36.4%) were treated with sorafenib, 23 patients (17.4%) received TACE, and another 23 patients (17.4%) were treated with a combination of TACE and sorafenib. Thirty-eight of 132 patients (28.8%) received no specific HCC treatment. In both groups, impaired liver function was the main reason for withholding HCC-specific treatment (Additional file 1: Figure S1). Further, there were no differences concerning portal vein invasion or thrombosis, intrahepatic tumor expansion or site and number of extrahepatic metastases between the different treatment approaches in both sub-groups.

Influence of HCC treatment on overall survival and prognostic factors

Median OS of all included patients was 5.0 [4.0 – 6.0] months. Patients who did not receive any HCC specific treatment had a median OS of 3 months [95% CI: 2.01 – 3.95] compared to patients who were treated with sorafenib (6 months [95% CI: 4.67 – 7.33], $p = 0.009$), with TACE (9 months [95% CI: 4.46 – 13.54], $p < 0.001$) and to those who were treated with a combination of TACE and sorafenib (16 months [95% CI: 9.94 – 22.10], $p = 0.002$) (Fig. 2). These results were confirmed in a multivariate Cox regression model showing that TACE (HR 0.50 [0.33 – 0.76], $p = 0.001$) and a combination of TACE and sorafenib (HR 0.39 [0.23-0.66], $p < 0.001$) were significant independent prognostic factors in patients with metastatic HCC (Table 2). These results were confirmed in the sub-groups (treatment before and after 2007).

In order to analyze the additional effect of sorafenib on OS in metastatic patients treated with TACE, a subgroup analysis including only patients who have either been treated with TACE ($n = 42$) or with a combination of TACE and sorafenib ($n = 23$) was performed. Multivariate Cox regression analysis revealed that additional treatment with sorafenib was not an independent prognostic factor. Intrahepatic tumor burden (HR 1.86 [0.99 – 3.47], $p = 0.053$) was an independent negative prognostic factor in these patients (Table 3).

Discussion

HCC is often diagnosed in an advanced stage with or without extrahepatic metastases. In these patients, curative treatment options are not available. According to the BCLC classification these patients are classified as BCLC stage C and sorafenib is recommended as the treatment of choice [5, 11, 20]. However, sorafenib treatment only leads to a modest improvement of OS of approximately 3 months [11]highlighting that new treatment approaches in patients with advanced HCC either with or without extrahepatic metastases are urgently needed. It has to be considered that 66-89% of advanced HCC patients do not die from extrahepatic metastatic disease but rather form intrahepatic HCC progression or cancer associated liver failure [10, 16]. These data provide the rationale for local intrahepatic treatment of HCC e.g. using TACE with the goal to improve OS due to delayed intrahepatic tumor progression. Therefore, we set out to analyze the effect of TACE on OS in patients with metastatic HCC.

47.4% of the included patients did not receive any HCC specific treatment. Apart from no available effective treatment option before 2007, the most important reason for withholding HCC treatmentwas the presence of impaired liver function. Multivariate Cox regression models revealed that liver function as indicated by the ALBI score, is an important predictor of OS in patients with metastatic HCC. These results support the importance of preserving liver function during HCC specific

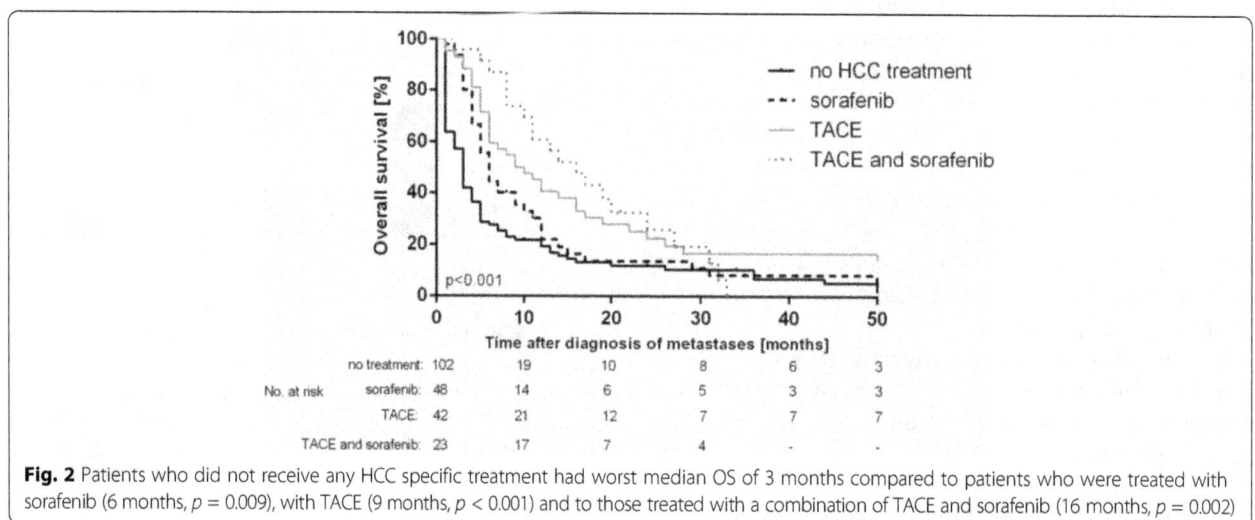

Fig. 2 Patients who did not receive any HCC specific treatment had worst median OS of 3 months compared to patients who were treated with sorafenib (6 months, $p = 0.009$), with TACE (9 months, $p < 0.001$) and to those treated with a combination of TACE and sorafenib (16 months, $p = 0.002$)

Table 2 Prognostic factors in patients with metastatic HCC

Parameters	Univariate			Multivariate		
	HR[1]	95% CI[2]	p	HR	95% CI	p
Age	0.99	0.98 - 1.01	0.745			
gender (male vs. female)	1.43	0.96 - 2.14	0.082			
Intrahepatic tumor expansion (multifocal vs. oligonodular)	1.74	1.23 - 2.47	0.002	1.63	1.11 - 2.42	0.014
Tumor size (cm)	1.00	0.97 - 1.04	0.889			
ECOG			0.127			
0	1					
1	1.04	0.69-1.58				
2	1.50	1.01-2.22				
Treatment			<0.001			0.007
No therapy	1			1		
Sorafenib	0.62	0.43 – 0.91	0.013	0.86	0.56 – 2.26	0.475
TACE	0.45	0.30 – 0.66	<0.001	0.54	0.35 – 0.84	0.006
TACE and sorafenib	0.41	0.25 – 0.68	<0.001	0.48	0.28 – 0.81	0.006
ALBI			<0.001			<0.001
ALBI 1	1			1		
ALBI 2	1.63	1.15 - 2.31	0.006	1.56	1.10 - 2.30	0.026
ALBI 3	3.33	2.15 - 5.15	<0.001	3.42	2.09 - 5.61	<0.001
viral vs. non-viral etiology	0.89	0.65 - 1.20	0.432			
Segmental portal vein thrombosis	1.12	0.97 - 1.29	0.128			
AFP > 400 ng/ml	1.51	1.13 - 2.01	0.005	1.50	1.10 - 1.92	0.010
BCLC (C vs. D)	5.15	3.31 - 8.02	<0.001	2.45	1.42 – 4.29	0.001
multiple metastases	0.96	0.69 - 1.33	0.797			

TACE is an independent prognostic factor in patients with metastatic HCC. Moreover, liver function represented by the ALBI score is also a strong prognostic factor indicating the importance of a preserved liver function for OS in these patients
Abbreviations: [1] HR hazard ratio, [2] 95% CI 95% confidence interval

treatment. Retrospective assessment of the Child score was often difficult due to inaccurate assessment of the highly subjective parameters ascites and hepatic encehalopathy. Being aware of this selection bias, we decided to use the ALBI grade for measurement of liver function as it has shown good prognostic effects in patients with liver cirrhosis and HCC [19, 21, 22]. Another important reason for choosing the ALBI grade for measurement of liver function was that the ALBI grade showed a better discriminatory capacity compared to the Child score in the estimation of the prognosis in our patient cohort (by means of Harrell's concordance index (0.64 vs. 0.57)).

As there had been no effective systemic chemotherapeutic therapy available for patients with advanced HCC before sorafenib, patients with metastatic disease were treated with TACE on an individual basis. As previous studies showed good evidence that prognosis of metastatic patients is mainly determined by intrahepatic HCC [13, 14], selected patients were treated with TACE even after sorafenib had been introduced. In many Asian centers, TACE is regularly performed in these patients even though there are no randomized controlled studies supporting this strategy

[23]. Zhao et al. reported a meta-analysis of patients with advanced HCC who were treated with TACE showing a median OS of 14.0 months in the TACE group and 9.7 months in the sorafenib group [15]. This meta analysis primarily included patients with vascular invasion and in only four studies patients with extrahepatic metastases had been analyzed and these results may not reflect the efficacy of TACE in metastatic patients. These inclusion criteria may explain why OS in our patients treated with TACE was lower with 9 months. Compared to systemic treatment with sorafenib, TACE was associated with better OS in patients with metastatic HCC. There might be a bias in our patient cohort due to inclusion of patients before sorafenib. Stratifying patients according to the time point of study inclusion (before and after introduction of sorafenib), the sub-group analyses showed that in both cohorts TACE was an independent prognostic factor. These results may be the rationale for focusing on intrahepatic treatment rather than on systemic treatment in patients with metastatic HCC.

Moreover, we set out to analyze if addition of sorafenib to TACE may result in better OS. In the recently published SPACE trial, addition of sorafenib to TACE did

Table 3 Prognostic factors in patients with metastatic HCC treated with TACE or TACE and sorafenib in combination

Parameters	Univariate			Multivariate		
	HR[1]	95% CI[2]	p	HR	95% CI	p
Age	1.01	0.98 – 1.04	0.725			
gender (male vs. female)	2.27	1.00 – 5.11	0.048	2.39	0.99 – 5.76	0.052
Intrahepatic tumor expansion (multifocal vs. oligododular)	1.95	1.07 – 3.55	0.028	1.86	0.99 – 3.47	0.031
Tumor size (cm)	1.02	0.95 - 1.10	0.527			
Sorafenib	0.89	0.51 – 1.56	0.688			
ALBI			0.769			
ALBI 1	1					
ALBI 2	1.24	0.69 – 2.24	0.468			
ALBI 3	1.16	0.46 – 2.94	0.761			
viral vs. non-viral etiology	1.03	0.60 – 1.76	0.923			
segmental portal vein thrombosis	2.10	1.04 – 4.24	0.038			
AFP > 400 ng/ml	1.16	0.68 - 2.00	0.582			
ECOG						
0	1					
1	0.91	0.43 – 1.95				
2	2.60	0.91 7.48				
multiple metastases	0.99	0.48 – 2.04	0.981			

Additional sorafenib treatment in patients with metastatic HCC treated with TACE did not result in an independent positive prognostic effect. BCLC was not entered in the Cox model as all patients were classified as BLCL C who were treated with TACE or TACE and sorafenib
Abbreviations: [1] HR hazard ratio, [2]95% CI 95% confidence interval

not result in a clinically relevant improved time to progression and OS in patients with intermediate HCC [24]. After adjusting for other important parameters in multivariate Cox regression models, the combined use of sorafenib and TACE had also no additional prognostic effect in our study. It has to be considered that only in 22.7% of our patients the recommended dose of 800 mg sorafenib daily has been administered. Further, treatment duration with sorafenib was short. Clearly, these factors may have limited the efficacy of sorafenib. However, reduced doses of sorafenib and short treatment durations somewhat reflect clinical reality with this drug [25].

Only few patients had been treated with DEB-TACE while most of our patients received cTACE. It is well known that in patients with cTACE higher systemic levels of the injected chemotherapeutic agent are observed compared to patients treated with DEB-TACE which may also have a therapeutic impact on extrahepatic metastases [26]. Therefore, further studies are warranted to eluciate this important question.

Taken together, intrahepatic tumor treatment with TACE was associated with a better OS compared to treatment with sorafenib and that the combination of bothwas no independet prognostic factor. Therefore,we suggestevaluatingthe technical feasibility of TACE in all metastatic patients. However, as many patients had been treated with several sessions of TACE before development

of metastases, the transarterial approach may be difficult and even not possible. In this settingstereotactic body radiation therapy (SBRT) has emerged as another innovative treatment possibility in patients with advanced HCC achieving local intrahepatic tumor control and first small studies have shown promising results [27–31]. Studies focusing on SBRT in metastatic HCC are urgently needed. Further, transarterial radioembolization with Yttrium-90 has shown good local tumor control rates compared to conventional transarterial chemoembolisation [32]. Therefore, this may be another possibility to achieve local intrahepatic tumor control in metastatic HCC and should be investigated in further prospective studies.

Noteworthy, our study has several limitations. The decision for treatment with TACE depended on many different parameters including intrahepatic tumor expansion, portal vein thrombosis, the performance status of the patients, liver function and also on the extent of the metastatic disease (patients with multiple metastases have rarely been treated). Considering these factors, retrospective analyses of OS according to different treatment approaches, are always associated with a significant detection bias and will result in overestimation of treatment efficacy. Due to the differences in baseline characteristics we performed multivariate Cox regression model to adjust for these possible confounders. Moreover, we used OS as the primary endpoint which includes cancer-related, liver-related deaths as well as other deaths. It may be important to link OS to the different causes of death, but due to the retrospective design of our study, we were not able to perform these analyses. For our multi-variate model, we only had 65 cases and due to the small sample size, this analysis may be biased and should be repeated with more patients in prospective, randomized studies. Further, we did not assess intrahepatic tumor response after TACE as imaging follow-up was only available in 39 patients.

Conclusion

Taken together, our data suggest that treatment with TACE in metastatic HCC patients with preserved liver function may be associated with better OS. Although these preliminary data have been derived from retrospective analyses, they may help to design prospective, randomized controlled trials to assess the efficacy of TACE in patients with metastatic HCC.

Abbreviations

95% CI: 95% confidence interval; AFP: Alpha-fetoprotein; BCLC: Barcelona Clinic Liver Classification; CT: Computerized tomography; HBV: Hepatitis B virus; HCC: Hepatocellular carcinoma; INR: International normalized ratio; MRI: Magnetic resonance imaging; NASH: Non-alcoholic steatohepatitis; OS: Overall survival; SBRT: Stereotactic body radiation therapy; TACE: Transarterial chemoembolisation

Acknowledgments

Not applicable.

Funding

The article processing charge was funded by the German Research Foundation (DFG) and the University of Freiburg in the funding programme Open Access Publishing.
DB is supported by the Berta-Ottenstein-Programme, Faculty of Medicine, University of Freiburg.

Authors' contributions

DB: study concept and design, acquisition of data, analysis and interpretation of data, statistical analyses, drafting of the manuscript; RS: acquisition of data; NG: acquisition of data, interpretation of the data, critical revision of the manuscript for important intellectual content; NB: critical revision of the manuscript for important intellectual content; TB: critical revision of the manuscript for important intellectual content, CNH: critical revision of the manuscript for important intellectual content, TBB: critical revision of the manuscript for important intellectual content; EG: critical revision of the manuscript for important intellectual content; LM: performed the transarterial chemoembolisation, critical revision of the manuscript for important intellectual content; RT: critical revision of the manuscript for important intellectual content, analysis and interpretation of data; MS: study concept and design, interpretation of data, drafting of the manuscript. All authors approved the final version of the article, including the authorship.

Consent for publication

Not applicable.

Competing interests

DB receives teaching and speaking fees from Bayer HealthCare.

Author details

[1]Department of Medicine II, Medical Center University of Freiburg, Faculty of Medicine, University of Freiburg, Hugstetter Str. 55, D-79106 Freiburg, Germany. [2]Berta-Ottenstein-Programme, Faculty of Medicine, University of Freiburg, Freiburg, Germany. [3]Department of Radiation Oncology, Medical Center University of Freiburg,Faculty of Medicine, University of Freiburg, Robert-Koch-Str. 3, D-79106 Freiburg, Germany. [4]Department of Radiology, Medical Center University of Freiburg, Faculty of Medicine, University of Freiburg, Hugstetter Str. 55, D-79106 Freiburg, Germany.

References

1. Hassan MM, Abdel-Wahab R, Kaseb A, et al. Obesity early in adulthood increases risk but does not affect outcomes of Hepatocellular carcinoma. Gastroenterology. 2015;149(1):119–29.
2. Mittal S, El-Serag HB. Epidemiology of hepatocellular carcinoma: consider the population. J Clin Gastroenterol. 2013;47(Suppl):S2–6.
3. El-Serag HB. Hepatocellular carcinoma. N Engl J Med. 2011;365(12):1118–27.
4. Hu H, Duan Z, Long X, et al. Sorafenib combined with transarterial chemoembolization versus transarterial chemoembolization alone for advanced-stage hepatocellular carcinoma: a propensity score matching study. PLoS One. 2014;9(5):e96620.
5. Forner A, Llovet JM, Bruix J. Hepatocellular carcinoma. Lancet. 2012; 379(9822):1245–55.
6. Llovet JM, Di Bisceglie AM, Bruix J, et al. Design and endpoints of clinical trials in hepatocellular carcinoma. J Natl Cancer Inst. 2008;100(10):698–711.
7. Katyal S, Oliver JH 3rd, Peterson MS, Ferris JV, Carr BS, Baron RL. Extrahepatic metastases of hepatocellular carcinoma. Radiology. 2000;216(3):698–703.
8. Shuto T, Hirohashi K, Kubo S, et al. Treatment of adrenal metastases after hepatic resection of a hepatocellular carcinoma. Dig Surg. 2001;18(4):294–7.
9. Si MS, Amersi F, Golish SR, et al. Prevalence of metastases in hepatocellular carcinoma: risk factors and impact on survival. Am Surg. 2003;69(10):879–85.
10. Uka K, Aikata H, Takaki S, et al. Clinical features and prognosis of patients with extrahepatic metastases from hepatocellular carcinoma. World J Gastroenterol. 2007;13(3):414–20.
11. Llovet JM, Ricci S, Mazzaferro V, et al. Sorafenib in advanced hepatocellular carcinoma. N Engl J Med. 2008;359(4):378–90.
12. Kalyan A, Nimeiri H, Kulik L. Systemic therapy of hepatocellular carcinoma: current and promising. Clin Liver Dis. 2015;19(2):421–32.
13. Kanda M, Tateishi R, Yoshida H, et al. Extrahepatic metastasis of hepatocellular carcinoma: incidence and risk factors. Liver Int. 2008;28(9):1256–63.
14. Natsuizaka M, Omura T, Akaike T, et al. Clinical features of hepatocellular carcinoma with extrahepatic metastases. J Gastroenterol Hepatol. 2005; 20(11):1781–7.
15. Zhao Y, Cai G, Zhou L, et al. Transarterial chemoembolization in hepatocellular carcinoma with vascular invasion or extrahepatic metastasis: a systematic review. Asia Pac J Clin Oncol. 2013;9(4):357–64.
16. Okusaka T, Okada S, Ishii H, et al. Prognosis of hepatocellular carcinoma patients with extrahepatic metastases. Hepato-Gastroenterology. 1997;44(13):251–7.
17. Bruix J, Sherman M. Management of hepatocellular carcinoma: an update. Hepatology. 2011;53(3):1020–2.
18. European Association For The Study Of The Liver, European Organisation For Research And Treatment Of Cancer. EASL-EORTC clinical practice guidelines: management of hepatocellular carcinoma. J Hepatol. 2012;56(4): 908–43.
19. Johnson PJ, Berhane S, Kagebayashi C, et al. Assessment of liver function in patients with hepatocellular carcinoma: a new evidence-based approach-the ALBI grade. J Clin Oncol. 2015;33(6):550–8.
20. Forner A, Gilabert M, Bruix J, Raoul JL. Treatment of intermediate-stage hepatocellular carcinoma. Nat Rev Clin Oncol. 2014;11(9):525–35.
21. Pinato DJ, Sharma R, Allara E, et al. The ALBI grade provides objective hepatic reserve estimation across each BCLC stage of hepatocellular carcinoma. J Hepatol. 2017;66(2):338–46.

22. Pinato DJ, Yen C, Bettinger D, et al. The albumin-bilirubin grade improves hepatic reserve estimation post-sorafenib failure: implications for drug development. Aliment Pharmacol Ther. 2017;45(5):714–22.

23. Omata M, Lesmana LA, Tateishi R, et al. Asian Pacific Association for the Study of the liver consensus recommendations on hepatocellular carcinoma. Hepatol Int. 2010;4(2):439–74.

24. Lencioni R, Llovet JM, Han G, et al. Sorafenib or placebo plus TACE with doxorubicin-eluting beads for intermediate stage HCC: the SPACE trial. J Hepatol. 2016;64(5):1090–8.

25. Al-Rajabi R, Patel S, Ketchum NS, et al. Comparative dosing and efficacy of sorafenib in hepatocellular cancer patients with varying liver dysfunction. J Gastrointest Oncol. 2015;6(3):259–67.

26. Varela M, Real MI, Burrel M, et al. Chemoembolization of hepatocellular carcinoma with drug eluting beads: efficacy and doxorubicin pharmacokinetics. J Hepatol. 2007;46(3):474–81.

27. Su TS, Liang P, Lu HZ, et al. Stereotactic body radiation therapy for small primary or recurrent hepatocellular carcinoma in 132 Chinese patients. J Surg Oncol. 2016;113(2):181–7.

28. Wang PM, Chung NN, Hsu WC, Chang FL, Jang CJ, Scorsetti M. Stereotactic body radiation therapy in hepatocellular carcinoma: optimal treatment strategies based on liver segmentation and functional hepatic reserve. Rep Pract Oncol Radiother. 2015;20(6):417–24.

29. Meng M, Wang H, Zeng X, et al. Stereotactic body radiation therapy: a novel treatment modality for inoperable hepatocellular carcinoma. Drug Discov Ther. 2015;9(5):372–9.

30. Feng M, Brunner TB, Ben-Josef E. Stereotactic body radiation therapy for liver cancer: effective therapy with minimal impact on quality of life. Int J Radiat Oncol Biol Phys. 2015;93(1):26–8.

31. Klein J, Dawson LA, Jiang H, et al. Prospective longitudinal assessment of quality of life for liver cancer patients treated with stereotactic body radiation therapy. Int J Radiat Oncol Biol Phys. 2015;93(1):16–25.

32. Padia SA, Johnson GE, Horton KJ, et al. Segmental yttrium-90 Radioembolization versus segmental Chemoembolization for localized Hepatocellular carcinoma: results of a single-center, retrospective, propensity score-matched study. J Vasc Interv Radiol. 2017 Jun;28(6):777–85.

4

Secondary sclerosing cholangitis in localized hepatobiliary tuberculosis simulating cholangiocarcinoma

Aleena Jain[1]*[iD], Rachana Chaturvedi[2], Chetan Kantharia[3], Amita Joshi[2], Mangesh Londhe[2] and Mayura Kekan[4]

Abstract

Background: Hepatobiliary tuberculosis includes miliary, tuberculous hepatitis or localized forms. The localised form is extremely uncommon and can mimic malignancy. Still rarer is its presentation as sclerosing cholangitis.

Case presentation: A 50 year male presented with acute onset jaundice, significant weight loss and elevated liver enzymes with clinico-radiological suspicion of cholangiocarcinoma. A left hepatectomy was done and dilated bile ducts filled with caseous necrotic material were seen intra-operatively. Histopathology suggested localized hepatobiliary tuberculosis with features of secondary sclerosing cholangitis.

Conclusion: Localised hepatobiliary tuberculosis can cause diagnostic difficulties and its possibility should be considered especially in endemic areas.

Keywords: Hepatobiliary, Tuberculosis, Sclerosing cholangitis, Cholangiocarcinoma

Background

Tuberculosis (TB) is a worldwide health problem and an important cause of morbidity and mortality, especially in developing nations. While pulmonary involvement is commonest, extra-pulmonary TB is also an important clinical problem. Abdominal TB is one of the most prevalent forms with gastrointestinal, splenic, pancreatic, hepatobiliary, peritoneal, omental, mesenteric and/or abdominal lymph node involvement. Manifestations can be non-specific and mimic other conditions, including malignancies [1].

Sclerosing cholangitis is a chronic cholestatic disease, characterized by inflammation, obliterative fibrosis of bile ducts, stricture formation and progressive biliary destruction leading to cirrhosis. It occurs in two forms; primary/idiopathic (commonly) and acquired/secondary. The causes of latter include immune disorders, ischemia, infections, parasites, infiltrative processes and metastasis [2].

Here we report a case of localized hepatobiliary TB (HBTB) causing secondary sclerosing cholangitis (SSC), which is very uncommon.

Case presentation

A 50 years male presented with jaundice since 10 days associated with significant loss of weight & appetite. Previous history of fever 1 month ago was present, for which he was diagnosed and treated as typhoid. He was treated for blood hypertension for 5 years with no previous history of surgery. There was no past history TB or TB contact. On examination, he was afebrile and icterus was present. Abdominal examination revealed soft, non-tender abdomen with no guarding, rigidity or organomegaly.

Hemogram was within normal. Sequential liver function tests were abnormal, with bilirubin values ranging 9–18.6 mg/dl, alkaline phosphatase 227-862 U/L, ALT 227-876 U/L and AST from 71 to 1043 U/L. AMA and viral markers (HBsAg/HCV/HCV/HAV/HIV) were negative. ECG and Chest X-ray were normal. Ultrasonography and CT scan showed mildly enlarged liver with asymmetric dilation of intra-hepatic bile duct and a

* Correspondence: aleena14189@gmail.com
[1]Department of Pathology, Seth GSMC & KEMH, Parel, Mumbai, India
Full list of author information is available at the end of the article

proximal concentric ill-defined mildly enhancing soft tissue lesion suggesting cholangiocarcinoma [Fig. 1a]. Magnetic resonance cholangio-pancreatography (MRCP) showed filling defect in bile ducts likely to be calculus, cast or sludge along with few enlarged periportal lymph nodes [Fig. 1b].

Because fast progression of the disease, left hepatectomy with hepaticojejunostomy was done and during surgery, caseous necrotic material was seen oozing out from dilated bile ducts. Specimen measuring 12 × 12 × 6 cm showed dilated and thickened hepatic ducts, few studded with stones, along with 0.5-1 cm sized yellowish white nodules in the adjacent liver parenchyma [Fig. 1c, d]. Remaining parenchyma was non-cirrhotic with focal greenish discoloration.

On microscopy, fibrous expansion of portal tracts with bile ductular proliferation [Fig. 2a], extensive periductal fibrosis with focal onion skinning [Fig. 2b] and occasional collagen nodule formation was observed [Fig. 2c]. Bile ducts revealed caseous material in lumen with mucosal ulceration, occasional ill-defined granulomas and dense chronic inflammation composed of lymphoplasmacytic infiltrate with sheets of macrophages [Fig. 2d, e]. Liver parenchyma exhibited focal necrotising epithelioid granulomas and cholestasis [Fig. 2f]. Ziehl-Neelsen staining and PCR for acid-fast bacilli (AFB) and gomori-methanamine-silver for fungus were negative.

A diagnosis of localised HBTB with SSC-like features was made for which a trial of anti-tubercular treatment (ATT) was given. Patient responded well and PET-CT after treatment completion showed no residual fixation.

Discussion

Liver is not fit for mycobacterium tuberculosis because of its low tissue oxygen tension. However, three types of HBTB have been defined: miliary, granulomatous disease (tuberculous hepatitis) and localised [3]. The commonest, generalized miliary, usually has no clinical features related to liver. Tuberculous hepatitis presents as fever, mild jaundice, with/without hepatomegaly and rare pulmonary involvement. The least common localised form, shows exclusive hepatobiliary tract involvement based on clinical, radiologic and laboratory examination, further confirmed on microbiology and histopathology [4]. Localised HBTB involves liver parenchyma, biliary tract or both with the latter two being rare even in endemic areas [4]. Ours was a case of localised HBTB with no gastrointestinal or pulmonary involvement.

Broadly, there are two forms of HBTB, diffuse and localised. The diffuse form occurs if the bacilli reach heaptic parenchyma via hepatic artery from lungs or through portal vein in case of gastrointestinal involvement. In localised form, bacilli may reach liver via lymphatics or through rupture of a tuberculous lymph node at porta [3, 5]. Biliary involvement can be secondary to AFB excretion into bile producing strictures or due to compression by enlarged nodes or hepatic granulomas, leading to obstructive jaundice [1]. In our case it was difficult to ascertain whether biliary involvement was secondary to hepatic parenchymal disease or due to enlarged periportal lymph nodes.

Bandopadhyay and Maithy have tabulated clinical features, laboratory abnormalities and outcome from seven

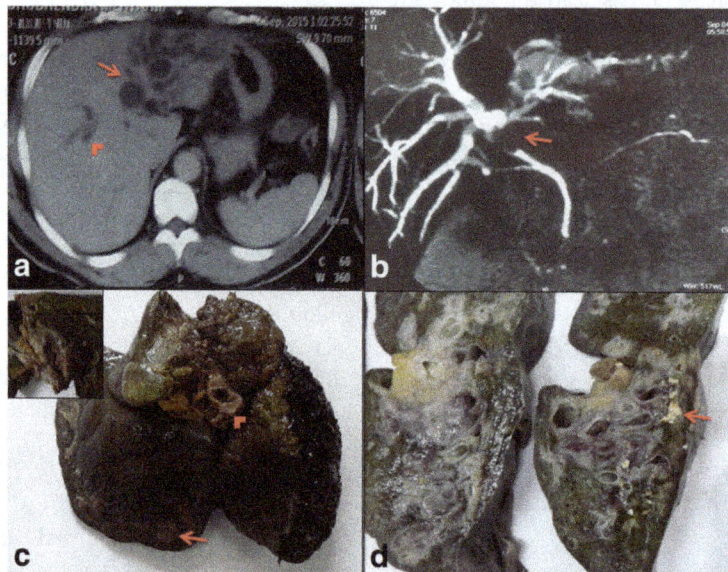

Fig. 1 a CT scan showing dilatation of left intrahepatic bile duct (arrow), more than right (arrowhead); **b** MRCP showing filling defect (arrow) in common hepatic duct; **c** Left hepatectomy showing yellow-white nodules (arrow) with dilated, thickened hepatic ducts (arrowhead). Large thick walled bile duct showing necrotic material (Inset); **d** Multiple dilated, thick walled hepatic ducts, few studded with stones (arrow)

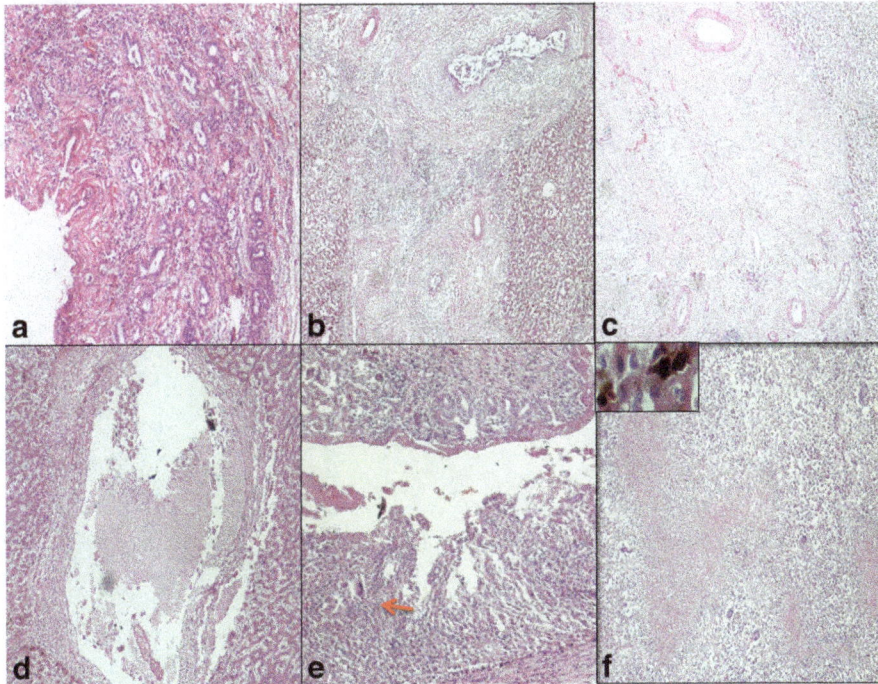

Fig. 2 a Bile ductular proliferation; **b** Fibrous expansion of portal tracts with onion skinning of bile ducts; **c** Absent bile duct with collagen nodule; **d** Bile duct filled with caseous material; **e** Ulcerated bile duct with granuloma (arrow); **f** Caseating hepatic granulomas. Adjacent liver parenchyma showing cholestasis (Inset) (H & E,× 400)

large series of HBTB and observed that fever was the most common symptom (50–90%) followed by abdominal pain (45–66%). Other features were jaundice, pruritis, loss of weight and appetitie. Hepatomegaly was the commonest abnormality on clinical examination [3]. Our patient had obstructive jaundice, weight loss and mild hepatomegaly. Though there is no specific age for HBTB, most patients are between 30 and 50 years, similar to ours (50 years) [3, 4].

It is often difficult to differentiate benign and malignant causes of biliary stricture because clinical, laboratory findings including LFTs and cholangiography are non-specific [5]. Treatment HBTB is mainly medical and surgery may be required if there is biliary involvement. In our case, clinical features and CT suggested cholangiocarcinoma, left hepatectomy with hepaticojejunostomy was indicated.

Grossly, liver can show nodules (tuberculoma/tubercular abscess) which may mimick primary or metastatic malignancy [1]. Biliary involvement can lead to diffuse thickening or strictures resembling primary sclerosing cholangitis or cholangiocarcinoma [5, 6]. In our case too, possibility of malignancy could not be ruled out on gross examination.

Microscopically, necrotizing caseating granulomas were observed in liver, which are considered pathognomic of TB. Bile ducts showed caseation in lumen, ulceration with dense chronic inflammation and vague

granulomas in the wall. Caseating granulomas have also occasionally been reported in Hodgkin disease, brucellosis and few fungal infections like coccidioidomycosis, with different clinical presentations [3].

SSC aetiologies are various, including infection. In HBTB, SSC-like changes have been described on cholangiography [5, 6]. However in our case, similar changes were seen on histology, which have not been previously described. The other causes of SSC were excluded on clinico-radiological examination.

The positivity of AFB stains and cultures varies from to 45 and 60% respectively. Diaz et al. found that at least 57% of hepatic tuberculosis granulomas were positive on PCR [7]. In our study, AFB and PCR were negative which might be related to presence of only focal granulomas with paucity of mycobacteria in the tissue. Culture was not available because the diagnosis was not suspected preoperatively. Many clinicians accept good clinical response to anti-TB drugs is an indirect reliable tool for TB diagnosis. In our case too, patient responded dramatically to ATT supporting HBTB diagnosis.

Conclusion

Atypical presentations of HBTB can lead to diagnostic difficulties; hence a high suspicion index is necessary for its diagnosis. Localised HBTB can cause SSC-like changes or stimulate malignant tumour.

Acknowledgements
NIL, no medical writer was involved.

Funding
NIL (for all authors).

Authors' contributions
AJa carried out concepts and design, literature search, participated in clinical study, data acquisition, data analysis and manuscript preparation will stand as guarantor also. RC carried out concepts and design, literature search, manuscript review. CK participated in clinical study, data acquisition and manuscript review. AJo carried out literature search, clinical study and data acquisition. All the authors read and approved the final manuscript.

Consent for publication
Written informed consent was obtained from the patient for publication of this case report and any accompanying images.

Competing interests
The authors declare that they have no competing interests.

Author details
[1]Department of Pathology, Seth GSMC & KEMH, Parel, Mumbai, India.
[2]Department of Pathology, Seth GSMC & KEMH, Mumbai, India. [3]G. I. Surgery, Seth GSMC & KEMH, Mumbai, India. [4]Department of Pathology, TNMC & Nair Ch hospital, Mumbai, India.

References
1. Chong VH, Lim KS. Hepatobiliary tuberculosis. Singap Med J. 2010;51(9):744–51.
2. Batts KP. Autoimmune and chronic cholestatic disorders of the liver. In: Odze and Goldblum surgical pathology of the GI tract, liver, biliary tract and pancreas; 3rd ed. 2014: Ch 47;1280-1282.
3. Bandopadhyay S, Maithy PK. Hepatobiliary tuberculosis. J Assoc Physician India. 2013;61:44–7.
4. Amarapurkar DN, Patel ND, Amarapurkar AD. Hepatobiliary tuberculosis in western India. Indian J Pathol Microbiol. 2008;51(2):175–81.
5. Jethwani U, et al. Tuberculosis of biliary tract: a rare cause of common bile duct stricture. OA Case Rep. 2013;2:53.
6. Ozin Y, et al. Sclerosing cholangitis-like changes in hepatobiliary tuberculosis. Turk J Gastroenterol. 2010;21:50–3.
7. Huang WT, et al. The nodular form of hepatic tuberculosis: a review with five additional new cases. J Clin Pathol. 2003;56:835.

5

Uneven acute non-alcoholic fatty change of the liver after percutaneous transhepatic portal vein embolization in a patient with hilar cholangiocarcinoma

Chun-Yi Tsai[*], Motoi Nojiri, Yukihiro Yokoyama, Tomoki Ebata, Takashi Mizuno and Masato Nagino

Abstract

Background: Portal vein embolization is essential for patients with biliary cancer who undergo extended hepatectomy to induce hypertrophy of the future remnant liver. Over 830 patients have undergone the portal vein embolization at our institution since 1990. Non-alcoholic fatty liver disease is an entity of hepatic disease characterized by fat deposition in hepatocytes. It has a higher prevalence among persons with morbid obesity, type 2 diabetes, and hyperlipidemia. Neither the mechanism of hepatic hypertrophy after portal vein embolization nor the pathophysiology of non-alcoholic fatty liver disease has been fully elucidated. Some researchers integrated the evident insults leading to progression of fatty liver disease into the multiple-hit hypothesis. Among these recognized insults, the change of hemodynamic status of the liver was never mentioned.

Case presentation: We present the case of a woman with perihilar cholangiocarcinoma who received endoscopic biliary drainage and presented to our institute for surgical consultation. A left trisectionectomy with caudate lobectomy and extrahepatic bile duct resection was indicated for curative treatment. To safely undergo left trisectionectomy, she underwent selective portal vein embolization of the liver, in which uneven acute fatty change subsequently developed. The undrained left medial sector of the liver with dilated biliary tracts was spared the fatty change. The patient underwent planned surgery without any major complications 6 weeks after the event and has since resumed a normal life. The discrepancies in fatty deposition in the different sectors of the liver were confirmed by pathologic interpretations.

Conclusion: This is the first report of acute fatty change of the liver after portal vein embolization. The sparing of the undrained medial sector is unique and extraordinary. The images and pathologic interpretations presented in this report may inspire further research on how the change of hepatic total inflow after portal vein embolization can be one of the insults leading to non-alcoholic fatty liver disease/ change.

Keywords: Non-alcoholic fatty liver disease, Portal vein embolization, Hilar cholangiocarcinoma, Biliary tract obstruction, Case report

* Correspondence: andreas3048@gmail.com
Division of Surgical Oncology, Department of Surgery, Nagoya University
Graduate School of Medicine, 65 Tsurumai-cho, Showa-ku, Nagoya 466-8550,
Japan

Background

Non-alcoholic fatty liver disease (NAFLD) is a specific entity of disease representing fat accumulation in hepatocytes that ranges from simple steatosis to necroinflammatory steatohepatitis [1, 2]. By definition, the diagnosis must be made in patients who have no evidence of excessive alcohol consumption. It is becoming one of the most common hepatic diseases in Western countries, with higher prevalence among persons with morbid obesity or type 2 diabetes [3, 4]. The pathogenesis of NAFLD is not fully elucidated, although several theories have been proposed. Regarding inflammatory steatohepatitis, or non-alcoholic steatohepatitis (NASH), the "two-hit hypothesis" postulates that an additional oxidative injury causes hepatocellular inflammation and fibrosis in patients with existing steatosis [5]. Many potential oxidative insults have been proposed as inducers of this process. Following the accumulation of studies, the more rational "multiple-hit hypothesis" which was composed of several parallel factors contributing to progression of fatty liver change has substituted the relatively simplified "two-hit hypothesis" [6]. Regard the two hypotheses, portal flow discrepancies have not been suggested as an underlying cause.

Patients with hilar cholangiocarcinoma usually present with obstructive jaundice at the time of diagnosis and require extended hepatectomy: hence, two procedures are required before the curative operation. The first is biliary drainage to decrease serum total bilirubin levels, and the second is portal vein embolization (PVE), which is necessary for the induction of hypertrophy of the future remnant liver [7, 8]. We have aggressively treated patients with biliary tract cancer and have used PVE without major complications in over 830 patients since 1990 [9, 10]. Although the hemodynamic changes, especially the changes of portal flow after PVE were enormous, none of these patients developed acute fatty change of the liver after PVE according to our database and literature review. The following case represents an even more extraordinary picture of uneven acute fatty change of the liver after PVE, in which the left medial sector of the liver with biliary tract obstruction was spared the changes. The changes between the affected and the unaffected segments are illustrated via images and confirmed by pathologic interpretations.

Case presentation

A 55-year-old women who was neither a smoker or heavy drinker fulfilling the criteria for alcoholism was admitted to a regional hospital due to jaundice for 2 weeks. She had underlying hyperlipidemia treated only with diet control. Her body-mass index (BMI) was 26.1 kg/m2. Laboratory tests revealed elevated liver enzymes and hyperbilirubinemia. Computed tomography (CT) demonstrated hilar obstruction with separate bile

duct dilatation in the bilateral lobes of the liver. Endoscopic retrograde cholangiopancreatography (ERCP) showed an infiltrating lesion at the bile duct bifurcation, and the diagnosis of hilar cholangiocarcinoma was made after simultaneous endoscopic biopsy. Endoscopic nasobiliary drainage (ENBD) and endoscopic biliary stenting (EBS) were also performed during the same procedure (Fig. 1). She was referred to our hospital for possible surgery. Left trisectionectomy plus caudate lobectomy with extrahepatic bile duct resection was deemed necessary to achieve R0 resection. The future liver remnant (FLR) volume (volume of the right posterior sector) was 423 ml (29.3%) by CT volumetry, and PVE was indicated to induce hypertrophy of the FLR.

The left and right anterior portal branches were embolized with fibrin and steel coils [9]. There were no complications after the procedure, and routine laboratory testing yielded results similar to those pre-PVE. Routine sonography of the liver was carried out on 5th day after PVE, which confirmed good portal flow in the right posterior sector and thrombosis of the embolized portal branches. The patient was readmitted 3 weeks after PVE for volumetric evaluation of the liver and an indocyanine green clearance (ICG) test. The volume of the right posterior sector had increased to 772 ml (41.3%) and the ICG-K was 0.194. Unexpectedly, a repeat CT showed diffuse fatty change of the liver parenchyma, except for the left medial sector where the bile ducts were incompletely drained (Fig. 2b). Serum laboratory parameters

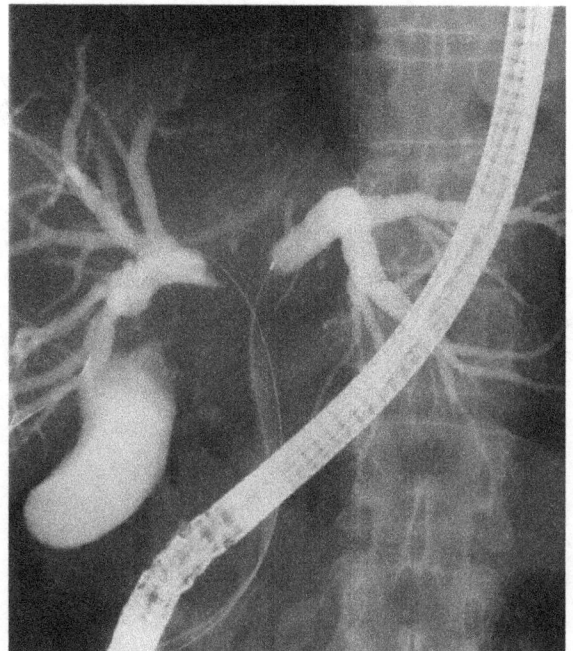

Fig. 1 Cholangiographic finding. Cholangiography after ERCP and ENBD showed that the bile ducts of segment IV of the liver were not opacified (drained)

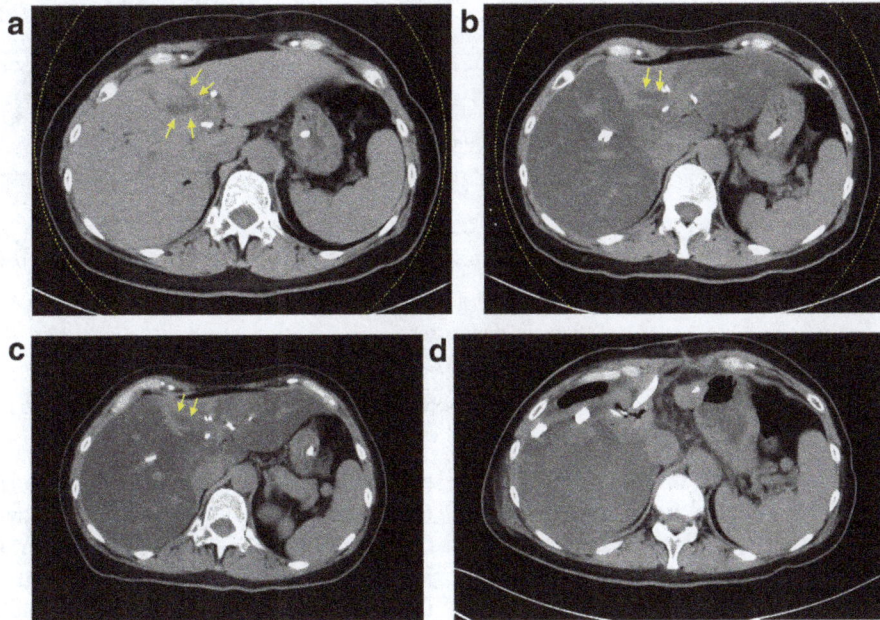

Fig. 2 CT of the liver at different stage. **a** CT of the liver before PVE. Yellow arrows, undrained (dilated) bile ducts (**b**) CT after PVE demonstrating acute fatty change of the liver and sparing of segment IV. Yellow arrows, undrained (dilated) bile ducts (**c**) CT 6 weeks after PVE (**d**) CT of the liver remnant 1 week after trisectionectomy

remained unchanged. Surgery was postponed for 3 weeks. The repeat CT still demonstrated uneven fat deposition in the liver (Fig. 2c).

Due to concern regarding cholangiocarcinoma progression, surgery was performed according to preoperative planning. Gross inspection on laparotomy revealed fatty change of the liver. The pathologic interpretation of the specimen showed different proportions of macrovesicular and microvesicular fat deposition, whereas the left medial sector showed only minimal changes (Fig. 3). The patient did not suffer hepatic dysfunction after surgery. A biliary fistula developed at the transection surface. She was discharged after resolution of the biliary fistula on postoperative day 62 and has since resumed a normal life. The course of treatment was summarized in the Table 1.

Discussion

There were two unusual observations in this case. First, to our knowledge, this is the first case of acute fatty change of the liver after PVE. Second, only the left medial sector of the liver, in which the biliary tracts were incompletely drained, was spared the fatty change, as demonstrated by both imaging and pathologic interpretation of the specimens. Although the mechanisms underlying these observations are unknown, they may have provided a connection between the change of hepatic inflow and the mechanism leading to progression of NAFLD.

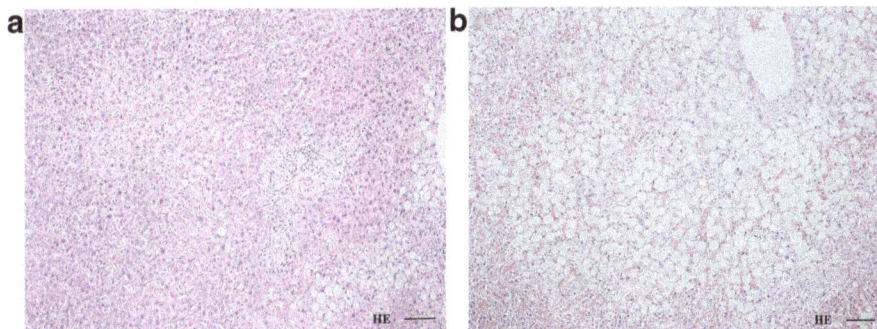

Fig. 3 Histologic aspect of different sectors of the liver. Microscopic pictures (100×, H&E stain, scale bar =100 µm) of fatty change in the medial sector (**a**) and lateral sector (**b**). Fat deposition is remarkable in the lateral sector

Table 1 Timeline

July 2015	Jaundice for 2 weeks
August 2015	MDCT, ERCP and biopsy confirmed hilar cholangiocarcinoma
	EBS and ENBD for biliary drainage
August 2015	PVE for left trisectionectomy
September 2015	Unevenly acute fatty change of the liver on MDCT
October 2015	Stationary of fatty change of the liver
	Operation: left trisectionectomy and caudate lobectomy with extrahepatic bile duct resection
	Surgical complication: biliary fistula
November 2015	Discharged from hospital
February 2016	Follow up without recurrence and sequela

MDCT multidetector computed tomography, *ERCP* endoscopic retrograde cholangiopancreaticography, *EBS* endoscopic biliary stent, *ENBD* endoscopic nasobiliary drainage, *PVE* portal vein embolization

NAFLD represents a broad spectrum of disease due to fat deposition in the liver, ranging from asymptomatic hepatic steatosis to necroinflammatory steatohepatitis leading to irreversible cirrhosis [11]. The manifestation of triglyceride accumulation may be due to excessive importation from the blood stream or diminished exportation and oxidation [12]. Steatosis could be detected on images; however, the diagnosis requires the specific histopathologic features demonstrated by biopsy of the liver. To delineate the mechanism of progression of NAFLD to NASH, the "multiple-hit hypothesis" that multiple parallel insults attack on genetic predisposing individuals was proposed to substitute the outdated "two-hit hypothesis" [13]. Regard the patient presented with extraordinary acute fatty deposition of the liver after PVE, which was confirmed by pathologic interpretations, we attempted to integrate the hemodynamic changes in her liver after PVE as one of the possible insults.

Based on a review of her disease course, PVE was the only major event before the uneven fatty changes of the liver. Since 1990, we have performed over 830 PVEs for patients with biliary tract cancer. This is the first patient to develop acute fatty change of the liver after PVE, either from our series or from the literature. PVE induces hemodynamic changes in both arterial and portal blood flow in both embolized and non-embolized hepatic tissue [14]. The volume of her right posterior sector increased from 423 ml (29.4%) to 772 ml (41.3%) after PVE. The volume of the entire liver increased from 1441 ml to 1869 ml after PVE. The effect of PVE was remarkable in this patient.

Alterations in portal and arterial flow secondary to acute biliary tract obstruction have been observed in dogs [15]. The phenomenon is discussed mostly in patients with obstructive jaundice who receive PVE because of its negative impact on FLR hypertrophy [14]. Based on this patient's CT results and the pathologic interpretations of the specimens, it was confirmed that the incompletely drained medial sector was spared or minimally affected by the acute fatty change after PVE. It was speculated that portal venous flow was substantially decreased because of the dilated bile duct in the Glisson's sheath before PVE. Therefore, total blood flow

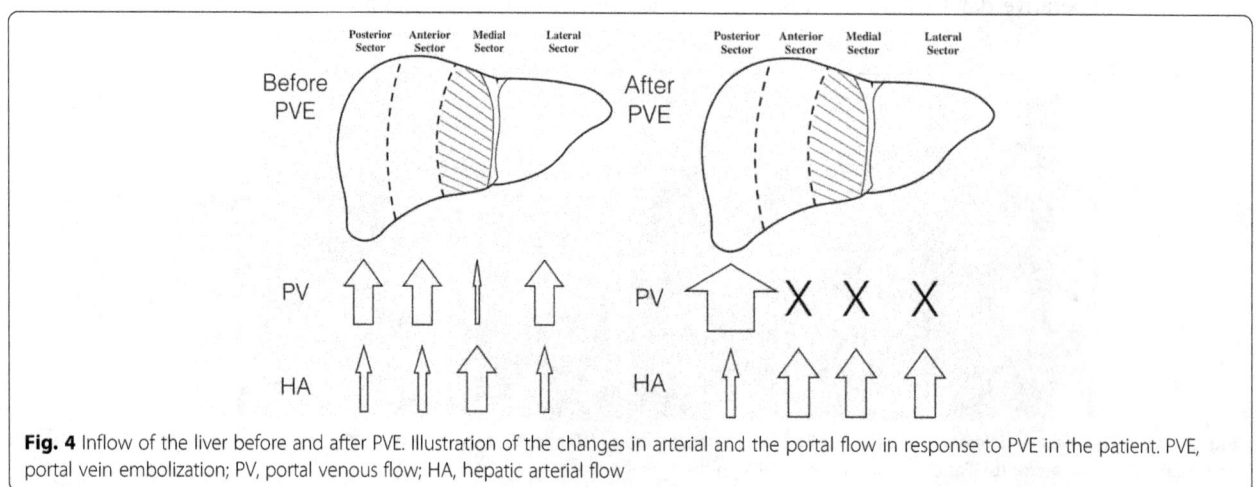

Fig. 4 Inflow of the liver before and after PVE. Illustration of the changes in arterial and the portal flow in response to PVE in the patient. PVE, portal vein embolization; PV, portal venous flow; HA, hepatic arterial flow

in the left medial sector did not change much after PVE, which is in contrast to the dramatic blood flow changes experienced by the other sectors. In the non-embolized right posterior sector (the FLR), portal venous flow increased to accommodate blood flow from the remainder of the gastrointestinal tract after PVE. In the embolized sectors, portal venous flow was shut down, and hepatic arterial flow was increased. Hepatic arterial flow accounts for 25% of total hepatic inflow in humans and increases correspondingly to maintain constant hepatic inflow when portal flow is altered, which is known as the hepatic arterial buffer response [16]. Figure 4 illustrates the indicative, non-quantified changes in both hepatic arterial and portal flow before and after PVE among different sectors of the liver. In summary, the left medial sector experienced the least change in total inflow stemming from dilated biliary trees (unrelieved obstruction).

Conclusion

In conclusion, the uneven fatty change of the liver in this patient was extraordinary and has never been reported. We surmised that differences in hepatic inflow led to uneven sparing with respect to fatty change of the liver. Although the mechanisms underlying NAFLD and hepatic hypertrophy after PVE involve more than mere hemodynamic changes [5, 14], this specific presentation may give a clue for further research on the hemodynamic change of the hepatic inflow as a potential insult leading to progression of NAFLD.

Abbreviations

CT: computed tomography; EBS: endoscopic biliary stenting; ENBD: endoscopic nasobiliary drainage; ERCP: endoscopic retrograde cholangiopancreatography; FLR: future liver remnant; ICG: indocyanine green; NAFLD: non-alcoholic fatty liver disease; NASH: non-alcoholic steatohepatitis; PVE: portal vein embolization

Acknowledgements

We acknowledge all the medical staffs that took care of the patient. We also acknowledge all the surgical staffs that helped the perioperative management.

Funding

There is no funding support for this manuscript.

Author's contributions

TE and TM designed the study and the concept. CT and M Nojiri performed acquisition of data. M Nojiri and YY analyzed the data with interpretation. CT and YY drafted the manuscript. M Nagino provided critical revision. All authors read and approved the final manuscript.

Consent for publication

The patient gave written consent to publish this case report and individual details.

Competing interests

There are no competing interest for any of the authors.

References

1. Petta S, Muratore C, Craxi A. Non-alcoholic fatty liver disease pathogenesis: the present and the future. Dig Liver Dis. 2009;41(9):615–25.
2. Chalasani N, Younossi Z, Lavine JE, Diehl AM, Brunt EM, Cusi K, Charlton M, Sanyal AJ, American Gastroenterological A, American Association for the Study of liver D, et al. The diagnosis and management of non-alcoholic fatty liver disease: practice guideline by the American Gastroenterological Association, American Association for the Study of Liver Diseases, and American College of Gastroenterology. Gastroenterology. 2012;142(7):1592–609.
3. Marchesini G, Brizi M, Morselli-Labate AM, Bianchi G, Bugianesi E, McCullough AJ, Forlani G, Melchionda N. Association of nonalcoholic fatty liver disease with insulin resistance. Am J Med. 1999;107(5):450–5.
4. Targher G, Bertolini L, Padovani R, Rodella S, Tessari R, Zenari L, Day C, Arcaro G. Prevalence of nonalcoholic fatty liver disease and its association with cardiovascular disease among type 2 diabetic patients. Diabetes Care. 2007;30(5):1212–8.
5. Dowman JK, Tomlinson JW, Newsome PN. Pathogenesis of non-alcoholic fatty liver disease. QJM. 2010;103(2):71–83.
6. Buzzetti E, Pinzani M, Tsochatzis EA. The multiple-hit pathogenesis of non-alcoholic fatty liver disease (NAFLD). Metabolism. 2016;65(8):1038–48.
7. Nagino M, Nimura Y, Kamiya J, Kondo S, Uesaka K, Kin Y, Kutsuna Y, Hayakawa N, Yamamoto H. Right or left trisegment portal vein embolization before hepatic trisegmentectomy for hilar bile duct carcinoma. Surgery. 1995;117(6):677–81.
8. Nagino M, Kamiya J, Kanai M, Uesaka K, Sano T, Yamamoto H, Hayakawa N, Nimura Y. Right trisegment portal vein embolization for biliary tract carcinoma: technique and clinical utility. Surgery. 2000;127(2):155–60.
9. Nagino M, Nimura Y, Kamiya J, Kondo S, Kanai M. Selective percutaneous transhepatic embolization of the portal vein in preparation for extensive liver resection: the ipsilateral approach. Radiology. 1996;200(2):559–63.
10. Nagino M, Kamiya J, Nishio H, Ebata T, Arai T, Nimura Y. Two hundred forty consecutive portal vein embolizations before extended hepatectomy for biliary cancer: surgical outcome and long-term follow-up. Ann Surg. 2006; 243(3):364–72.
11. Angulo P. Nonalcoholic fatty liver disease. N Engl J Med. 2002;346(16): 1221–31.
12. Donnelly KL, Smith CI, Schwarzenberg SJ, Jessurun J, Boldt MD, Parks EJ. Sources of fatty acids stored in liver and secreted via lipoproteins in patients with nonalcoholic fatty liver disease. J Clin Invest. 2005;115(5):1343–51.
13. Tilg H, Moschen AR. Evolution of inflammation in nonalcoholic fatty liver disease: the multiple parallel hits hypothesis. Hepatology. 2010;52(5):1836–46.
14. Yokoyama Y, Nagino M, Nimura Y. Mechanisms of hepatic regeneration following portal vein embolization and partial hepatectomy: a review. World J Surg. 2007;31(2):367–74.
15. Kanda H, Nimura Y, Yasui A, Uematsu T, Kamiya S, Machiki Y, Kitagawa Y, Shionoya S. Hepatic blood flow after acute biliary obstruction and drainage in conscious dogs. Hepato-Gastroenterology. 1996;43(7):235–40.
16. Lautt WW. Mechanism and role of intrinsic regulation of hepatic arterial blood flow: hepatic arterial buffer response. Am J Phys. 1985;249(5 Pt 1): G549–56.

6

Relationship of sarcopenia with steatohepatitis and advanced liver fibrosis in non-alcoholic fatty liver disease

Rui Yu[1*†] (ID), Qiangwei Shi[2†], Lei Liu[3] and Lidong Chen[1]

Abstract

Background: Several studies have emerged indicating that sarcopenia is associated with nonalcoholic fatty liver disease, we aimed to systematically review and quantify the association between sacropenia and the histological severity of nonalcoholic fatty liver disease.

Methods: Pubmed, the Cochrane Library and EMBASE were searched (until August 2017) for studies examining the relationship of sarcopenia with steatohepatitis and advanced liver fibrosis in nonalcoholic fatty liver disease. Pooled odds ratios were estimated by fixed effects models.

Results: Three articles met our inclusion criteria, with a total of 3226 individuals. Two of the studies examined the association between sacropenia and steatohepatitis, a significant association was documented between sarcopenia and steatohepatitis (OR = 2.35, 95%CI 1.45, 3.81). All of the three studies assessed the association between sarcopenia and advanced liver fibrosis, a significant association between sarcopenia and advanced liver fibrosis (OR = 2.41, 95%CI 1.94, 2.98). No significant heterogeneity was detected among studies in all comparisons. These results remained essentially unchanged after excluding any of the studies in the sensitivity analysis.

Conclusions: Sarcopenia in patients with nonalcoholic fatty liver disease is associated with a higher likelihood of having steatohepatitis or advanced liver fibrosis. Demonstration of the role of sarcopenia in nonalcoholic fatty liver disease development in future studies could have important therapeutic implications.

Keywords: Sarcopenia, Nonalcoholic fatty liver disease, Meta-analysis, Steatohepatitis, Liver fibrosis

Background

Non-alcoholic fatty liver disease (NAFLD) has become the predominant cause for chronic liver disease in the Western countries and is estimated to impact more than 30% of Americans [1] and Chinese [2], with the prevalence continuously rising. Globally, the prevalence of NAFLD is rising as a result of increasingly sedentary lifestyle, globalization of Western diet and increasing frequency of obesity [3]. NAFLD comprises of a wide spectrum of disease including simple steatosis, non-alcoholic steatohepatitis (NASH), from liver fibrosis to cirrhosis, liver failure and hepatocellular carcinoma. It is generally recognised that the presence of histologic NASH is associated with worse outcomes compared to no-NASH NAFLD and the general population [4, 5]. Several studies have shown that NAFLD with advanced fibrosis is a significant predictor of mortality from cardiovascular diseases [6] as well as of liver-related events [7]. Thus, early assessment and intervention of this high-risk subjects may reduce the burden associated with these diseases.

Sarcopenia is characterised by generalised and progressive loss of skeletal muscle mass and strength, frequently associated with poor quality of life, physical disability and death [8]. Previously, it was regarded as consequence of ageing; but recently, studies identified it as a progressive disease frequently associated with

---

* Correspondence: yurui312@163.com

†Equal contributors

[1]Department of Gastroenterology, The First Affiliated Hospital of Zhengzhou University, Zhengzhou, China

Full list of author information is available at the end of the article

multisystem disorders [9]. As both diseases - sarcopenia and NAFLD – share similar mediator such as insulin resistance, increased inflammation and physical inactivity, many studies have emerged over the past few years examining the relationship of sarcopenia with the presence of NAFLD [10, 11] and its severity [12–15]. In our study, we aimed to systematically review and quantify the association between sacropenia and the histological severity of NAFLD. We hypothesised that sacropenia was associated with steatohepatitis and advanced liver fibrosis in non-alcoholic fatty liver disease.

Methods

Search strategy

Relevant studies were identified by a PubMed, EMBASE, and the Cochrane Library literature search with the following terms: ("sarcopenia" MeSH or "sarcopenia" or "sarcopenic obesity" or "muscle wasting") and ("non-alcoholic fatty liver disease" MeSH or "fatty liver" MeSH or "non-alcoholic fatty liver disease" or "fatty liver" or "steatohepatitis" or "NASH" or "NAFLD"). Moreover, we examined the reference lists of relevant reviews and original papers. The information contained in this report is based on articles published before August 2017.

Study selection

We developed strict criteria for categorizing the studies by two independent reviewers (QWS and RY). We included all studies that reported data on sarcopenia with steatohepatitis or liver fibrosis of NAFLD. We excluded studies that examined other types of liver disease (viral hepatitis,alcoholic liver disease, toxin-induced liver injury, hepatocellular carcinoma); studies without original data; in vitro or animal studies; and papers absent or inadequate information about sarcopenia, study population, or not enough information to calculate the odds ratio (OR) and 95% confidence intervals (CI).

Data extraction

Data were extracted independently by two investigators (QWS and RY) and then cross-checked. When data were unclear or required assumptions to be made, a third investigators (LL) was consulted so that a consensus could be reached before recording an entry in the database. We abstracted key study characteristics of selected publications, including country, publication year, participant characteristics (age, gender, ethnicity), study design, method of diagnosis of sarcopenia, NAFLD, liver steatosis and fibrosis. The quality of reporting was assessed by an evaluation system modified from the Newcastle-Ottawa Scale (NOS) [16], the meta-analysis was conducted following the Meta-analysis of Observational Studies in Epidemiology (MOOSE) guidelines [17].

Statistical analysis

All analyses were performed using Stata software (v. 12. 0; Stata, College Station, TX). $P < 0.05$ was considered significant. In all analyses, pooled ORs and 95% CIs were calculated. The significance of the pooled OR was calculated by the Z-test. A fixed effect model (Inverse Variance) was chosen in the present study. The study heterogeneity was assessed using the Cochran's Q statistic and I^2 statistic, considering a Q statistic $P < 0.1$ or $I^2 > 50\%$ as significant heterogeneity. Owing to the limited number of studies included in each analysis, publication bias was not assessed.

The sensitivity analyses were also conducted to assess the consistency of results and to investigate the influence of one study on the overall meta analysis. It was carried out by sequential omission of individual studies.

Results

Search results

The search strategy yielded 286 studies. Seventeen of these 286 were considered of potential value, and we retrieved full texts for further evaluation. After detailed assessment and exclusion, 3 studies were included (Fig. 1). The main characteristics of the studies analyzed are summarized in Table 1. The publication year of the studies ranged from 2016 to 2017. Of the 3 studies included, 2 rest in Asia [13, 14], one originated in Europe [12].

Article characteristics

NAFLD was ascertained by liver biopsy in two studies [12, 13], and by non-invasive prediction models in one study [15]. The sarcopenia was diagnosed by the skeletal muscle mass index (SMI), which was evaluated by bioelectric impedance analysis (BIA) in two of the studies [12, 13], by dual energy Xray absorptiometry (DXA) in one [15]. Meta-analyses involved 3226 individuals for liver fibrosis and 465 individuals for NASH. The quality of included studies according to NOS is presented in Table 1, no study was excluded on the basis of poor NOS score (Additional file 1).

Meta-analysis

For NASH, two studies examined the association between sarcopenia and NASH. Both two studies showed a direct relationship between sarcopenia and and NASH. Overall, we found a significant association between sarcopenia and NASH (OR = 2.35, 95%CI 1.45, 3.81). The Cochran's Q statistic and I^2 statistic did not show heterogeneity among the studies ($P > 0.1$; Fig.2).

For liver fibrosis, a total of 3 studies examined the association between sarcopenia and advanced liver fibrosis (ALF). Figure 3 shows the pooled ORs for ALF. From three studies analyzed, all of them showed a direct relationship between sarcopenia and and ALF. Overall, we found a significant association between sarcopenia and

Table 1 Characteristics of studies included in meta-analysis on sarcopenia with steatohepatitis and liver fibrosis

Year	First Author	Design	NAFLD (N)/ Total (N)	Country	Age (Years)	Gender (% Male)	Method of diagnosis of sarcopenia	Method of diagnosis of NAFLD	Method of diagnosis of liver fibrosis	Study quality[1]
2017	Petta [12]	Cross-sectional	225/225	Italy	48.3	62.7	BIA	Liver biopsy	Liver biopsy	8
2017	Koo [13]	Cross-sectional	240/309	Korea	53	46.9	BIA	Liver biopsy	Liver biopsy	9
2016	Lee [15][a]	Cross-sectional	2761/2761	Korea	55.8	55	DXA	NLFS [32]	NFS [33]	6

BIA, Bioelectric impedance analysis, DXA Dual energy X-ray absorptiometry, LSM liver stiffness measurement, NLFS NAFLD liver fat score, NFS The NAFLD fibrosis score
[a]NAFLD and liver fibrosis was defined using different prediction models, data of the first method was caculated and presented
[1]Methodological quality of included studies assessed using a method based in the 9-star Newcastle-Ottawa Scale

ALF (OR = 2.41, 95%CI 1.94, 2.98). The Cochran's Q statistic and I^2 statistic did not show heterogeneity among the studies ($P > 0.1$; Fig.3).

In the sensitivity analysis, after excluding any of the studies, there were only minimal changes in the comparisons between groups.

Discussion

A significant direct association was found between sarcopenia and NASH (OR = 2.35, 95%CI 1.45, 3.81) or ALF (OR = 2.41, 95%CI 1.94, 2.98) in this systematic review and meta-analysis including more than 3000 NAFLD patiens. Several hypotheses could be put forward to

further explain the complex inter-relationships between sarcopenia and NAFLD.

Skeletal muscle plays a key role in insulin resistance as a primary tissue contributing to whole body insulin-mediated glucose uptake [18], muscle depletion reduces the predominant cellular target for insulin action, inducing glucose intolerance and accelerating gluconeogenesis, which conversely, will promote proteolysis and muscle wasting. Moreover, insulin resistance results in lipolysis and accordingly generation of free fatty acids, which can easily be taken by both muscle and liver [19, 20]. The insulin resistance-mediated muscle depletion mass and thus the less uptake of free fatty acids by muscle will further result in exposure to and increased uptake in free fatty acids by liver [21].

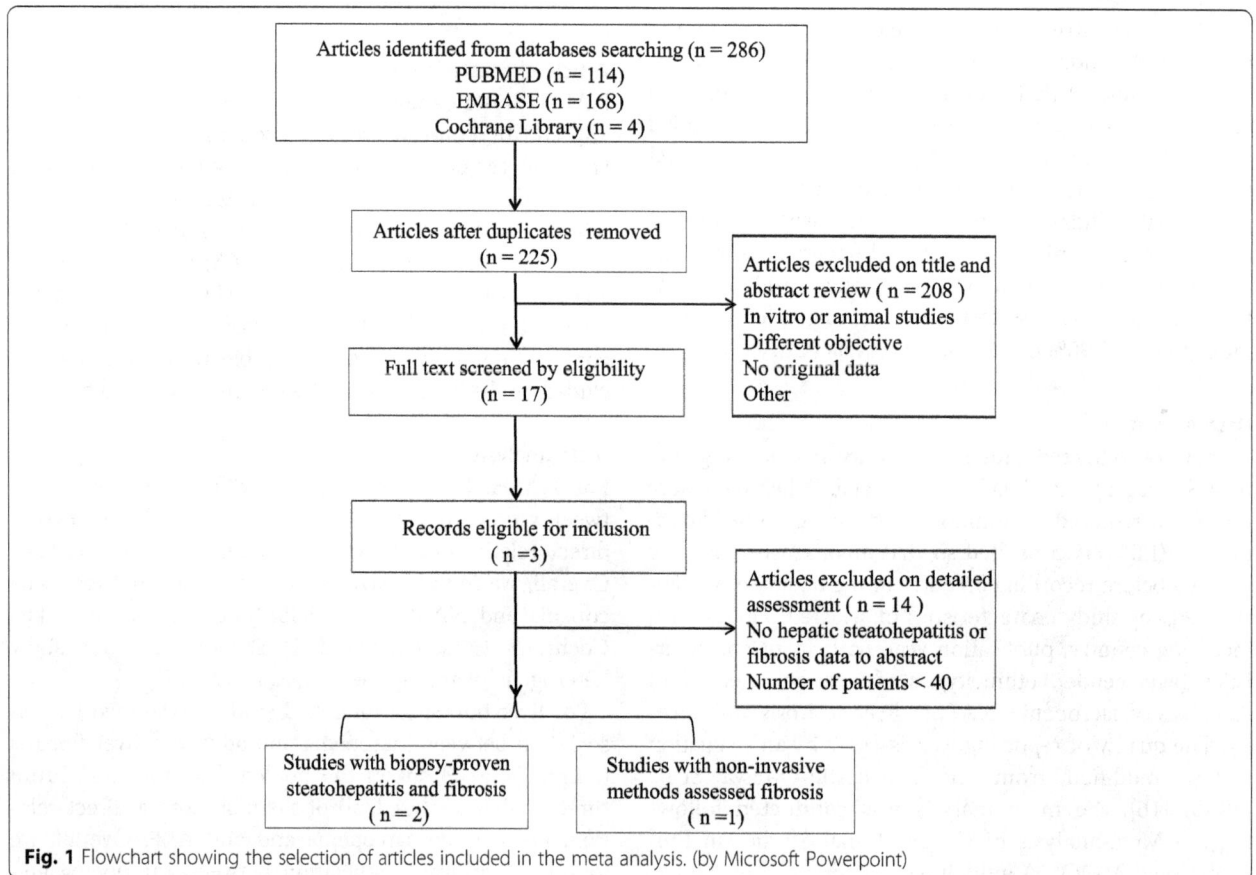

Fig. 1 Flowchart showing the selection of articles included in the meta analysis. (by Microsoft Powerpoint)

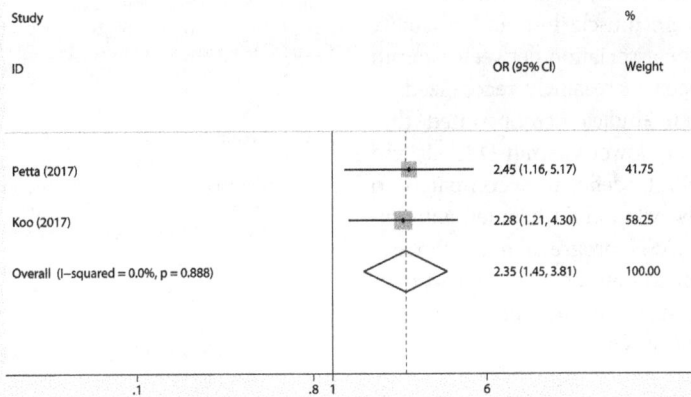

Fig. 2 Forest plot of the meta-analysis performed to investigate the association between sarcopenia and NASH. (by Stata and Adobe Illustrator)

Growth hormone (GH) and insulin-like growth factor-1 (IGF-1) is another potential link between sarcopenia and NAFLD. GH and IGF-I play important roles in linear growth in childhood, and continue to have essential metabolic fuctions throughout whole life. GH and IGF-1 are key effectors of changes in muscle mass. It has been well-described that abdominal and visceral obesity have strong influence on the suppression of GH secretion, and obese patients with the lowest GH secretion presenting the most severe metabolic complications; reduced GH and IGF-1 levels seen in patients with obesity, may be detrimental to both skeletal muscle and liver, contributing to ectopic fat storage [22]. Growing evidence has revealed that GH as well as IGF-I also play important roles in the liver, GH/IGF-1 axis impairment seems to be associated to the risk of both developing to sarcopenic obesity and ectopic fat storage in the liver [23–25].

Chronic inflammation and oxidative stress have been shown to prompt muscle wasting [26]. The interaction of several intracellular signaling pathways may affect the balance between protein synthesis and breakdown, inducing apoptosis, which cause the primary pathology of muscle wasting [27]. Oxidative stress and chronic inflammation also can result in a stress response of hepatocytes, leading to the development of NASH and progression of fibrosis [28].

Additionally, the link between sarcopenia and NAFLD severity may partially owing to the vitamin D deficiency frequently found in patients with liver diseases. Growing evidence has established a close association between vitamin D status and sarcopenia. Some data suggest that

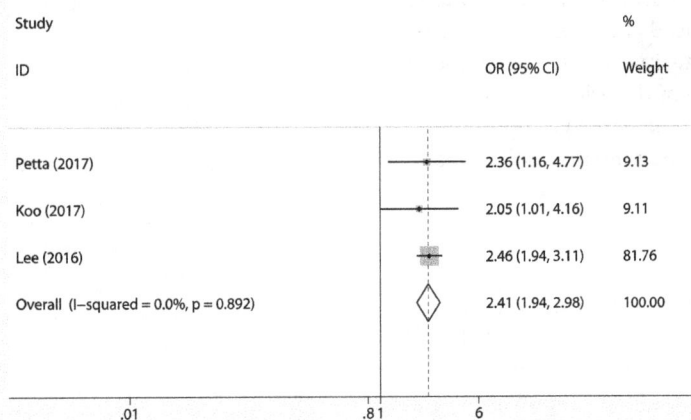

Fig. 3 Forest plot of the meta-analysis performed to investigate the association between sarcopenia and ALF. (by Stata and Adobe Illustrator)

vitamin D deficiency may impair muscle function and is associated with sarcopenia, furthermore, low vitamin D status is associated with lower muscle mass, poorer muscle function, and predicts more severe muscle loss and disability development [29]. As well, the association between vitamin D levels and NAFLD has been increasingly recognized. A meta-analysis with seventeen studies demonstrated that NAFLD patients had significant lower vitamin D levels and higher probability of vitamin D deficiency, compared to controls [30]. In vitro study, vitamin D supplementation was shown to ameliorate NASH progression in choline-deficient and iron-supplemented l-amino acid-defined diet-induced NASH model [31], suggesting a potential role of vitamin D in the development of NAFLD.

Overall, the overlap in the pathophysiology of sarcopenia and NAFLD make it challenging to determine whether sarcopenia is a risk factor for NASH, or it is a complication of NASH. The two entities are so intricately inter-meshed that the presence of either one may increases the risk for the other. Clinicians should have an increased awareness of sarcopenia to diagnose it in patients with NAFLD, and should intervene early in these high-risk patients. Further studies are needed to assess intervention in sarcopenia and the development of pharmacologic intervention that addresses both conditions.

To our knowledge, this is the first meta-analysis to investigate sarcopenia with steatohepatitis and advanced liver fibrosis in NAFLD. Another strength of this study was that only high quality articles based on NOS quality assessment were included. The limitations of the study need to be considered: (a) all studies included are of cross-section nature, thus a cause-effect relationship between sarcopenia and NAFLD severity cannot be drawn. (b) Two of the studies used liver biopsy-the gold standard, while another study used noninvasive markers to identify NAFLD cases and advanced histology, the different method for NAFLD diagnosis may result in increased risk of publication bias. (c) some of the original studies did not provide ORs adjusted for potentially important confounders, such as BMI, age, and presence of diabetes.

Conclusions

In summary, this meta-analysis demonstrated that sarcopenia was associated with the severity of NAFLD. The possible causal relationship between sarcopenia and the severity of NAFLD, which needs to be proven by future prospective studies, may offer attractive therapeutic opportunities for treatment of NAFLD.

Abbreviations
ALF: advanced liver fibrosis; BIA: bioelectric impedance analysis; CI: confidence intervals; DXA: dual energy Xray absorptiometry; GH: growth hormone; IGF-1: insulin-like growth factor-1; NAFLD: Non-alcoholic fatty liver disease; NASH: non-alcoholic steatohepatitis; NOS: Newcastle-Ottawa Scale; OR: odds ratio; SMI: skeletal muscle mass index

Authors' contributions
RY acquisition of data, analysis and interpretation of data, drafting the article, final approval; QWS acquisition of data, analysis and interpretation of data, drafting the article, final approval; LL interpretation of data, revising the article, final approval. LDC interpretation of data, revising the article, final approval.

Competing interests
The authors declare that they have no competing interests.

Author details
[1]Department of Gastroenterology, The First Affiliated Hospital of Zhengzhou University, Zhengzhou, China. [2]Department of Cardiology, The First Affiliated Hospital of Zhengzhou University, Zhengzhou, China. [3]Department of Nasology, The First Affiliated Hospital of Zhengzhou University, Zhengzhou, China.

References
1. Williams CD, Stengel J, Asike MI, Torres DM, Shaw J, Contreras M, Landt CL, Harrison SA. Prevalence of nonalcoholic fatty liver disease and nonalcoholic steatohepatitis among a largely middle-aged population utilizing ultrasound and liver biopsy: a prospective study. Gastroenterology. 2011;140(1):124–31.
2. Wong VW, Chu WC, Wong GL, Chan RS, Chim AM, Ong A, Yeung DK, Yiu KK, Chu SH, Woo J, et al. Prevalence of non-alcoholic fatty liver disease and advanced fibrosis in Hong Kong Chinese: a population study using proton-magnetic resonance spectroscopy and transient elastography. Gut. 2012; 61(3):409–15.
3. Loomba R, Sanyal AJ. The global NAFLD epidemic. Nat Rev Gastroenterol Hepatol. 2013;10(11):686–90.
4. Soderberg C, Stal P, Askling J, Glaumann H, Lindberg G, Marmur J, Hultcrantz R. Decreased survival of subjects with elevated liver function tests during a 28-year follow-up. Hepatology. 2010;51(2):595–602.
5. Ekstedt M, Franzen LE, Mathiesen UL, Thorelius L, Holmqvist M, Bodemar G, Kechagias S. Long-term follow-up of patients with NAFLD and elevated liver enzymes. Hepatology. 2006;44(4):865–73.
6. Kim D, Kim WR, Kim HJ, Therneau TM. Association between noninvasive fibrosis markers and mortality among adults with nonalcoholic fatty liver disease in the United States. Hepatolog. 2013;57(4):1357–65.
7. Angulo P, Kleiner DE, Dam-Larsen S, Adams LA, Bjornsson ES, Charatcharoenwitthaya P, Mills PR, Keach JC, Lafferty HD, Stahler A, et al. Liver fibrosis, but no other histologic features, is associated with long-term outcomes of patients with nonalcoholic fatty liver disease. Gastroenterology. 2015; 149(2):389–97.
8. Cruz-Jentoft AJ, Baeyens JP, Bauer JM, Boirie Y, Cederholm T, Landi F, Martin FC, Michel JP, Rolland Y, Schneider SM, et al. Sarcopenia: European consensus on definition and diagnosis: report of the European working group on sarcopenia in older people. Age Ageing. 2010;39(4):412–23.
9. The Lancet Diabetes Endocrinology. Sarcopenia: a fate worth challenging. The Lancet Diabetes & Endocrinology. 2014;2(3):183.
10. Lee YH, Jung KS, Kim SU, Yoon HJ, Yun YJ, Lee BW, Kang ES, Han KH, Lee HC, Cha BS. Sarcopaenia is associated with NAFLD independently of obesity and insulin resistance: Nationwide surveys (KNHANES 2008-2011). J Hepatol. 2015;63(2):486–93.
11. Kim HY, Kim CW, Park CH, Choi JY, Han K, Merchant AT, Park YM. Low skeletal muscle mass is associated with non-alcoholic fatty liver disease in Korean adults: the fifth Korea National Health and nutrition examination survey. Hepatobiliary Pancreat Dis Int. 2016;15(1):39–47.
12. Petta S, Ciminnisi S, Di Marco V, Cabibi D, Camma C, Licata A, Marchesini G,

Craxi A. Sarcopenia is associated with severe liver fibrosis in patients with non-alcoholic fatty liver disease. Aliment Pharmacol Ther. 2017;45(4):510–8.

13. Koo BK, Kim D, Joo SK, Kim JH, Chang MS, Kim BG, Lee KL, Kim W. Sarcopenia is an independent risk factor for non-alcoholic steatohepatitis and significant fibrosis. J Hepatol. 2017;66(1):123–31.

14. Yamaguchi A, Ebinuma H, Nakamoto N, Miyake R, Shiba S, Taniki N, Wakayama Y, Chu PS, Saito H, Kanai T. The association between sarcopenia and liver fibrosis progression in non-alcoholic fatty liver disease: assessment by non-invasive transient elastography and bioelectrical impedance body composition analyzer. Hepatology. 2015;1296A:62.

15. Lee YH, Kim SU, Song K, Park JY, Kim DY, Ahn SH, Lee BW, Kang ES, Cha BS, Han KH. Sarcopenia is associated with significant liver fibrosis independently of obesity and insulin resistance in nonalcoholic fatty liver disease: Nationwide surveys (KNHANES 2008-2011). Hepatology. 2016;63(3):776–86.

16. Stang A. Critical evaluation of the Newcastle-Ottawa scale for the assessment of the quality of nonrandomized studies in meta-analyses. Eur J Epidemiol. 2010;25(9):603–5.

17. Stroup DF, Berlin JA, Morton SC, Olkin I, Williamson GD, Rennie D, Moher D, Becker BJ, Sipe TA, Thacker SB. Meta-analysis of observational studies in epidemiology: a proposal for reporting. Meta-analysis of observational studies in epidemiology (MOOSE) group. JAMA. 2000;283(15):2008–12.

18. DeFronzo RA, Jacot E, Jequier E, Maeder E, Wahren J, Felber JP. The effect of insulin on the disposal of intravenous glucose. Results from indirect calorimetry and hepatic and femoral venous catheterization. Diabetes. 1981;30(12):1000–7.

19. Jocken JW, Goossens GH, Boon H, Mason RR, Essers Y, Havekes B, Watt MJ, van Loon LJ, Blaak EE. Insulin-mediated suppression of lipolysis in adipose tissue and skeletal muscle of obese type 2 diabetic men and men with normal glucose tolerance. Diabetologia. 2013;56(10):2255–65.

20. Jocken JW, Langin D, Smit E, Saris WH, Valle C, Hul GB, Holm C, Arner P, Blaak EE. Adipose triglyceride lipase and hormone-sensitive lipase protein expression is decreased in the obese insulin-resistant state. J Clin Endocrinol Metab. 2007;92(6):2292–9.

21. Mayerson AB, Hundal RS, Dufour S, Lebon V, Befroy D, Cline GW, Enocksson S, Inzucchi SE, Shulman GI, Petersen KF. The effects of rosiglitazone on insulin sensitivity, lipolysis, and hepatic and skeletal muscle triglyceride content in patients with type 2 diabetes. Diabetes. 2002;51(3):797–802.

22. Berryman DE, Glad CA, List EO, Johannsson G. The GH/IGF-1 axis in obesity: pathophysiology and therapeutic considerations. Nat Rev Endocrinol. 2013;9(6):346–56.

23. Takahashi Y. Essential roles of growth hormone (GH) and insulin-like growth factor-I (IGF-I) in the liver. Endocr J. 2012;59(11):955–62.

24. Koehler E, Swain J, Sanderson S, Krishnan A, Watt K, Charlton M. Growth hormone, dehydroepiandrosterone and adiponectin levels in non-alcoholic steatohepatitis: an endocrine signature for advanced fibrosis in obese patients. Liver Int. 2012;32(2):279–86.

25. Poggiogalle E, Lubrano C, Gnessi L, Mariani S, Lenzi A, Donini LM. Fatty liver index associates with relative sarcopenia and GH/ IGF- 1 status in obese subjects. PLoS One. 2016;11(1):e0145811.

26. Phillips T, Leeuwenburgh C. Muscle fiber specific apoptosis and TNF-alpha signaling in sarcopenia are attenuated by life-long calorie restriction. FASEB J. 2005;19(6):668–70.

27. Meng SJ, Yu LJ. Oxidative stress, molecular inflammation and sarcopenia. Int J Mol Sci. 2010;11(4):1509–26.

28. Tilg H, Moschen AR. Evolution of inflammation in nonalcoholic fatty liver disease: the multiple parallel hits hypothesis. Hepatology. 2010;52(5):1836–46.

29. Lappe JM, Binkley N. Vitamin D and Sarcopenia/Falls. J Clin Densitom. 2015;18(4):478–82.

30. Eliades M, Spyrou E, Agrawal N, Lazo M, Brancati FL, Potter JJ, Koteish AA, Clark JM, Guallar E, Hernaez R. Meta-analysis: vitamin D and non-alcoholic fatty liver disease. Aliment Pharmacol Ther. 2013;38(3):246–54.

31. Nakano T, Cheng YF, Lai CY, Hsu LW, Chang YC, Deng JY, Huang YZ, Honda H, Chen KD, Wang CC, et al. Impact of artificial sunlight therapy on the progress of non-alcoholic fatty liver disease in rats. J Hepatol. 2011;55(2):415–25.

32. Kotronen A, Peltonen M, Hakkarainen A, Sevastianova K, Bergholm R, Johansson LM, Lundbom N, Rissanen A, Ridderstrale M, Groop L, et al. Prediction of non-alcoholic fatty liver disease and liver fat using metabolic and genetic factors. Gastroenterology. 2009;137(3):865–72.

33. Angulo P, Hui JM, Marchesini G, Bugianesi E, George J, Farrell GC, Enders F, Saksena S, Burt AD, Bida JP, et al. The NAFLD fibrosis score: a noninvasive system that identifies liver fibrosis in patients with NAFLD. Hepatology. 2007;45(4):846–54.

7

The early outcomes of candidates with portopulmonary hypertension after liver transplantation

Bingsong Huang[1†], Yi Shi[1†], Jun Liu[2†], Paul M. Schroder[3], Suxiong Deng[1], Maogen Chen[1], Jun Li[1], Yi Ma[1*] and Ronghai Deng[1*]

Abstract

Background: Portopulmonary hypertension (PPH) was once regarded as a contraindicaton to liver transplantation (LT). However, growing evidence has indicated that PPH patients undergoing LT may show similar outcomes compared to those without PPH, and researchers have recommended it not be an absolute contraindication. Given this controversy, we aimed to identify and review the current evidence on this topic and to provide a comparison of the outcomes after LT between candidates with PPH and those without.

Methods: We systematically searched the MEDLINE, EMBASE and Cochrane Library databases for all studies that compared the outcomes of PPH patients and those without PPH after LT. All studies reporting outcomes of PPH patients versus those without PPH (Control) were further considered for inclusion in this meta-analysis. Odds ratios (OR) and 95% confidence intervals (CI) were calculated to compare the pooled data between PPH and Control groups.

Results: Eleven retrospective trials and one prospective, randomized, controlled trial, involving 37,686 transplant recipients were included. The PPH patients had increased 1-year mortality with an OR of 1.59 (95% CI = 1.26–2.01, $P = 0.0001$) compared to the control group. There was no significant difference in graft loss and 30-day mortality after LT between the two groups.

Conclusions: Patients with PPH who underwent LT had increased 1-year mortality compared to those without PPH, while graft loss and 30-day mortality were similar. Nevertheless, LT may be a reasonable therapeutic option for some patients with PPH, but further studies are needed to identify those select patients with PPH who would benefit most from LT.

Keywords: Portopulmonary hypertension, Liver transplantation, Meta-analysis

Background

Portopulmonary hypertension (PPH) is defined by the presence of the following features in patients with portal hypertension: mean pulmonary arterial pressure (mPAP) determined by Portopulmonary hypertension (PPH) is defined by the presence of the following features in patients with portal hypertension: mean pulmonary arterial pressure (mPAP) determined by right-heart catheterisation of > 25 mmHg at rest or > 30 mmHg

during exercise, elevated pulmonary vascular resistance (PVR) > 3 wood units (240 dynes/s per cm-5), and normal pulmonary artery wedge pressure (PAWP) < 15 mmHg. [1–3]. PPH represents a serious complication of portal hypertension and is regarded as a contraindication to liver transplantation (LT) by some experts. It is a relatively common pathologic state in the setting of end-stage liver disease (ESLD), especially cirrhosis, with a reported incidence ranging from 1 to 10% to as high as 39% in patients receiving LT [4–6].

The pathophysiology of the relationship between portal hypertension and pulmonary hypertension is poorly understood. Some researchers consider the development of pulmonary hypertension in the ESLD population

* Correspondence: anhuimayi2002@163.com; mddrh81@163.com

†Bingsong Huang, Yi Shi and Jun Liu contributed equally to this work.

[1]Organ Transplant Center, the First Affiliated Hospital, Sun Yat-sen University, No. 58 Zhongshan 2nd Road, Guangzhou 510080, China

Full list of author information is available at the end of the article

dependent upon the presence of significant portal hypertension, but the mechanisms by which portal hypertension cause pulmonary hypertension remain unclear [7]. Others maintain that the elevation of mPAP represents a hyperdynamic state of blood circulation and that this elevation in mPAP eventually leads to portal hypertension [4, 8–11]. The true pathophysiology likely represents a combination of factors including the patient's underlying disease process and relevant comorbidities that determine the dominant causes of these high-pressure states.

Recently growing evidence suggests that PPH should no longer be considered an absolute contraindication to LT unless PPH is severe and associated with right ventricular dysfunction [6, 12, 18, 19]. Newer retrospective comparisons between patients with PPH and those without who underwent LT showed similar mortality between the two groups or slightly higher rates of death in PPH group that did not reach statistical significance [13, 14]. In 2012, a prospective controlled study showed that there were no significant differences between the PPH group and the control group in terms of six-month patient and graft survivals (100% vs. 88.9, 100% vs. 100%, respectively) [15].

The role of LT in patients with PPH has long been debated. Given the current controversy, in this meta-analysis, we aimed to combine data from all published studies to reevaluate the outcomes of the LT patients with preoperative PPH and give some suggestions for the management of PPH patients waiting for LT.

Methods
Data sources and searches
We searched the PubMed/Medline, Embase and Cochrane library databases using the terms "Portopulmonary hypertension" OR "Pulmonary hypertension" AND "Liver transplantation." The search included all studies published up to February 2017. Publications were limited to those reporting results from human subjects. Review articles were excluded after limit filtering. To prevent missing relevant publications on the topic, we also performed manual searches of the references of the relevant publications.

Study selection: Inclusion and exclusion criteria
Only those reporting outcomes of LT patients preoperatively diagnosed with PPH were included. Overlapping cohort studies from the same institution were excluded to avoid duplication. Studies lacking a control group or whose populations included subjects with other pulmonary diseases were excluded since other pulmonary disease processes can cause pulmonary hypertension. Studies comparing outcomes between the PPH patients with LT and without LT were also excluded. Studies for which the data

could not be extracted for analysis such as those reporting outcomes only in figure format (without description or tables) were excluded. Case reports whose data had poor homogeneity and studies examining patients who received multi-organ transplants were also excluded.

Quality assessment and data extraction
Publications were reviewed and two independent investigators extracted data with disagreements being resolved through discussion and consensus. The primary outcome was overall one-year patient survival rates. Secondary outcomes included early (30 days post-LT) patient and graft survival rates. The Newcastle-Ottawa quality assessment scale (Additional file 1: Table S1) [16] was applied to assess the quality of all included trials. A study can be awarded a maximum of one star for each numbered item within the Selection and Outcome categories. A maximum of two stars can be given for Comparability. Articles scoring five stars or more were considered to be of high quality. In addition, a RCT trial included was assessed by the Jadad score [17] in which case a score of at least 4 indicated a high methodological quality.

Data synthesis and analysis
Pooled odds ratios (OR) were used to evaluate the event rates, and the results were reported with 95% confidence intervals (CI). A P value < 0.05 was considered a significant difference in the values between the two groups. Heterogeneity through all the included studies was evaluated by χ^2 and I^2 statistical tests. Heterogeneity was considered significant when $P < 0.05$ or $I^2 > 50\%$, and a random effect model was adopted. A random effect model is a kind of hierarchical linear model, which assumes that the data set being analyzed consists of a hierarchy of different populations whose differences relate to that hierarchy. When $P > 0.05$ for χ^2 or $I^2 < 50\%$ for I^2 statistical tests, indicating low statistical heterogeneity in both cases, a fixed effect model was used. A fixed effect model is a statistical model that represents the observed quantities in terms of explanatory variables that are treated as if the quantities were non-random. A funnel plot was used to assess publication bias. A funnel plot is designed to check the existence of publication bias in systematic reviews and meta-analyses. The largest studies will be near the average while small studies will be spread on both sides of the average. Variation can indicate publication bias. All statistical analyses for the current study were performed with Review Manager (RevMan Version 5.3.5, The Nordic Cochrane Centre, The Cochrane Collaboration, 2014).

Results

Search results and included studies

The PRISMA flow diagram and results based on the search strategies and selection criteria described above are outlined in Fig. 1. Briefly, 2260 articles were initially identified. Among those references, 2218 studies were excluded after screening titles. The remaining 42 publications reporting results after LT for patients with PPH underwent more extensive review. Nineteen of these studies had no data available and were excluded from this meta-analysis. Five studies involved multiple organ transplantation, 4 studies lacked a control (no-PPH) group, one study was a case report, and one study was a manuscript reporting guidelines, which were also excluded. A total of 12 studies meeting all criteria were included in this meta-analysis, and the study characteristics are shown in Table 1. No evidence of publications bias among the included studies was found by means of a funnel plot (data not shown). A total of 507 LT recipients with PPH and 37,179 LT patients without PPH were included in this meta-analysis.

Hemodynamic parameters in the PPH group

The diagnosis of PPH is made from measurements during right heart catheterization with mPAP of > 25 mmHg, PVR > 240 dynes·s·cm – 5, and PAWP < 15 mmHg, and this definition was relatively consistent among the trials included in this meta-analysis. Some of the articles used a higher threshold of mPAP for diagnosis (mPAP> 30 mmHg) and inclusion in the PPH group [18, 19]. Others such as the DeMartino 2017 article, only included patients with moderate to severe PPH (mPAP> 35 mmHg and PVR greater than 240 PVR dynes·s·cm – 5) [4]While many studies used a single value of mPAP to serve as inclusion criteria for their PPH group, some further separated the PPH group into three grades of PPH: mild, moderate, and severe with considerable variation in the distinction between the

three subgroups among the trials included in this meta-analysis. The hemodynamic parameters of the PPH groups in each of the studies are shown in Table 2.

Primary outcome
1-year mortality

Ten studies involving 453 LT recipients with PPH and 37,105 LT recipients without PPH reported 1-year survival rates after transplantation. The results of the SRTR study (2014 Salgia, et al.) showed a higher 1-year mortality rate in PPH patients compared to patients without PPH ($P = 0.005$) [6]. In the remaining 9 studies [5, 13, 15–19], there was no significant difference in 1-year mortality rates between the two groups. The combined 1-year mortality rate was 26.0% for the PPH group and 12.7% for the control group. There was no significant heterogeneity identified among the 10 studies ($\chi^2 = 7.25$, $p = 0.61$, $I^2 = 0\%$). A fixed effect model was used, which showed that the OR for mortality at 1 year after LT was 1.59 (95% CI $=1.26–2.01$; $P = 0.0001$) for the PPH group compared to the control group (Fig. 2). Thus, one-year mortality after LT was significantly higher in the PPH group compared to the control group.

Secondary outcomes
30-day mortality

There were 3 studies that reported 30-day mortality after LT. Overall, the mortality within 30 days of LT surgery was 12.8% for the control group and 17.9% for the PPH group. No heterogeneity was identified across the 3 studies ($\chi^2 = 2.68$, $P = 0.26$; $I^2 = 25\%$), thus a fixed effect model was adopted. The OR for 30-day mortality in liver recipients with PPH versus those without was 1.42 (95% CI = 0.60–3.35, $P = 0.42$), which was not statistically significant (Fig. 3). These data show no significant

Table 1 Characteristics of the PPH trials

References	Institute	Sample size		Study periods	Recipients age	MELD score		NOS star level
		PPH	No-PPH			PPH	No-PPH	
DeMartino(2017) [4]	USA(single center)	31	269	2010–2013	57 (50–62)	32 (25–38)	25 (20–29)	66
Rajaram(2016) [13]	USA(single center)	13	20	2005–2015	52(37–62)	21.0 ± 9.2	24.7 ± 9.5	
Bozbac(2015) [17]	Turkey(single center)	47	156	2004–2015	42.1 ± 14.1	N/A[b]	N/A	6
Salgia (2014) [6]	SRTR[a]	78	34,240	2002–2010	54 (49–60)	14 (11–18)	18 (13–25)	6
Mangus(2013) [16]	USA(single center)	102	1161	2001–2010	53 (18–76)	22(9–40)	18 (6–40)	7
Yassen(2012) [15] ▲	Egypt(single center)	9	10	2008–2011	50.3	17 ± 5	14 ± 2	◆5
Pietri(2010) [14]	Italy(single center)	24	24	2003–2008	54(49–60)	25.0 ± 12.0	22.0 ± 10.9	6
Saner (2006) [7]	Germany(single center)	23	48	2004–2005	49.6	N/A	N/A	6
Veloso(2004) [21]	Brazil(single center)	31	26	1999–2001	46	N/A	N/A	6
Starkel (2002) [18]	UK(single center)	38	107	1997–1999	49.2	N/A	N/A	6
Ramsay(1997) [32]	USA(single center)	103	1103	1984–1995	N/A	N/A	N/A	5
Taura(1996) [19]	Spain(single center)	8	15	N/A	45.2	N/A	N/A	5

▲, random controlled, double-blind study; ◆Jadad **score**
[a]SRTR, Scientific Registry of Transplant recipients
[b]N/A, non-available

2260 Articles identified by database searching

--> 1129 duplicates removed

1131 Articles remained

--> 1089 excluded after screening titles, including:

329 basic science articles

255 reviews or commentaries

181 not relevant to PPH

172 focused on clinical reports

152 involved patients without LT

42 Articles remained

--> 30 excluded after abstract and full text review, including:

19 no data available

5 involved multi-organ transplant

4 had no control group

1 case report

1 guideline manuscript

12 Articles remained

Fig. 1 PRISMA flow diagram showing selection of articles for review

difference in 30-day mortality after LT between those with PPH and those without.

Graft loss rates

Another secondary endpoint that was examined was graft loss at 1 year after transplantation in order to understand the influence of initial PPH on the success of the transplant. Three of the studies reported graft loss rate. There was no heterogeneity detected among the three studies that reported one year graft loss rates ($\chi^2 = 2.45$, $P = 0.12$; $I^2 = 59\%$), thus a random effect model was implemented for further comparison. The OR for one-year graft loss was 1.71 (95% CI =0.97–3.00, $P = 0.06$) in the patients with PPH compared to those without (Fig. 4). Therefore, patients without PPH demonstrated significantly better one-year graft survival after LT than those that had PPH prior to transplant.

Discussion

In this manuscript we aimed to provide a comprehensive meta-analysis comparing the early outcomes after LT between candidates with PPH and those without. A total of twelve studies with 37,688 patients were included in this meta-analysis. The primary outcome of 1-year mortality was significantly higher in those with PPH, while 30-day mortality was no different from controls. In addition, those with PPH had significantly higher rates of graft loss at 1 year after LT. To our knowledge this is the first comprehensive, systematic review of the available data on this topic and therefore provides important insight into the controversy regarding the benefit of LT in patients with PPH.

Patients with liver disease are at higher risk for pulmonary vascular conditions such as PPH due to systemically high intravascular flow and increased pulmonary venous volume. In a communication from the French

Table 2 Hemodynamics condition of PPH group

References	Grade of PPH(mmHg),n			Mean mPAP(mmHg)
DeMartino(2017) [4]	> 35			38(range,35–46)
	31			
Rajaram(2016) [13]	> 25			45.51 ± 2.1
	13			
Bozbac(2015) [17]	> 30			44.2 ± 7.8
	47			
Salgia (2014) [6]	25–35(treated PPH)			N/A
	78			
Mangus(2013) [16]	25–30(low mild)	30–34(high mild)	> 35(moderate)	N/A
	63	30	9	
Yassen(2012) [15]	25–34(mild)	35–44(moderate)		30.1 ± 11.4
	6	3		
Pietri(2010) [14]	25–34(mild)	> 35(moderate)		N/A
	21	3		
Saner (2006) [7]	25–34(mild)	35–44(moderate)	> 45(severe)	N/A
	16	5	2	
Veloso(2004) [21]	> 25			31.48 ± 4.42
	31			
Starkel (2002) [18]	25–34(mild)	> 35(moderate to severe)		N/A
	31	7		
Ramsay(1997) [32]	30–44(mild)	45–59(moderate)	> 60(severe)	N/A
	81	14	7	
Taura(1996) [19]	> 25			33.4(range-28-38)
	8			

pulmonary arterial hypertension (PAH) registry ($n = 154$, where only 33% had been treated with PAH-specific therapies), Le Pavec, et al. [20] described 1-, 3-, and 5-year survivals of 88, 75 and 68%, respectively, for PPH patients. Causes of death in this study were equally distributed between right ventricle failure due to progressive PPH and direct complications from liver cirrhosis. If no therapy is implemented, the prognosis of PPH is very poor with 5-year survival of 4–14% reported at some centers [18, 21].

Current pharmacologic treatment options for PPH include oral and intravenous vasodilator therapy such as prostacyclin analogues, phosphodiesterase 5-inhibitors, and endothelin receptor antagonists [1]. Nevertheless, the available data supporting the use of these specific therapies in PPH are only presented in case series and uncontrolled observational studies.

The therapeutic potential of LT in PPH has also been demonstrated, as Bozbas, et al. showed

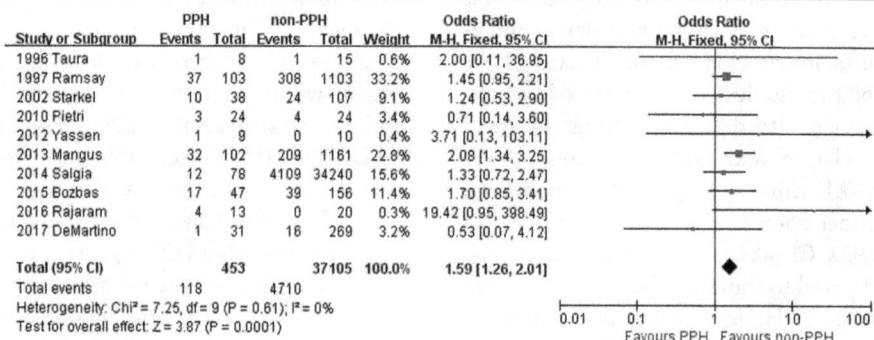

Fig. 2 Patient mortality at 1 year

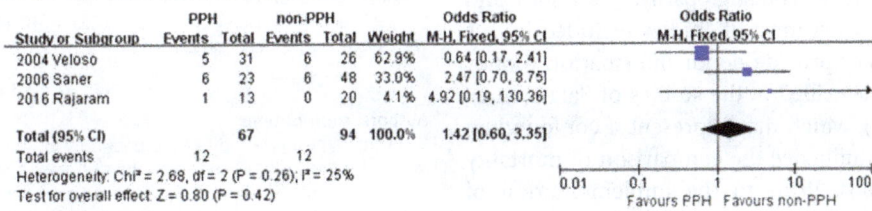

Fig. 3 Patient mortality at 30 days

significant reductions in mPAPs after LT in patients with PPH [17]. However, due to poor outcomes reported early on in the experience of LT for patients with PPH, it was considered a contraindication to LT by many transplant centers [22–25]. More recent evidence from retrospective data in multiple centers suggests that unless PPH is severe and associated with right ventricular dysfunction, it should no longer be considered an absolute contraindication to liver transplant [4, 6, 17, 26]. Indeed, Ramsay, et al. reviewed 1205 LT recipients involving 102 PPH patients, the 3-year mortality rates of the no-PPH, mild PPH, moderate PPH and severe PPH groups were 28, 33, 35, and 71%, respectively [18]. They concluded that patients with severe PPH likely had pathological changes in the pulmonary vasculature that were irreversible even after LT, as severe PPH was associated with a much higher perioperative mortality rate. A retrospective study from the UNOS SRTR database reported 123 PPH patients [6], seventy-eight of them underwent LT, whose 1- and 3-year survival were 85 and 81%. The other 45 had not been transplanted and 11 of them died on the waitlist, which indicated 3-year survival for PPH patients on the waitlist was about 75. 6%. Based in part on these data, the United States organ allocation policy gives higher priority to perform LT in PPH patients if hemodynamics are expected to significantly improved and meet standardized Model for end-stage liver disease (MELD) exception guidelines [4, 27, 28]. Because of the important prognostic implications demonstrated by these studies along with these changes in organ allocation policies, the American Association for the Study of Liver Disease and the International Liver Transplantation Society recommended all patients evaluated for LT be screened

for PPH by transthoracic echocardiogram (TTE), with confirmatory testing by right heart catheterization (RHC) [3, 8, 29, 30].

The overall mortality at 1 year after LT in our meta-analysis is comparable to the individual analyses with 26% mortality in the PPH group. However, this data includes multiple degrees of PPH as demonstrated in our analysis of the hemodynamic status of the patients included in each of the studies. The individual studies such as the Ramsay, et al. and Saner, et al. that defined three groups mild, moderate, and severe PPH prior to LT can help to determine and select the appropriate patient population that would have outcomes similar to those without PPH. Identifying threshold values of mPAP in PPH patients that predict poorer outcomes after transplant or provide guidance about which patients would benefit from specific treatment of their PPH prior to LT will be useful questions for future work in this field. Determination of these values and novel ways of evaluating prognosis after LT in the population of patients with PPH also has broader implications for organ allocation policy in this patient population.

There are multiple limitations inherent to this meta-analysis. The majority of the studies that were included for analysis are retrospective, observational studies. In addition, all but four of the studies had relatively small sample sizes of participants, which may have precluded an accurate assessment of heterogeneity. Donor factors such as preoperative condition of the donor, age, cold and warm ischemia time, and donation type have a great impact on the post-operative outcomes of LT recipients. For instance, donation after cardiac death (DCD) LT has worse long-term outcomes compared to donation after brain death (DBD) LT, with an increase in biliary

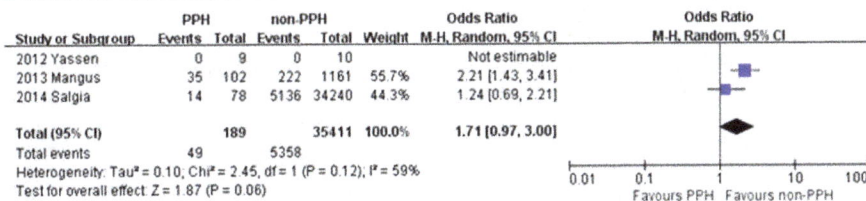

Fig. 4 Graft loss at one year

complications, ischemic cholangiopathy, graft loss and mortality [31]. However, most of studies included in this meta-analysis did not provide donor information (donor baseline was only described in the studies of Salgia, et al. and Mangus, et al.), which may represent a confounding variable that could influence the comparison of mortality rates between groups. Prior to the implementation of TTE as a valuable tool in identifying patients with PPH, this technology was not routinely used to screen LT candidates for these phenomena. Therefore, a portion of candidates who suffered from PPH may be missing from our analysis, especially in those studies that reported data from earlier times. In addition, the follow-up time in our analysis was relatively short (only out to 1 year), which may not be representative of the long-term outcomes for these patients after LT. Also, there were only 3 studies (with relatively small sample sizes) reporting 30-day mortality so drawing conclusions based on this analysis is difficult. Due to the wide distribution of study periods and the advances in technology and operative techniques over these time periods, a degree of bias related to these temporal changes in management may have been present and was not accounted for in the analysis. Lastly, a few of the studies had no available baseline data such as MELD score and age of patients included calling into question the quality of those studies. However, all the studies were evaluated by the Newcastle-Ottawa quality assessment scale or similar evaluation method and determined to be of sufficient quality for this meta-analysis.

Conclusion

There is an increase in 1-year patient mortality and graft loss after LT in candidates with PPH. Thus, PPH remains an important risk factor that should continue to be screened for in LT candidates. It is likely that different grades of PPH exist some of which are amenable to treatment, and select patients with PPH are likely to benefit more than others from LT. Therefore, more randomized controlled trials with a larger sample sizes and long term follow-up are needed to evaluate the long-term outcomes in these patients as well as to refine the selection of patients with PPH who would benefit most from LT.

Abbreviations

CI: Confidence intervals; DBD: Donation after brain death; DCD: Donation after cardiac death; ESLD: End-stage liver disease; HR: Hazard ratio; LT: Liver transplantation; MELD: Model for end-stage liver disease; OR: Pooled odds ratios; PAH: Pulmonary arterial hypertension; PAP: Pulmonary arterial pressure; PPH: Portopulmonary hypertension; RHC: Right heart catheterization; SRTR: Scientific registry of transplant recipients; TTE: Transthoracic echocardiogram

Funding

This work was in part supported by the National Natural Science Foundation of China (81770410 and 81401324), Scientific Program for Young teacher of Sun Yat-sen University(16ykpy05), the National Natural Science Foundation of China, China (81370574, and 81670591), Guangdong Natural Science Foundation, China (2016A030311028), and the Science and Technology Program of Guangzhou, China (201704020073).

Authors' contributions

BSH writing the article and takes responsibility for the integrity of the work as a whole. YM and RHD conceived the study, and participated in its design. YS performed the assessment of quality and collection of data. JL (Jun Liu), JL (Jun Li), and SXD participated in data collection.PMS and MGC give critical revision of the article. All authors read and approved the final manuscript.

Competing interests

The authors declare that they have no competing interests

Author details

[1]Organ Transplant Center, the First Affiliated Hospital, Sun Yat-sen University, No. 58 Zhongshan 2nd Road, Guangzhou 510080, China. [2]Department of Respiratory, the First People's Hospital affiliated to Guangzhou Medical University, Guangzhou 510080, China. [3]Department of Surgery, Duke University Medical Center, 10 Duke Medicine Circle Durham, Durham, NC 27710, USA.

References

1. Hoeper MM, Krowka MJ, Strassburg CP. Portopulmonary hypertension and hepatopulmonary syndrome. Lancet. 2004;363(9419):1461–8.
2. Cosarderelioglu C, Cosar AM, Gurakar M, Pustavoitau A, Russell SD, Dagher NN, Gurakar A. Portopulmonary hypertension and liver transplant: recent review of the literature. Exp Clin Transplant. 2016;14(2):113–20.
3. Krowka MJ, Fallon MB, Kawut SM, Fuhrmann V, Heimbach JK, Ramsay MA, Sitbon O, Sokol RJ. International liver transplant society practice guidelines: diagnosis and Management of Hepatopulmonary Syndrome and Portopulmonary Hypertension. Transplantation. 2016;100(7):1440–52.
4. DeMartino ES, Cartin-Ceba R, Findlay JY, Heimbach JK, Krowka MJ. Frequency and outcomes of patients with increased mean pulmonary artery pressure at the time of liver transplantation. Transplantation. 2017;101(1):101–6.
5. Krowka M. Pulmonary hemodynamics and perioperative cardiopulmonary-related mortality in patients with Portopulmonary hypertension undergoing liver transplantation. LIVER TRANSPLANT. 2000;6(4):443–50.
6. Salgia RJ, Goodrich NP, Simpson H, Merion RM, Sharma P. Outcomes of liver transplantation for Porto-pulmonary hypertension in model for end-stage liver disease era. DIGEST DIS SCI. 2014;59(8):1976–82.
7. Saner FH, Nadalin S, Pavlakovi G, Gu Y, SWMO D, Gensicke J, Fruhauf NR, Paul A, Radtke A, Sotiropoulos GC, et al. Portopulmonary hypertension in the early phase following liver transplantation. Transplantation. 2006;82(7):887–91.
8. Raevens S, Colle I, Reyntjens K, Geerts A, Berrevoet F, Rogiers X, Troisi RI, Van Vlierberghe H, De Pauw M. Echocardiography for the detection of portopulmonary hypertension in liver transplant candidates: an analysis of cutoff values. Liver Transpl. 2013;19(6):602–10.
9. Iqbal CW, Krowka MJ, Pham TH, Freese DK, El YM, Ishitani MB. Liver transplantation for pulmonary vascular complications of pediatric end-stage liver disease. J Pediatr Surg. 2008;43(10):1813–20.
10. Warnaar N, Molenaar IQ, Colquhoun SD, Slooff MJ, Sherwani S, de Wolf AM, Porte RJ. Intraoperative pulmonary embolism and intracardiac thrombosis complicating liver transplantation: a systematic review. J Thromb Haemost. 2008;6(2):297–302.
11. Ashfaq M, Chinnakotla S, Rogers L, Ausloos K, Saadeh S, Klintmalm GB, Ramsay M, Davis GL. The impact of treatment of portopulmonary hypertension on survival following liver transplantation. Am J Transplant. 2007;7(5):1258–64.
12. Swanson KL, Wiesner RH, Nyberg SL, Rosen CB, Krowka MJ. Survival in portopulmonary hypertension: Mayo Clinic experience categorized by treatment subgroups. Am J Transplant. 2008;8(11):2445–53.
13. Rajaram P, Parekh A, Fisher M, Kempker J, Subramanian R. Comparison of post-liver transplantation outcomes in Portopulmonary hypertension and pulmonary venous hypertension: a single-center experience. Transplant Proc. 2017;49(2):338–43.

14. De Pietri L, Montalti R, Begliomini B, Reggiani A, Lancellotti L, Giovannini S, Di Benedetto F, Guerrini G, Serra V, Rompianesi G, et al. Pulmonary hypertension as a predictor of postoperative complications and mortality after liver transplantation. Transplant Proc. 2010;42(4):1188–90.

15. Yassen AM, Elsarraf WR, Elsadany M, Elshobari MM, Salah T, Sultan AM: The impact of Portopulmonary hypertension on intraoperative right ventricular function of living donor liver transplant recipients. Anesth Analg. 2012;1: 689–93.

16. Mangus RS, Kinsella SB, Marshall GR, Fridell JA, Wilkes KR, Tector AJ. Mild to moderate pulmonary hypertension in liver transplantation. J Surg Res. 2013;184(2):1150–6.

17. Savas BS, Eroglu S, Oner EF, Moray G, Haberal M. Pulmonary hypertension improves after Orthotopic liver transplant in patients with chronic liver disease. Exp Clin Transplant. 2015;13(Suppl 3):115–9.

18. Starkel P, Vera A, Gunson B, Mutimer D. Outcome of liver transplantation for patients with pulmonary hypertension. Liver Transpl. 2002;8(4):382–8.

19. Taura P, Garcia-Valdecasas JC, Beltran J, Izquierdo E, Navasa M, Sala-Blanch J, Mas A, Balust J, Grande L, Visa J. Moderate primary pulmonary hypertension in patients undergoing liver transplantation. Anesth Analg. 1996;83(4):675–80.

20. Herve P, Le Pavec J, Sztrymf B, Decante B, Savale L, Sitbon O. Pulmonary vascular abnormalities in cirrhosis. Best Pract Res Clin Gastroenterol. 2007;21(1):141–59.

21. Veloso CA, Boin IFS, Dragosavac D, Leonardi LS, Figueiredo LC, Araújo S, Terzi RGG. Retrospective analysis of patients who developed pulmonary hypertension during the early postoperative period after liver transplantation. TRANSPL P. 2004;36(4):938–40.

22. De Wolf AM, Begliomini B, Gasior TA, Kang Y, Pinsky MR. Right ventricular function during orthotopic liver transplantation. Anesth Analg. 1993;76(3):562-568.

23. Krowka MJ, Mandell MS, Ramsay MAE, Kawut SM, Fallon MB, Manzarbeitia C, Pardo M, Marotta P, Uemoto S, Stoffel MP, et al. Hepatopulmonary syndrome and portopulmonary hypertension: a report of the multicenter liver transplant database. LIVER TRANSPLANT. 2004;10(2):174–82.

24. Fukazawa K, Poliac LC, Pretto EA. Rapid assessment and safe management of severe pulmonary hypertension with milrinone during orthotopic liver transplantation. Clin Transpl. 2010;24(4):515–9.

25. Koch DG, Caplan M, Reuben A. Pulmonary hypertension after liver transplantation: case presentation and review of the literature. Liver Transpl. 2009;15(4):407–12.

26. Bozbas SS, Eyuboglu FO, Arslan NG, Ergur FO, Karakayali H, Haberal M. The prevalence and the impact of portopulmonary hypertension on postoperative course in patients undergoing liver transplantation. Transplant Proc. 2009;41(7):2860–3.

27. Lentine KL, Villines TC, Axelrod D, Kaviratne S, Weir MR, Costa SP. Evaluation and Management of Pulmonary Hypertension in kidney transplant candidates and recipients: concepts and controversies. Transplantation. 2017;101(1):166–81.

28. Krowka MJ, Wiesner RH, Heimbach JK. Pulmonary contraindications, indications and MELD exceptions for liver transplantation: a contemporary view and look forward. J Hepatol. 2013;59(2):367–74.

29. Murray KF, Carithers RJ. AASLD practice guidelines: evaluation of the patient for liver transplantation. Hepatology. 2005;41(6):1407–32.

30. Ford HJ, Aris RM, Andreoni K. Screening for portopulmonary hypertension with transthoracic echocardiography: implications for early mortality associated with liver transplantation. Am J Respir Crit Care Med. 2009;180(4):378. 378-379

31. O'Neill S, Roebuck A, Khoo E, Wigmore SJ, Harrison EM. A meta-analysis and meta-regression of outcomes including biliary complications in donation after cardiac death liver transplantation. Transpl Int. 2014;27(11):1159–74.

32. Ramsay MA, Simpson BR, Nguyen AT, Ramsay KJ, East C, Klintmalm GB. Severe pulmonary hypertension in liver transplant candidates. Liver Transpl Surg. 1997;3(5):494–500.

Hepcidin levels correlate to liver iron content, but not steatohepatitis, in non-alcoholic fatty liver disease

Joel Marmur[1,2], Soheir Beshara[3], Gösta Eggertsen[3], Liselotte Onelöv[3], Nils Albiin[4], Olof Danielsson[5], Rolf Hultcrantz[1] and Per Stål[1]* (iD)

Abstract

Background: One-third of patients with non-alcoholic fatty liver disease (NAFLD) develop dysmetabolic iron overload syndrome (DIOS), the pathogenesis of which is unknown. Altered production of the iron-regulatory peptide hepcidin has been reported in NAFLD, but it is unclear if this is related to iron accumulation, lipid status or steatohepatitis.

Methods: Eighty-four patients with liver disease, 54 of which had iron overload, underwent liver biopsy ($n = 66$) and/or magnetic resonance imaging ($n = 35$) for liver iron content determination. Thirty-eight of the patients had NAFLD, 29 had chronic liver disease other than NAFLD, and 17 had untreated genetic hemochromatosis. Serum hepcidin was measured with ELISA in all patients and in 34 controls. Hepcidin antimicrobial peptide (*HAMP*) mRNA in liver tissue was determined with real-time-quantitative PCR in 36 patients.

Results: Serum hepcidin was increased similarly in NAFLD with DIOS as in the other chronic liver diseases with iron overload, except for genetic hemochromatosis. *HAMP* mRNA in liver tissue, and serum hepcidin, both correlated to liver iron content in NAFLD patients ($r^2 = 0.45$, $p < 0.05$ and $r^2 = 0.27$, $p < 0.05$ respectively) but not to body mass index, NAFLD activity score or serum lipids. There was a good correlation between *HAMP* mRNA in liver tissue and serum hepcidin ($r^2 = 0.39$, $p < 0.01$).

Conclusions: In NAFLD with or without dysmetabolic iron overload, serum hepcidin and *HAMP* mRNA in liver correlate to body iron content but not to the degree of steatohepatitis or lipid status. Thus, the dysmetabolic iron overload syndrome seen in NAFLD is not caused by an altered hepcidin synthesis.

Keywords: Hepcidin, Iron overload, Non-alcoholic fatty liver disease

Background

Non-alcoholic fatty liver disease (NAFLD) is the most prevalent liver disease worldwide, with an association to obesity, insulin resistance and the metabolic syndrome [1–3]. Approximately one-third of patients with NAFLD develop elevated serum ferritin and hepatic iron overload, a condition known as the "dysmetabolic iron overload syndrome" (DIOS) [4, 5]. The underlying mechanisms for DIOS are unknown. Increased iron stores could be of pathogenic importance in NAFLD, since it may increase the risk of hepatocyte ballooning, inflammation and fibrosis, which are features of liver damage seen in non-alcoholic steatohepatitis (NASH) which is the more severe form of NAFLD [6–8].

The body's iron balance is regulated by hepcidin, a 25 amino-acid peptide that inhibits iron uptake in the gut and iron recycling from macrophages, consequently decreasing iron levels in plasma [9]. An inappropriately low hepcidin synthesis has been reported in NAFLD [10, 11] which could facilitate iron uptake and predispose for DIOS, but results are not consistent [12, 13]. Hepcidin levels in NAFLD are difficult to elucidate, since both obesity and diabetes may increase hepcidin production [12, 14, 15]. For example, in morbidly obese subjects, hepcidin is released from adipose tissue [12, 13, 15, 16], which may lead to anemia and entrapment of iron in

* Correspondence: per.stal@ki.se
[1]Unit of Liver Diseases, Department of Upper GI, C1-77 Huddinge, Karolinska University Hospital, Karolinska Institutet, 141 86 Stockholm, Sweden
Full list of author information is available at the end of the article

reticuloendothelial cells [9]. Thus, in NAFLD data is conflicting whether or not hepcidin predominantly correlates to body iron stores [16, 17], to features of the metabolic syndrome [18, 19] or the hepatic inflammation seen in steatohepatitis (NASH). In a recent study, hepatic iron measured by magnetic resonance imaging was found to be the major determinant of serum ferritin in NAFLD [20]. In a large study on individuals with metabolic syndrome, results suggested that that the iron regulatory feedback on hepcidin synthesis was preserved in these patients [21].

The aim of the present study was to elucidate whether body iron stores, steatohepatitis or lipid status in NAFLD correlated to hepcidin synthesis. For this purpose, we compared serum hepcidin levels and hepatic hepcidin antimicrobial peptide (HAMP) gene expressions in NAFLD patients with various degrees of iron overload, to those of patients with other forms of acquired or genetic iron overload. We aimed to include patients with various hepcidin levels, and therefore we included untreated hereditary hemochromatosis patients (with a known hepcidin deficiency) as well as patients with iron overload associated to other chronic liver diseases, presumably having elevated serum hepcidin levels. We correlated our findings to iron indices, liver biopsy features, anthropometric data, and lipid parameters.

Methods

Patient data collection and investigations

All patients referred to the Unit of Liver Diseases at the Karolinska University Hospital for liver biopsy due to chronic liver disease and/or hemochromatosis, and with an elevated serum ferritin, between January 2008 and April 2013, were asked to participate in the study. Hyperferritinemia was defined as a serum ferritin > 350 µg/L. In addition, patients with chronic liver disease and normal iron parameters undergoing liver biopsy were enrolled for comparison. All patients were over 18 years of age and had given written informed consent. One patient was excluded due to iron deficiency. No patients included had been subject to treatment with iron reduction therapy before entering the study.

A total of 84 patients were enrolled (26 females, 58 males), of which 62 had elevated ferritin levels and 23 a normal serum ferritin concentration. Thirty-eight of the 84 patients had NAFLD, 17 had untreated hereditary hemochromatosis (HH), and 29 had various other causes of chronic liver disease (CLD), such as autoimmune liver disease, alcoholic liver disease, chronic viral hepatitis, alpha-1-antitrypsin deficiency, cryptogenic cirrhosis, porphyria cutanea tarda, methotrexate-induced liver fibrosis, or the hemochromatosis phenotype but without the C282Y or H63D mutations. All these other etiologies (except NAFLD and HFE-associated HH) were thus grouped

together as CLD. NAFLD was defined as either Grade 1 or more steatosis in the liver biopsy according to Kleiner et al. [22], or a bright liver with increased echogenicity at abdominal ultrasound investigation. Among the 17 patients with HH, 12 were HFE C282Y homozygotes and five were C282Y/H63D compound heterozygotes. In the group of 29 patients with chronic liver disease, eight had a normal iron content in the liver, and 21 had iron overload, and were classified as "chronic liver disease with iron overload" (CLD-IO). One of these had received oral iron substitution for several years; however, none had been treated with parenteral iron substitution or blood transfusions. Amongst the 21 patients classified as CLD-IO, ten had a clinical phenotype of hemochromatosis (elevated serum ferritin and transferrin saturation, and hepatic iron overload) but without homozygosity for the HFE C282Y mutation or compound heterozygosity for the C282Y and H63D mutations, and without alcohol overconsumption. The other 19 CLD patients had alcohol overconsumption (> 30 g/day) (n = 9), primary biliary cholangitis (n = 2), hepatitis C (n = 1), alpha-1-antitrypsin deficiency (n = 1), porphyria cutanea tarda (n = 1), cryptogenic cirrhosis (n = 2), or methotrexate-treated psoriasis (n = 3). None of the patients with HH, NAFLD or CLD with the clinical phenotype of hemochromatosis had reported a previous or current alcohol consumption exceeding 20 g/day. Two CLD-IO patients (with alpha-1-antitrypsin deficiency and alcohol overconsumption, respectively) were heterozygous for the H63D mutation, and one (with alcohol overconsumption) was heterozygous for the C282Y mutation.

Iron overload was defined as a histologic iron score of ≥1 or an estimated iron content > 40 µmol/g on magnetic resonance imaging (MRI) investigation (see below). The patient groups are displayed in Table 1.

Liver biopsy was performed in 66 out of the 84 patients. MRI was used for iron assessment in 35 cases, and in 14 of these, histology was lacking. In 21 cases, there was both histology and MRI. In four cases (two HH homozygotes, one HH compound heterozygote, and one with CLD and normal ferritin) both liver histology and MRI was lacking.

Data collection from controls

A total of 40 healthy controls, recruited from hospital staff, participated in the study. None had a history of liver disease. Written consent was given. Of the controls, six individuals were excluded (elevated transaminases in one case, compound heterozygosity of the HFE gene and elevated serum ferritin in one case, iron deficiency with serum ferritin < 15 µg/L in three cases, and elevated ferritin (413 µg/L) in one case). The remaining 34 controls were included in the study (Table 1).

Biochemical data was collected at the time of enrollment in the study. Blood samples were drawn before 10

Table 1 Clinical and laboratory data for patients and controls

	Control N = 34	NAFLD N = 22	NAFLD with DIOS N = 16	CLD N = 8	CLD-IO N = 21	Compound heterozygous HH N = 5	Homozygous HH N = 12
Gender (F/M)	19/15	8/14	5/11	4/4	6/15	1/4	2/10
Age (y)	40 ± 10*	54 ± 16	59 ± 10	57 ± 8	58 ± 8	59 ± 9	51 ± 6
BMI (kg/m^2)	23.3 ± 2.6*	30.4 ± 4.2#	28.1 ± 2.4	27.3 ± 5.1	27.0 ± 4.2	29.0 ± 3.5	28.2 ± 4.8
Hemoglobin (g/L)	142 ± 11	150 ± 15	149 ± 17	140 ± 10	140 ± 17	158 ± 15	154 ± 12
ALT (U/L)	18 ± 6*	94 ± 76	59 ± 41	71 ± 59	53 ± 29	41 ± 35	82 ± 35
CRP (mg/L)	1.1 ± 0.4	3.0 ± 2.9	1.8 ± 0.9	2.8 ± 3.0	3.8 ± 5.5	3.6 ± 4.0	3.3 ± 2.7
Serum ferritin (μg/L)	94 ± 87	304 ± 248	816 ± 285¤	454 ± 688	1304 ± 1295¤	878 ± 408¤	1753 ± 998¤
Transferrin saturation (%)	0.28 ± 0.11	0.28 ± 0.09	0.39 ± 0.09	0.31 ± 0.15	0.50 ± 0.21§	0.46 ± 0.10§	0.76 ± 0.21*
Hepatic iron score	N.D.	0.11 ± 0.21	2.19 ± 0.95¤	0.29 ± 0.27	2.98 ± 1.22¤	3.38 ± 0.75¤	4.35 ± 0.63¤

CLD chronic liver disease, IO iron overload, HH hereditary hemochromatosis, NAFLD non-alcoholic fatty liver disease, DIOS dysmetabolic iron overload syndrome.
Values denote mean ± S.D
*$P < 0.05$ vs. all other groups
#$p < 0.05$ vs. Control, CLD, CLD-IO
¤$p < 0.05$ vs. Control, NAFLD, CLD
§$p < 0.05$ vs. Control, NAFLD, DIOS, CLD, homozygous HH

A.M. in the morning. Subjects were not fasting but had had a light breakfast. Routine blood chemistry analyses as well as *HFE* mutation analysis were performed on all subjects at the Department of Clinical Chemistry at Karolinska University Hospital. Body mass index was calculated using the formula: weight in kilogram / (height in meters) ^{2}.

Quantitative assay of hepcidin in serum samples

Freshly drawn samples from the 84 patients and 34 controls were centrifuged and serum was stored at − 70 °C until analysis. Samples were analyzed for hepcidin by a competitive ELISA kit (Bachem, Peninsula Laboratories, LLC, CA, United States) as reported previously [23]. Reference ranges established in 83 normal subjects showed hepcidin levels that ranged 8–76 and 2–50 μg/L for men and women, respectively (2.5–97.5 percentiles). The results were significantly different between genders. As internal controls, pooled sera of 7 and 6 samples representing low (≈0.4 μg/L) and normal (≈3 μg/L) levels respectively were frozen at − 70 °C. Control sera were run in 6 replicates at each assay. The intra-assay variation showed CVs of 18% for low and 13% for normal controls, while inter-assay CVs were 18 and 19%, respectively. The lower limit of detection, calculated as 3 SD above the lowest standard, was 0.05 μg/L and linearity for this kit was determined as between 0,2–5 μg/L (2–50 μg/L for samples diluted 1:10). Samples outside linearity limits were rerun using proper dilution factor, and all samples were run in duplicate.

Analysis of IL-6 and TNFα

IL-6 and TNFα were measured using Bio-plex Pro Human Cytokine Group 1 kit (Bio-rad Laboratories, Hercules, CA, USA) according to the manufacturer's instructions.

Briefly, plasma/serum was diluted 1:4 using Bio-plex sample diluents. To obtain the nine point (including blank) standard curve, the kit standard was reconstituted and diluted fourfold. The 10× IL-6 and TNFα coupled beads were diluted in kit assay buffer and added to all standard and sample wells. The plate was incubated on shaker 30 min. After washing IL-6 and TNFα biotinylated detection antibodies were added and the plate was incubated as above. In the final step, PE-conjugated Streptavidin was added and the plate was run on a Magpix instrument (Luminex Corporation, Austin TX, USA) and analyzed with xPonent software (Luminex).

Analysis of HAMP mRNA in liver biopsies

Sixty-six patients underwent liver biopsy, and tissue from 39 of these was collected for hepcidin mRNA analysis. Tissues were immediately immersed in RNAlater and stored at − 70°C until processed. Total RNA was successfully retrieved from 36 of the 39 utilized liver biopsies with a dry weight of 0.3–5.9 mg using the RNAqueous -4PCR kit (Ambion PN AM1914). Recovered quantities of RNA ranged from 13 to 200 ng/μL. The quality and quantity of the extracted RNA was verified with the Bio-Rad Experion 700–7000 electrophoresis system, and only samples with an RQI > 8 were included in the study. cDNA synthesis was carried out with the High Capacity Reverse Transcriptase Kit (Applied Biosystems), using 65–930 ng of total RNA per sample. Determination of specific mRNA levels was performed as described previously [23].

Histologic examination of liver biopsy samples

Liver biopsy samples were revalued by an experienced pathologist (O.D.) blinded to clinical data. Samples from NAFLD-patients were evaluated for the degree of steatosis (0–3), lobular inflammation (0–3) and hepato-cellular ballooning (0–2) according to Kleiner et al. [22]. The unweighted sum of these three variables were used to calculate the NAFLD activity score (NAS). Patients with NAS ≥5 were diagnosed with NASH.

Siderosis was determined for all patients semi-quantitatively on histopathologic examination of Perls' stained liver biopsy samples adapted from Deugnier et al. [24] to match available levels of magnification.

An iron score from 0 to 4 for iron in hepatocytes was determined as follows: [0] granules absent or barely dis-cernible at a magnification of 400X; [1] barely discern-ible granules at a magnification of 200X but easily confirmed at a magnification of 400X; [2] discrete gran-ules at 100X magnification; [3] discrete granules easily confirmed at magnification of 40X, but barely discernible at a magnification of 20X; [4] granules obvious at a mag-nification of 20X, and barely visible for the naked eye. RES-iron was also determined and scored as [0] none, [1] mild, [2] or more than mild, as described by Nelson et al. [25]. These two scores were transformed into a histologic iron score (HIS) ranging from 0 to 5, compris-ing the score for iron in hepatocytes (0–4), plus one point for RES iron in those cases where it had been de-termined as more than mild, or a half point where it has been determined as mild. Iron overload was defined as a histologic iron score of ≥1.

Magnetic resonance imaging (MRI)

MRI was used for detection and quantification of liver iron overload in 35 patients and correlated to histology in 21 of these (Fig. 1). The liver iron was assessed semi-quantitatively as described by Gandon et al. [26].

In the correlation analyses of serum hepcidin to liver iron content, MRI iron was approximated to histologic liver iron (HIS) score based on the correlation estimated from Fig. 1: < 40 μmol iron/g tissue = HIS 0; 40–74 μmol/g = HIS 1; 75–129 μmol/g = HIS 2; 130–179 μmol/g = HIS 3; 180–239 μmol/g = HIS 4; ≥240 μmol iron/g tissue = HIS 5.

Statistical analyses

The relationship between two categorical variables was examined with Chi^2-test or Fisher's exact test (when ap-plicable). Numerical values of laboratory parameters were analyzed using one-way ANOVA and validated for equal variance and normal distribution. Kruskal-Wallis ANOVA was used when the assumptions did not hold. The correlation between two numerical variables was analyzed with simple linear regression validated for lin-earity, variance between observations and for normal distribution. In the cases where the assumptions did not hold the Spearman's rank order correlation was used in-stead. Multiple linear regression was used for variables that were significantly correlated to serum hepcidin in the simple linear regression. A p-value < 0.05 was con-sidered statistically significant.

Results

Clinical and laboratory data

The distribution of patients, and clinical and laboratory data of patients and controls are demonstrated in Table 1. Controls were significantly younger than pa-tients, and had lower BMI, ALT and serum ferritin

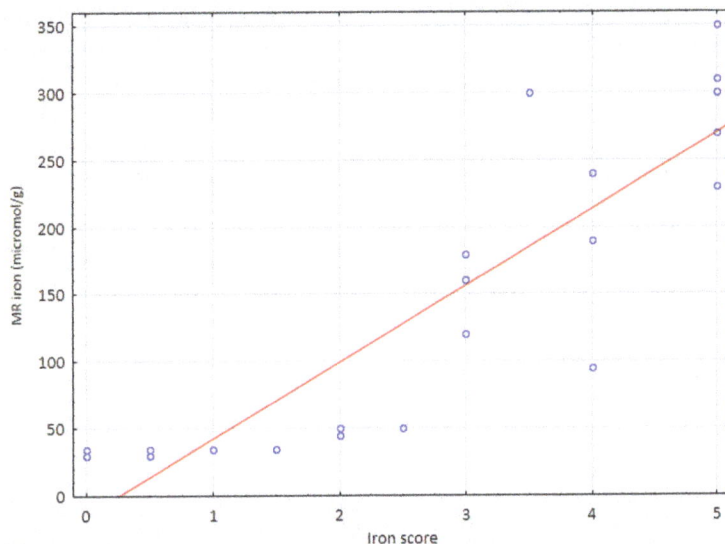

Fig. 1 Graph demonstrating the correlation between MRI iron content (μmol/g) and histological iron score in 21 patients in whom both MRI and liver biopsy was performed. There was a good correlation between these variables ($r^2 = 0.77$; $p < 0.01$)

levels. BMI was highest in the NAFLD patient group. Transferrin saturation was significantly increased in patients with homozygous HH, and in the 10 CLD-IO patients with a HH phenotype without HFE mutations, compared with the other patient groups and controls. Hepatic iron score did not differ significantly between patients with DIOS and CLD-IO.

Distribution of HFE mutations

The distribution of *HFE* mutations are shown in Table 2. Among patients with chronic liver disease and iron overload (CLD-IO), four were heterozygous for C282Y, two homozygous and one heterozygous for H63D. The H63D mutation was significantly more frequent in patients with NAFLD as compared with the controls ($p < 0.05$).

Correlation analysis of histologic iron score and hepatic iron content determined by MRI

Simple linear regression showed a good correlation between histologic iron score and hepatic iron content determined by MRI, as demonstrated in Fig. 1 ($r^2 = 0.77$, $p < 0.01$).

Serum hepcidin and hepcidin mRNA in liver biopsies

Serum hepcidin values for the different patient groups and controls are shown in Fig. 2. Serum hepcidin levels were significantly increased in patients with NAFLD with DIOS and in those with chronic liver disease with iron overload (CLD-IO) compared with the other groups. The ratios between serum hepcidin and ferritin are shown in Fig. 3. As expected, this ratio was significantly reduced in homozygous HH compared with the other groups. Among patients with CLD-IO, this ratio was slightly lower in those with alcoholic liver disease (ALD) or hepatitis C (0.049 ± 0.034) as compared with those without alcohol overconsumption (0.058 ± 0.032), or DIOS patients (0.070 ± 0.037), although these differences were not statistically significant.

Figure 4 shows the ratios between serum hepcidin and hepatic iron score, which was similar in patients with CLD-IO and DIOS, and reduced in those with homozygous HH. The hepcidin/iron score ratio was slightly lower in those with ALD or hepatitis C (18.7 ± 8.1) as compared with those without alcohol overconsumption (22.4 ± 10.2), or DIOS (30.8 ± 23.7), however not statistically significant. There was a significant correlation between serum hepcidin levels and hepatic *HAMP* mRNA ($r^2 = 0.39$, $p < 0.01$).

Clinical, laboratory and histological findings in patients with NAFLD with or without DIOS (Table 3)

Serum hepcidin, serum transferrin saturation and hepatic iron score were all significantly higher in NAFLD with DIOS as compared with NAFLD without DIOS ($p < 0.05$). Serum levels of triglycerides or total cholesterol did not differ significantly between the groups. Levels of TNF-α and IL-6 were highest in NAFLD without DIOS and elevated serum ferritin (difference not statistically significant). *HAMP* mRNA in liver tissue correlated to the hepatic iron score ($r^2 = 0.45$, $p < 0.05$) but not to NAFLD activity score ($r^2 = 0.003$, $p < 0.89$). Serum hepcidin correlated significantly to serum ferritin ($r^2 = 0.20$, $p < 0.01$) and serum transferrin saturation ($r^2 = 0.17$, $p < 0.01$) but not to BMI, TNF-α, IL-6, triglycerides or cholesterol. In multiple linear regression analysis only ferritin correlated significantly to serum hepcidin levels when adjusted for other variables. There was no significant difference in stage of fibrosis, grade of steatosis, ballooning, lobular inflammation or NAFLD activity score between the groups (Table 3).

Discussion

In the present study, we demonstrate that in NAFLD patients, hepcidin in serum and *HAMP* mRNA in liver tissue correlate significantly to body iron stores, regardless if they are expressed as serum ferritin or liver iron content. Furthermore, there was no correlation to the degree of steatohepatitis (defined as NAFLD activity score), to lipid parameters (serum cholesterol or triglycerides), body mass index, or C-reactive protein. We found that serum hepcidin levels in NAFLD patients with dysmetabolic iron overload (DIOS) are similar to those found in other liver

Table 2 *HFE* genotypes in patients and controls

	wt/wt	C282Y/wt	C282Y/C282Y	C282Y/H63D	H63D/wt	H63D/H63D
Controls ($n = 34$)	26	4	–	–	4	–
NAFLD with normal iron stores ($n = 22$)[a]	13	1	–	–	6*	1
NAFLD with DIOS ($n = 16$)	12	2	–	–	2	–
CLD ($n = 8$)[b]	4	–	–	–	2	–
CLD-IO ($n = 21$)	14	4	–	–	1	2
Compound heterozygous HH ($n = 5$)	–	–	–	5	–	–
Homozygous HH ($n = 12$)	–	–	12	–	–	–

CLD chronic liver disease, *IO* iron overload, *HH* hereditary hemochromatosis, *NAFLD* non-alcoholic fatty liver disease, *DIOS* dysmetabolic iron overload
*$p < 0.05$ in patients with NAFLD vs. controls
[a]one missing value
[b]two missing values

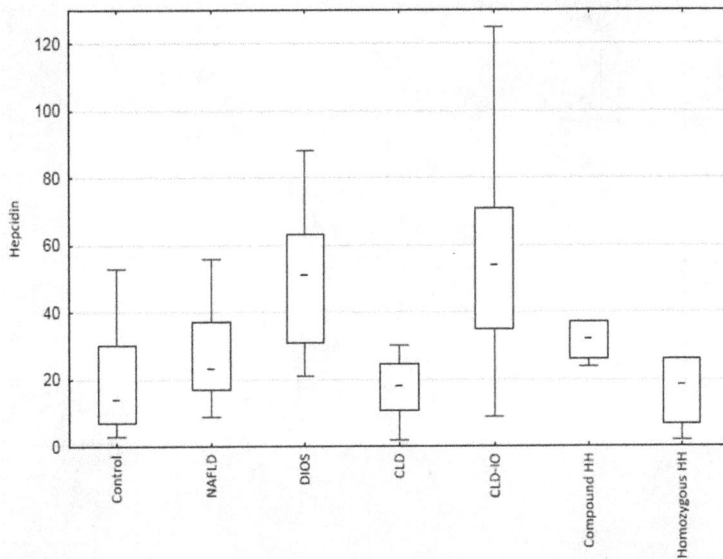

Fig. 2 Serum hepcidin levels (µg/L) in the different patient groups. The box plots show the median, the interquartile range and the min-max values. Hepcidin levels were significantly increased in chronic liver disease with iron overload (CLD-IO) and non-alcoholic fatty liver disease with dysmetabolic iron overload (NAFLD-DIOS) compared with the other groups (Kruskal-Wallis ANOVA, $p < 0.05$)

diseases with iron overload (CLD-IO), except for hereditary hemochromatosis, in which patients have an inherited hepcidin deficiency. In our patient cohort without morbid obesity, hepatic *HAMP* mRNA levels showed a good correlation to the serum hepcidin values measured by ELISA. When calculating the hepcidin levels in relation to serum ferritin (Fig. 3) or to the liver iron score (Fig. 4), patients with DIOS had overall similar ratios as patients with CLD-IO, although those with

alcoholic liver disease and hepatitis C had a trend to somewhat lower levels. Others have demonstrated that hepatic iron is the major determinant of serum ferritin levels in NAFLD, results in line with the present study [20]. Together, these findings point at an adequate hepcidin synthesis in NAFLD in relation to iron stores, and the iron accumulation in DIOS cannot be explained by hepcidin deficiency, in contrast to what is seen in hereditary hemochromatosis.

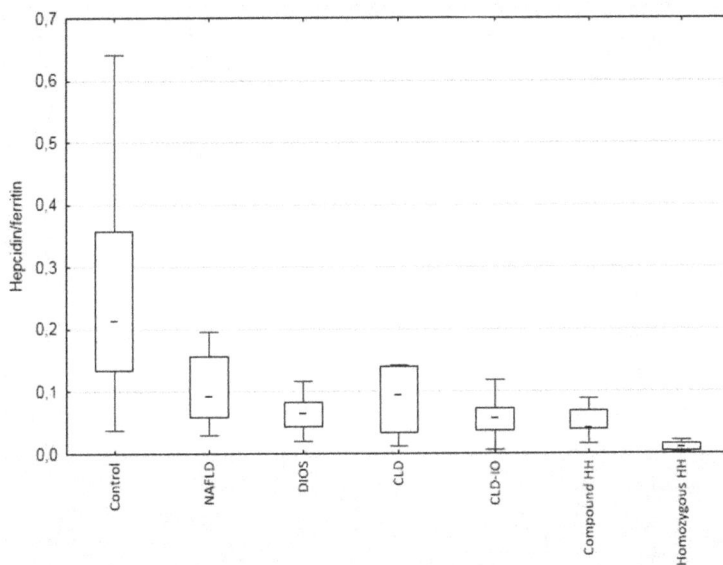

Fig. 3 The ratios between serum hepcidin (µg/L) and serum ferritin (µg/L). Patients with homozygous HH had significantly lower ratios compared with the other groups (Kruskal-Wallis ANOVA, $p < 0.05$)

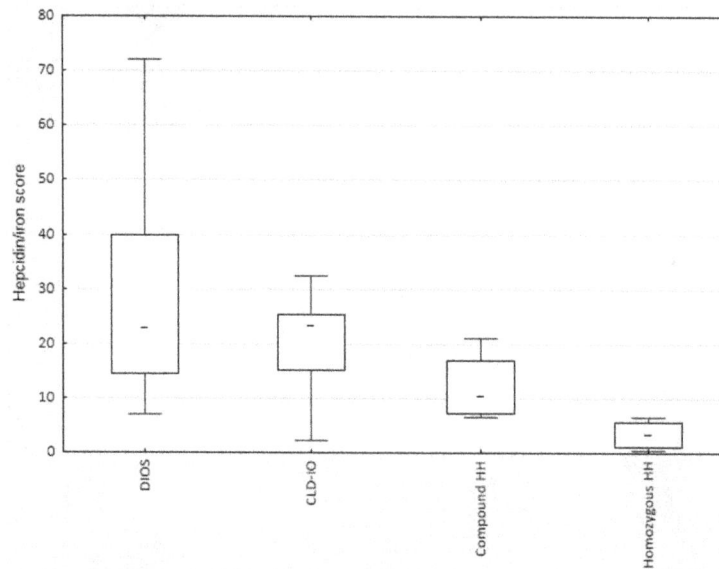

Fig. 4 The ratios between serum hepcidin (µg/L) and hepatic iron contents ("iron score"). The calculation of iron scores is described in Methods. Patients with homozygous HH had significantly lower ratios compared with the other groups (Kruskal-Wallis ANOVA, $p < 0.05$)

Some other previous studies have presented conflicting results. Barisani et al. found an inadequate hepcidin production for a given level of iron status in NAFLD patients compared to controls, although not as low as in beta-thalassemia or hereditary hemochromatosis [11]. In contrast, several other studies found hepcidin levels to correlate to iron parameters in NAFLD and DIOS [17, 21, 27, 28]. Senates et al. found an association between serum hepcidin and cholesterol and triglycerides levels, but not with iron parameters [18], which contrasts with our findings. In obesity, hepcidin can be produced by adipose tissue [13, 28], possibly through activation of hemojuvelin gene expression [29]. Thus, in morbidly obese patients undergoing bariatric surgery, hepcidin

Table 3 Clinical, laboratory and liver biopsy findings in patients with NAFLD with and without dysmetabolic iron overload syndrome (DIOS), and normal vs. elevated serum ferritin, respectively

	NAFLD without DIOS (n = 22)		NAFLD with DIOS (n = 16)
	With serum ferritin < 350 µg/L (n = 15)	With serum ferritin > 350 µg/L (n = 7)	
Serum hepcidin (µg/L)	24 ± 19	37 ± 13	53 ± 28*
Serum ferritin (µg/L)	156 ± 78*	621 ± 170	816 ± 285
Transferrin saturation (%)	28 ± 8	25 ± 10	39 ± 9#
Liver iron score	0.03 ± 0.13	0.14 ± 0.24	2.13 ± 0.92*
CRP (mg/L)	2.7 ± 2.2	3.7 ± 4.2	1.8 ± 0.91
Plasma-triglycerides (mmol/L)	2.89 ± 1.09	1.83 ± 1.09	1.95 ± 0.90
Plasma cholesterol (mmol/L)	5.18 ± 0.96	5.25 ± 0.84	5.25 ± 0.71
TNF-α (ng/L)	6.27 ± 5.13	137 ± 316	8.37 ± 5.82
IL-6 (ng/L)	2.47 ± 1.71	32.3 ± 62.7	2.36 ± 1.02
NAS	4.5 ± 1.8	3.6 ± 1.7	4.4 ± 1.8
Steatosis (grade)	2.07 ± 0.80	2.00 ± 1.00	2.72 ± 0.65
Ballooning	1.07 ± 0.59	0.80 ± 0.84	0.63 ± 0.67
Lobular inflammation	1.20 ± 0.86	1.00 ± 0.71	1.00 ± 1.00
Portal inflammation	0.27 ± 0.46	0.60 ± 0.55	0.18 ± 0.40
Fibrosis	1.33 ± 0.90	2.00 ± 1.00	2.72 ± 0.65

Values denote mean ± S.D
*=p < 0.05 (vs. the other groups)
= p < 0.05 (vs. NAFLD with serum ferritin > 350 µg/L)

levels correlate to the grade of obesity, but not to the degree of fat in the liver tissue [12, 15]. Likewise, the presence of NASH did not alter the expression of *HAMP* mRNA in adipose tissue [13]. Low-grade inflammation associated with obesity could lead to elevation of both serum ferritin and hepcidin levels. In inflammatory conditions, elevated serum hepcidin would diminish iron uptake and mobilization, possibly causing entrapment of iron in Kupffer cells [19]. However, none of our patients were morbidly obese, and the strong correlation between hepcidin in serum and *HAMP* mRNA in liver tissue in the present study indicates a negligible contribution from adipose tissue to hepcidin synthesis in our cohort.

It has been reported that hepcidin levels were depressed in patients with chronic hepatitis C [30] or alcoholic liver disease [31], suggesting that hepcidin deficiency play a role in the iron accumulation seen in these conditions. As compared to NAFLD-DIOS in our cohort, we found a somewhat lower hepcidin-to-ferritin and hepcidin-to-iron score ratios in patients with alcoholic liver disease and hepatitis C, although the present study was underpowered to detect a true difference in this regard. This finding is in line with the view that there is an adequate hepcidin synthesis in NAFLD-DIOS, why other explanations for the iron accumulation in this condition have to be sought for [16].

We did not find an increased frequency of *C282Y* or *H63D* mutations in NAFLD patients with DIOS as compared to patients with other liver diseases, or healthy controls. However, the *H63D* mutation was enriched in NAFLD patients with normal iron stores, indicating that this mutation may play a role in NAFLD pathogenesis, as suggested previously [17].

Eighteen of our 84 patients did not agree to undergo liver biopsy. In these cases, iron assessment was instead performed by magnetic resonance imaging (MRI), which is considered to be an accurate method to quantify iron overload in the range 60–375 µmol/g [32]. It is not influenced by steatosis or fibrosis and in patients with cirrhosis it may be even more accurate than biopsy [26]. In 21 cases, we performed both liver biopsy and MRI, obtaining a good correlation in cases with a hepatic iron score of 2 or more.

The strength of the present study is that hepcidin was measured both in serum and as *HAMP* mRNA in liver tissue, the correlations of which were excellent. Furthermore, iron content was assessed both with MRI and liver biopsy, and NAFLD patients were compared with other patient cohorts with various degree of iron overload, including genetic hemochromatosis who has an inherited hepcidin deficiency. The major limitation of the study is the small cohort, making it underpowered to perform sub-analyses of various patient groups, e.g. NAFLD without DIOS, alcoholic liver disease or hepatitis C. Also, the smaller size and the younger age of the control

group in the present study, relative to the patient cohort, is a limitation when comparing serum hepcidin levels in liver disease patients and healthy controls.

Future studies need to focus on hepcidin-independent mechanisms for the iron-loading seen in NAFLD with DIOS. Hitherto published data indicate that activated iron regulatory protein-1 and increased expression of duodenal divalent metal transporter-1 have been found in NASH [33]. Also, bone morphogenic protein-binding endothelial regulator [34] and hepatocyte nuclear factor-4alpha [35] have been reported to influence iron absorption, and in mice, a high fat diet by itself could increase iron absorption [36]. An impairment in the ability of hepcidin to inhibit iron absorption was demonstrated in DIOS, suggesting hepcidin resistance in this condition [37]. Nevertheless, it is unknown if the iron loading seen in up to one-third of patients with NAFLD is a consequence of the altered lipid metabolism, or an altered expression of iron-regulatory genes, or a combination of both. This topic warrants future research.

Conclusions
In conclusion, we found that in patients with non-alcoholic fatty liver disease with or without dysmetabolic iron overload, serum hepcidin correlates to iron indices such as serum ferritin, transferrin saturation and liver iron contents, but not to body mass index, NAFLD activity score, or lipid parameters. Hepcidin levels in NAFLD-DIOS are similar to those found in other liver diseases with iron overload, except for genetic hemochromatosis. These data indicate that NAFLD-DIOS is a condition with an adequate hepcidin synthesis and preserved iron-regulatory feedback.

Abbreviations
ALD: Alcoholic liver disease; CLD: Chronic liver disease; CLD-IO: Chronic liver disease with iron overload; DIOS: Dysmetabolic iron overload syndrome; HAMP: Hepcidin antimicrobial peptide; HH: Hereditary hemochromatosis; MRI: Magnetic resonance imaging; NAFLD: Non-alcoholic fatty liver disease; NASH: Non-alcoholic steatohepatitis

Acknowledgements
We are grateful to Terri Lindholm for MRI iron quantification expertise, and Pia Loqvist, Ingrid Ackzell, and Eva Berglund for blood and tissue sampling and excellent patient care.

Funding
This study was supported by grants from the Swedish Society of Medicine (Bengt Ihre's fund and Swedish Gastroenterology Fund), the Karolinska Institutet (Ruth and Richard Julins Foundation) and from the Stockholm County Council (ALF project 20150403).

Authors' contributions
Study conception and design: PS, JM. Acquisition of data: JM, PS, SB, GE, LO, NA, OD. Statistical analysis: PS. Analysis and interpretation of data: All authors.

Drafting of manuscript: JM, PS. Critical revision: All authors. Guarantor of article: PS. All authors approved the final version of the article, including the authorship list.

Competing interests

The authors declare that they have no competing interests.

Author details

[1]Unit of Liver Diseases, Department of Upper GI, C1-77 Huddinge, Karolinska University Hospital, Karolinska Institutet, 141 86 Stockholm, Sweden. [2]Unit of Gastroenterology and Hepatology, Department of Medicine, Ersta Hospital, Karolinska Institutet, Stockholm, Sweden. [3]Unit of Clinical Chemistry, Department of Laboratory Medicine, Karolinska University Hospital, Karolinska Institutet, Stockholm, Sweden. [4]Department of Radiology, Ersta Hospital, Karolinska Institutet, Stockholm, Sweden. [5]Unit of Pathology, Department of Laboratory Medicine, Karolinska University Hospital, Karolinska Institutet, Stockholm, Sweden.

References

1. Vernon G, Baranova A, Younossi ZM. Systematic review: the epidemiology and natural history of non-alcoholic fatty liver disease and non-alcoholic steatohepatitis in adults. Aliment Pharmacol Ther. 2011;34(3):274–85.
2. Marchesini G, Brizi M, Bianchi G, Tomassetti S, Bugianesi E, Lenzi M, McCullough AJ, Natale S, Forlani G, Melchionda N. Nonalcoholic fatty liver disease: a feature of the metabolic syndrome. Diabetes. 2001;50(8):1844–50.
3. Loomba R, Sanyal AJ. The global NAFLD epidemic. Nat Rev Gastroenterol Hepatol. 2013;10(11):686–90.
4. Nelson JE, Klintworth H, Kowdley KV. Iron metabolism in nonalcoholic fatty liver disease. Curr Gastroenterol Rep. 2012;14(1):8–16.
5. Datz C, Felder TK, Niederseer D, Aigner E. Iron homeostasis in the metabolic syndrome. Eur J Clin Investig. 2013;43(2):215–24.
6. Manousou P, Kalambokis G, Grillo F, Watkins J, Xirouchakis E, Pleguezuelo M, Leandro G, Arvaniti V, Germani G, Patch D, et al. Serum ferritin is a discriminant marker for both fibrosis and inflammation in histologically proven non-alcoholic fatty liver disease patients. Liver Int. 2011;31(5):730–9.
7. Kowdley KV, Belt P, Wilson LA, Yeh MM, Neuschwander-Tetri BA, Chalasani N, Sanyal AJ, Nelson JE, Network NCR. Serum ferritin is an independent predictor of histologic severity and advanced fibrosis in patients with nonalcoholic fatty liver disease. Hepatology. 2012;55(1):77–85.
8. Fracanzani AL, Valenti L, Bugianesi E, Vanni E, Grieco A, Miele L, Consonni D, Fatta E, Lombardi R, Marchesini G, et al. Risk of nonalcoholic steatohepatitis and fibrosis in patients with nonalcoholic fatty liver disease and low visceral adiposity. J Hepatol. 2011;54(6):1244–9.
9. Corradini E, Pietrangelo A. Iron and steatohepatitis. J Gastroenterol Hepatol. 2012;27(Suppl 2):42–6.
10. Siddique A, Nelson JE, Aouizerat B, Yeh MM, Kowdley KV, Network NCR. Iron deficiency in patients with nonalcoholic fatty liver disease is associated with obesity, female gender, and low serum hepcidin. Clin Gastroenterol Hepatol. 2014;12(7):1170–8.
11. Barisani D, Pelucchi S, Mariani R, Galimberti S, Trombini P, Fumagalli D, Meneveri R, Nemeth E, Ganz T, Piperno A. Hepcidin and iron-related gene expression in subjects with Dysmetabolic hepatic Iron overload. J Hepatol. 2008;49(1):123–33.
12. Vuppalanchi R, Troutt JS, Konrad RJ, Ghabril M, Saxena R, Bell LN, Kowdley KV, Chalasani N. Serum hepcidin levels are associated with obesity but not liver disease. Obesity. 2014;22(3):836–41.
13. Bekri S, Gual P, Anty R, Luciani N, Dahman M, Ramesh B, Iannelli A, Staccini-Myx A, Casanova D, Ben Amor I, et al. Increased adipose tissue expression of hepcidin in severe obesity is independent from diabetes and NASH. Gastroenterology. 2006;131(3):788–96.
14. Jiang F, Sun ZZ, Tang YT, Xu C, Jiao XY. Hepcidin expression and iron parameters change in type 2 diabetic patients. Diabetes Res Clin Pract. 2011;93(1):43–8.
15. Auguet T, Aragones G, Berlanga A, Martinez S, Sabench F, Binetti J, Aguilar C, Porras JA, Molina A, Del Castillo D, et al. Hepcidin in morbidly obese women with non-alcoholic fatty liver disease. PLoS One. 2017;12(10): e0187065.
16. Ruivard M, Laine F, Ganz T, Olbina G, Westerman M, Nemeth E, Rambeau M, Mazur A, Gerbaud L, Tournilhac V, et al. Iron absorption in dysmetabolic iron overload syndrome is decreased and correlates with increased plasma hepcidin. J Hepatol. 2009;50(6):1219–25.
17. Nelson JE, Brunt EM, Kowdley KV. Nonalcoholic steatohepatitis clinical research N: lower serum hepcidin and greater parenchymal iron in nonalcoholic fatty liver disease patients with C282Y HFE mutations. Hepatology. 2012;56(5):1730–40.
18. Senates E, Yilmaz Y, Colak Y, Ozturk O, Altunoz ME, Kurt R, Ozkara S, Aksaray S, Tuncer I, Ovunc AO. Serum levels of hepcidin in patients with biopsy-proven nonalcoholic fatty liver disease. Metab Syndr Relat Disord. 2011;9(4):287–90.
19. Aigner E, Weiss G, Datz C. Dysregulation of iron and copper homeostasis in nonalcoholic fatty liver. World J Hepatol. 2015;7(2):177–88.
20. Ryan JD, Armitage AE, Cobbold JF, Banerjee R, Borsani O, Dongiovanni P, Neubauer S, Morovat R, Wang LM, Pasricha SR, et al. Hepatic iron is the major determinant of serum ferritin in NAFLD patients. Liver Int. 2018;38(1):164–73.
21. Martinelli N, Traglia M, Campostrini N, Biino G, Corbella M, Sala C, Busti F, Masciullo C, Manna D, Previtali S, et al. Increased serum hepcidin levels in subjects with the metabolic syndrome: a population study. PLoS One. 2012; 7(10):e48250.
22. Kleiner DE, Brunt EM. Nonalcoholic fatty liver disease: pathologic patterns and biopsy evaluation in clinical research. Semin Liver Dis. 2012;32(1):3–13.
23. Dahlfors G, Stal P, Hansson EC, Barany P, Sisowath C, Onelov L, Nelson D, Eggertsen G, Marmur J, Beshara S. Validation of a competitive ELISA assay for the quantification of human serum hepcidin. Scand J Clin Lab Invest. 2015;75(8):652–8.
24. Deugnier Y, Turlin B. Pathology of hepatic iron overload. World J Gastroenterol. 2007;13(35):4755–60.
25. Nelson JE, Wilson L, Brunt EM, Yeh MM, Kleiner DE, Unalp-Arida A, Kowdley KV. Nonalcoholic steatohepatitis clinical research N: relationship between the pattern of hepatic iron deposition and histological severity in nonalcoholic fatty liver disease. Hepatology. 2011;53(2):448–57.
26. Gandon Y, Olivie D, Guyader D, Aube C, Oberti F, Sebille V, Deugnier Y. Non-invasive assessment of hepatic iron stores by MRI. Lancet. 2004; 363(9406):357–62.
27. Handa P, Vemulakonda AL, Maliken BD, Morgan-Stevenson V, Nelson JE, Dhillon BK, Hennessey KA, Gupta R, Yeh MM, Kowdley KV. Differences in hepatic expression of iron, inflammation and stress-related genes in patients with nonalcoholic steatohepatitis. Ann Hepatol. 2017;16(1):77–85.
28. Coimbra S, Catarino C, Santos-Silva A. The role of adipocytes in the modulation of iron metabolism in obesity. Obes Rev. 2013;14(10):771–9.
29. Luciani N, Brasse-Lagnel C, Poli M, Anty R, Lesueur C, Cormont M, Laquerriere A, Folope V, LeMarchand-Brustel Y, Gugenheim J, et al. Hemojuvelin: a new link between obesity and iron homeostasis. Obesity. 2011;19(8):1545–51.
30. Fujita N, Sugimoto R, Takeo M, Urawa N, Mifuji R, Tanaka H, Kobayashi Y, Iwasa M, Watanabe S, Adachi Y, et al. Hepcidin expression in the liver: relatively low level in patients with chronic hepatitis C. Mol Med. 2007;13(1–2):97–104.
31. Harrison-Findik DD, Schafer D, Klein E, Timchenko NA, Kulaksiz H, Clemens D, Fein E, Andriopoulos B, Pantopoulos K, Gollan J. Alcohol metabolism-mediated oxidative stress down-regulates hepcidin transcription and leads to increased duodenal iron transporter expression. J Biol Chem. 2006; 281(32):22974–82.
32. Olthof AW, Sijens PE, Kreeftenberg HG, Kappert P, van der Jagt EJ, Oudkerk M. Non-invasive liver iron concentration measurement by MRI: comparison of two validated protocols. Eur J Radiol. 2009;71(1):116–21.
33. Hoki T, Miyanishi K, Tanaka S, Takada K, Kawano Y, Sakurada A, Sato M, Kubo T, Sato T, Sato Y, et al. Increased duodenal iron absorption through up-regulation of divalent metal transporter 1 from enhancement of iron regulatory protein 1 activity in patients with nonalcoholic steatohepatitis. Hepatology. 2015;62(3):751–61.

34. Hasebe T, Tanaka H, Sawada K, Nakajima S, Ohtake T, Fujiya M, Kohgo Y. Bone morphogenetic protein-binding endothelial regulator of liver sinusoidal endothelial cells induces iron overload in a fatty liver mouse model. J Gastroenterol. 2017;52(3):341-351.

35. Shi W, Wang H, Zheng X, Jiang X, Xu Z, Shen H, Li M. HNF-4alpha negatively regulates Hepcidin expression through BMPR1A in HepG2 cells. Biol Trace Elem Res. 2017;176(2):294–304.

36. Dongiovanni P, Lanti C, Gatti S, Rametta R, Recalcati S, Maggioni M, Fracanzani AL, Riso P, Cairo G, Fargion S, et al. High fat diet subverts hepatocellular iron uptake determining dysmetabolic iron overload. PLoS One. 2015;10(2):e0116855.

37. Rametta R, Dongiovanni P, Pelusi S, Francione P, Iuculano F, Borroni V, Fatta E, Castagna A, Girelli D, Fargion S, et al. Hepcidin resistance in dysmetabolic iron overload. Liver Int. 2016;36(10):1540–8.

9

Taurocholic acid is an active promoting factor, not just a biomarker of progression of liver cirrhosis: evidence from a human metabolomic study and in vitro experiments

Zhimin Liu[1†], Zhifeng Zhang[1†], Mei Huang[1†], Xiaoping Sun[2], Bojia Liu[1], Qiyang Guo[1], Qingshan Chang[2] and Zhijun Duan[1*]

Abstract

Background: Previous studies have indicated that bile acid is associated with progression of liver cirrhosis. However, the particular role of specific bile acid in the development of liver cirrhosis is not definite. The present study aims to identify the specific bile acid and explore its possible mechanisms in promoting liver cirrhosis.

Methods: Thirty two cirrhotic patients and 27 healthy volunteers were enrolled. Age, gender, Child-Pugh classification and serum of patients and volunteers were collected. Liquid chromatography tandem mass spectrometry (LC-MS) was utilized to determine concentrations of 12 bile acids in serum. Principal component analysis, fold change analysis and heatmap analysis were used to identify the most changed bile acid. And pathway analysis was used to identify the most affected pathway in bile acid metabolism. Spearman rank correlation analysis was employed to assess correlation between concentrations of bile acids and Child-Pugh classification. Hepatic stellate cells (LX-2) were cultured in DMEM. LX-2 cells were also co-cultured with HepG2 cells in the transwell chambers. LX-2 cells were treated with Na+/taurocholate in different concentrations. Western blot was used to evaluate the expression of alpha smooth muscle actin (α-SMA), type I collagen, and Toll-like receptor 4 (TLR4) in LX-2 cells.

Results: Concentrations of 12 bile acids in serum of patients and healthy volunteers were determined with LC-MS successively. Principal component analysis, fold change analysis and heatmap analysis identified taurocholic acid (TCA) to be the most changed bile acid. Pathway analysis showed that TCA biosynthesis increased significantly. Spearman rank correlation analysis showed that concentration of TCA in serum of cirrhotic patients was positively associated with Child-Pugh classification. TCA increased the expression of α-SMA, type I collagen, and TLR4 in LX-2 cells. Moreover, the above effect was strengthened when LX-2 cells were co-cultured with HepG2 cells.

Conclusions: Increased TCA concentration in serum of liver cirrhotic patients is mainly due to increased bile acid biosynthesis. TCA is an active promoter of the progression of liver cirrhosis. TCA promoting liver cirrhosis is likely through activating hepatic stellate cells via upregulating TLR4 expression. TCA is a potential therapeutic target for the prevention and treatment of liver cirrhosis.

Keywords: Taurocholic acid, Liver cirrhosis, Hepatic stellate cell, Metabolomics

* Correspondence: cathydoctor@sina.com
†Zhimin Liu, Zhifeng Zhang and Mei Huang contributed equally to this work.
[1]Second department of Gastroenterology, First Affiliated Hospital of Dalian Medical University, Dalian 116011, China
Full list of author information is available at the end of the article

Background

Liver cirrhosis is the end stage liver disease resulting from continuous intra-hepatic inflammation and extracellular matrix (ECM) accumulation caused by uncontrolled chronic liver diseases. Liver cirrhosis is a global health problem. One epidemiological study conducted in US veterans showed that the prevalence of liver cirrhosis in 2013 was 1.06%, and the prevalence of liver cirrhosis had doubled from 2001 to 2013 [1]. Due to high prevalence of hepatitis B virus (HBV) infections, liver cirrhosis is also a common disease in China [2]. Moreover, liver cirrhosis can cause complications including variceal bleeding, hepatic encephalopathy and hepatorenal syndrome, which are life-threatening to cirrhotic patients. One systemic analysis estimated that global death attributed to liver cirrhosis was over 1 million [3]. Thus liver cirrhosis has rendered a great burden on health care system globally. To date, the optimal prevention and treatment of liver cirrhosis mainly depends on curing or controlling the primary diseases including hepatitis B, hepatitis C, alcoholic liver disease (ALD), primary biliary cholangitis (PBC), primary sclerosing cholangitis (PSC) and autoimmune hepatitis (AIH). Moreover, most chronic liver diseases can only be controlled but not cured. Risk factors affecting the development and progression of liver cirrhosis are multifactorial. Treatment of liver cirrhosis should be comprehensive. So identifying novel risk factors and potential therapeutic targets for prevention and treatment of liver cirrhosis is of great significance to both clinicians and drug developers.

Bile acids are synthesized in hepatocytes by cytochrome P450 (CYP) from cholesterol through classical and alternative pathways [4, 5]. In the classical pathway, cholesterol is hydroxylated by CYP7A1, CYP8B1, and CYP27A1 and converted to cholic acid (CA) and chenodeoxycholic acid (CDCA). In the alternative pathway, cholesterol is hydroxylated by CYP7A1 to produce 27-hydroxycholesterol, 27-hydroxycholesterol is then converted to CDCA through 7α-hydroxylation by CYP7B1. Bile acyl-CoA synthetase (BACS) and bile acid-CoA:amino acid Nacyltransferase (BAAT) subsequently conjugate taurine or glycine to CA or CDCA to produce taurochenodeoxycholic acid (TCDCA), glycocholic acid (GCA), taurocholic acid (TCA) and glycochenodeoxycholic acid (GCDCA). Because CA, CDCA, TCDCA, GCA, TCA and GCDCA are all synthesized in hepatocytes, these bile acids are termed primary bile acids. Primary bile acids are secreted by hepatocytes into intestinal lumen, and metabolized by enzymes of intestinal bacteria to form secondary bile acids.

Because cholestasis is very common in end stage liver cirrhosis, researchers postulated that serum bile acids might be associated with progression of liver cirrhosis. Metabolomic study can reveal difference of the profiling of bile acids between patients and healthy controls. One metabolomic study indicated that TCA, TCDCA, GCA

and glycoursodeoxycholic acid (GUDCA) were the most elevated bile acids in serum of liver cirrhotic patients, and concentrations of these bile acids were positively correlated with Child–Pugh scores [6]. Another metabolomic study showed that TCA, TCDCA, GCDCA, GCA, GUDCA and CDCA in the serum of acute decompensated cirrhotic patients were significantly higher than those in the serum of patients with compensated cirrhosis, and bile acids could serve as makers for risk stratification of cirrhotic patients to develop new onset acute decompensation [7]. However, previous metabolomic studies only evaluated diagnostic and prediction value of specific bile acid in progression of liver cirrhosis, and did not explore and verify specific bile acid to be a potential therapeutic target for liver cirrhosis. The present study aims to identify the specific bile acid and explore its possible mechanisms in promoting liver cirrhosis, and to find a potential therapeutic target for liver cirrhosis.

Methods

Clinical samples

Blood samples were collected from 32 patients with liver cirrhosis in the First Affiliated Hospital of Dalian Medical University from March 2013 to March 2015. Blood samples were also collected from 27 healthy volunteers in healthy examination center of the First Affiliated Hospital of Dalian Medical University during the same period. Before blood collection, all the patients and healthy volunteers fasted overnight. Venous blood was collected in the morning, then serum was collected through centrifugation of venous blood. All serum samples were stored at − 80 °C. Diagnosis of cirrhosis was based on a combination of clinical manifestations, laboratory tests and imaging presentations (typical cirrhotic morphological changes, splenomegaly and portal hypertension) in CT scanning or MRI scanning. Hepatocellular carcinoma, intrahepatic cholangiocarcinoma, carcinomas outside of liver, heart failure, renal diseases and metabolic diseases were excluded from our study. All the healthy volunteers were free of liver diseases, heart diseases, renal diseases and metabolic diseases as verified by laboratory tests and ultrasonography. Age, gender, clinical data, laboratory data and imaging data were retrieved from medical records.

Ethics, consent and permissions

The collections of human serum samples were approved by the Ethics Committee of First Affiliated Hospital of Dalian Medical University (No:LCKY2016–34). And written informed consent was obtained from each cirrhotic patient and healthy volunteer.

Target bile acid detection

Bile acid standards including lithocholic acid (LCA), hyodeoxycholic acid (HDCA), CDCA, deoxycholic acid

(DCA), ursodeoxycholic acid (UDCA), CA, GCA, tauro-lithocholic acid (TLCA), TCDCA, taurodeoxycholic acid (TDCA), tauroursodeoxycholic acid (TUDCA) and TCA were purchased from Sigma. Bile acid standards were diluted to different gradient concentrations. The collected serum samples stored at $-80\ ^\circ C$ were thawed at $4\ ^\circ C$. Each 50 μL serum sample mixed with 10 μL internal standard solution and 300 μL cold protein precipitation liquid (a methanol solution containing 0.1% ammonia) was centrifuged, and 200 μL supernatant was collected and dried under nitrogen. Each dried bile acid extract was dissolved with 50 μL methanol, and then was filtered. Liquid chromatography of Waters I-Class coupled to Waters Xevo TQ-S (IVD) mass spectrometer with an ESI source was used to analyze each bile acid extract and the diluted bile acid standards. Chromatographic separation was performed using ACQUITY UPLC BEH Phenyl Column (2.1 × 50 mm, 2.5 μm). The injection volume of sample was 5 μl. Quality control samples were prepared by mixing all of the dissolved bile acid extracts. During LC-MS analysis, one quality control sample was utilized to ensure data quality every 30 injections. Multiple reaction monitor (MRM) was used to collect data. Standard reference curves were depicted with diluted gradient concentrations of bile acid standards and the corresponding peak areas. The quantitative determination of 12 bile acids in human serum samples was calculated from the corresponding standard reference curves.

Cell culture

Hepatic stellate cell line LX-2 was purchased from the Cell Bank of the Xiangya Central Experiment Laboratory of Central South University (Changsha, China). Human hepatoma cell line HepG2 was purchased from American Type Culture Collection (ATCC, Manassas, VA). Cells were cultured in Dulbecco's Modified Eagle's Medium (DMEM) (Gibco) supplemented with 10% fetal bovine scrum (FBS) (Gibco) and antibiotics (100 IU/ml penicillin and 100 mg/ml streptomycin) in an incubator with humidified air containing 5% $CO2$ at $37\ ^\circ C$. Co-culture of the LX-2 and HepG2 cells in the transwell chambers was according to the method in a previous study [8].

Cell proliferation assay

LX-2 cells were plated into 96-well plates at a density of 2×10^4 cells/ml per well and incubated for 24 h, then incubated with Na+/taurocholate (Sigma) in different concentrations (50 μM, 75 μM, 100 μM and 150 μM) for another 24 h. Phosphate buffered saline (PBS) was as the control solution in cell proliferation assay. Cell proliferation was analyzed with Cell Counting Kit (Dojindo) according to the manufacturer's protocols.

Western blotting assay

LX-2 cells were treated with Na+/taurocholate (Sigma) (50 μM and100μM) dissolved in DMEM without FBS for 24 h. LX-2 cells co-cultured with HepG2 cells were also treated with Na+/taurocholate (Sigma) (50 μM and 100 μM) dissolved in DMEM without FBS for 24 h. Total cellular proteins were extracted with a protein exaction kit (Beyotime Biotechnology) according to the manufacturer's protocols. BCA Protein Assay Kit (Beyotime Biotechnology) was used for quantification of exacted proteins. After separated with SDS-PAGE, the proteins were transferred to a PVDF membrane. The PVDF membrane was blocked with 5% skim milk in Tris-buffered saline containing 0.05% Tween-20 (TTBS). The membranes were then incubated with the primary antibodies against Toll-like receptor4 (TLR4) (Santa Cruz Biotechnology), alpha Tubulin (α-Tubulin) (Proteintech), Collagen Type I (Proteintech) and smooth muscle actin (α-SMA) (Proteintech) overnight at $4\ ^\circ C$, and subsequently incubated with the secondary antibody for 2 h at $37\ ^\circ C$. Protein band was detected with the enhanced chemiluminescence (Advansta) method and imaged with a Bio-Rad ChemiDoc MP imaging system. Intensity of the α-Tubulin band was as the internal reference.

Statistical analyses

Principal component analysis (PCA), fold change analysis, partial least squares discriminant analysis (PLS-DA), heat-map analysis and pathway analysis were used to analyze bile acid metobolomic data of human serum samples. PCA, fold change analysis, PLS-DA, heatmap analysis and pathway analysis were conducted with MetaboAnalyst (http://www.metaboanalyst.ca/) according to the manual of analysis provided in the website [9]. Unpaired t test was employed to determine the difference of ages between cirrhotic patients and healthy controls. Chi-square test was utilized to determine the difference of gender between cirrhotic patients and healthy controls. Spearman correlation analysis was used to evaluate the association between concentrations of bile acids and Child-Pugh classification. Cell experimental data were presented as mean and standard deviation (SD). One-way ANOVA analysis and least significant difference (LSD) test were employed to determine the difference of means among three groups. Unpaired t test was employed to determine the difference of means between two groups. $P < 0.05$ was considered statistically significant. One-way ANOVA analysis, Chi-square test, Spearman correlation and unpaired t test were performed with the SPSS16.0 statistical software package (SPSS Inc., Chicago, IL, USA).

Results

Characteristics of liver cirrhotic patients and healthy controls

Thirty two liver cirrhotic patients and 27 healthy controls were enrolled in this study. Age and gender distributions between cirrhotic patients and healthy controls were not statistically significant. The causes of liver cirrhosis included HBV infection (13 patients), ALD (six patients), PBC (seven patients). And six patients were diagnosed with cryptogenic cirrhosis. Twelve cirrhotic patients were classified as Child-Pugh A, 17 cirrhotic patients were classified as Child-Pugh B, and three cirrhotic patients were classified as Child-Pugh C. The detailed characteristics of liver cirrhotic patients and healthy controls were presented in Table 1.

Target bile acid metabolomic analysis

Qualification and quantification of 12 bile acids in serum of liver cirrhotic patients and healthy controls were performed with LC-MS successively. Data normalization was recommended by MetaboAnalyst to reduce any systematic bias within a given data set and to improve overall data consistency so that meaningful biological comparisons can be made, and bell-shaped distribution of the appearance of characteristic graphical summary indicated the proper normalization [9]. In our study, the appearance of characteristic graphical summary of data became bell-shaped distribution after a log transformation (Fig. 1a).

PCA was used to visualize general clustering and trend of bile acids between groups. Both two dimension scores plot and three dimension scores plot showed that there was a distinguished classification between the observation clustering of liver cirrhosis group and that of healthy control group (Fig. 1b and c). PLS-DA was able to identify the most important biomarker between groups. PLS-DA also discriminated the observation clustering of liver cirrhosis group from that of healthy control group (Fig. 1d and e). PLS-DA showed that two components model was the optimal model (Fig. 1h). Importance in projection (VIP) analysis of PLS-DA indicated that TCA was the most important metabolite in component one and component two (Fig. 1f and g).

Heatmap analysis showed that TCA, TCDCA, TUDCA, GCA, UDCA, CDCA, CA, TLCA, TDCA, HDCA and

LCA were increased in liver cirrhotic patients as compared with healthy controls (Fig. 2a). Fold change analysis indicated that TCA was the most changed bile acid in liver cirrhotic patients, and DCA was the least changed bile acid in liver cirrhotic patients, as illustrated in Table 2. Unpaired t test showed that all the 12 bile acids in the liver cirrhosis group were significantly changed as compared with those in the control group, as illustrated in Table 3.

Pathway analysis was also used to identify the significantly changed metabolic pathway in bile acid metabolization according to the KEGG pathway database. Impact value more than 0.1 and hits value more 3 were used as the threshold to identify the significantly changed metabolic pathway [10]. Pathway analysis showed that primary bile acid synthesis was increased in liver cirrhosis (Fig. 2b and Table 4). Moreover, TCA was the most important metabolite in the increased primary bile acid synthesis in liver cirrhosis (Fig. 2c).

Spearman correlation analysis between child-Pugh classification and concentrations of twelve bile acids

Spearman correlation analysis showed that concentrations of TCA, GCA and TCDCA were significantly positively correlated with Child-Pugh classification ($P < 0.0001$) (Fig. 2d). Spearman correlation analysis indicated that concentrations of LCA, HDCA, CDCA, UDCA, CA, TLCA, TDCA and TUDCA were not correlated with Child-Pugh classification ($P > 0.05$) (Fig. 2d).

Effects of TCA on proliferation of hepatic stellate cell

In order to evaluate the effect of TCA on liver cirrhosis, we evaluated the effect of TCA on proliferation of LX-2 cells. Proliferation assay showed that TCA (50 μM, 75 μM, 100 μM and 150 μM) increased proliferation of LX-2 cells significantly (Fig. 3a). Moreover, the effect of TCA on proliferation of LX-2 was dose-dependent (Fig. 3a).

Effects of TCA on expression of collagen type I, α-SMA and TLR4

Collagen Type I expression and α-SMA expression were indicators of the activation level of stellate cells [11]. According to the concentrations of TCA in proliferation assay of LX-2 cells, we selected 50 μM and 100 μM TCA to treat LX-2 cells. Western blot showed that expression of Collagen Type I and α-SMA was increased by TCA treatment as compared with the control (Fig. 3b and Fig. 3c). Moreover, effect of TCA on the expression of Collagen Type I and α-SMA was also dose-dependent (Fig. 3b and c).

Accumulating evidences showed that TLR4 promoted hepatic stellate cell activation by down-regulating the TGF-β pseudoreceptor BAMBI in order to render hepatic stellate cell sensitive to TGF-β signaling [12, 13]. So we

Table 1 Characteristics of liver cirrhotic patients and healthy controls

	Liver cirrhosis	Healthy control	P
Male/Female	18/14	9/18	0.134
Age(years)	59.00 ± 12.92	51.78 ± 18.99	0.089
Child Pugh class A	12	–	–
Child Pugh class B	17	–	–
Child Pugh class C	3	–	–
Hepatitis B virus infection	13	–	–
Alcoholic liver disease	6	–	–
Primary biliary cholangitis	7	–	–
Cryptogenic cirrhosis	6	–	–

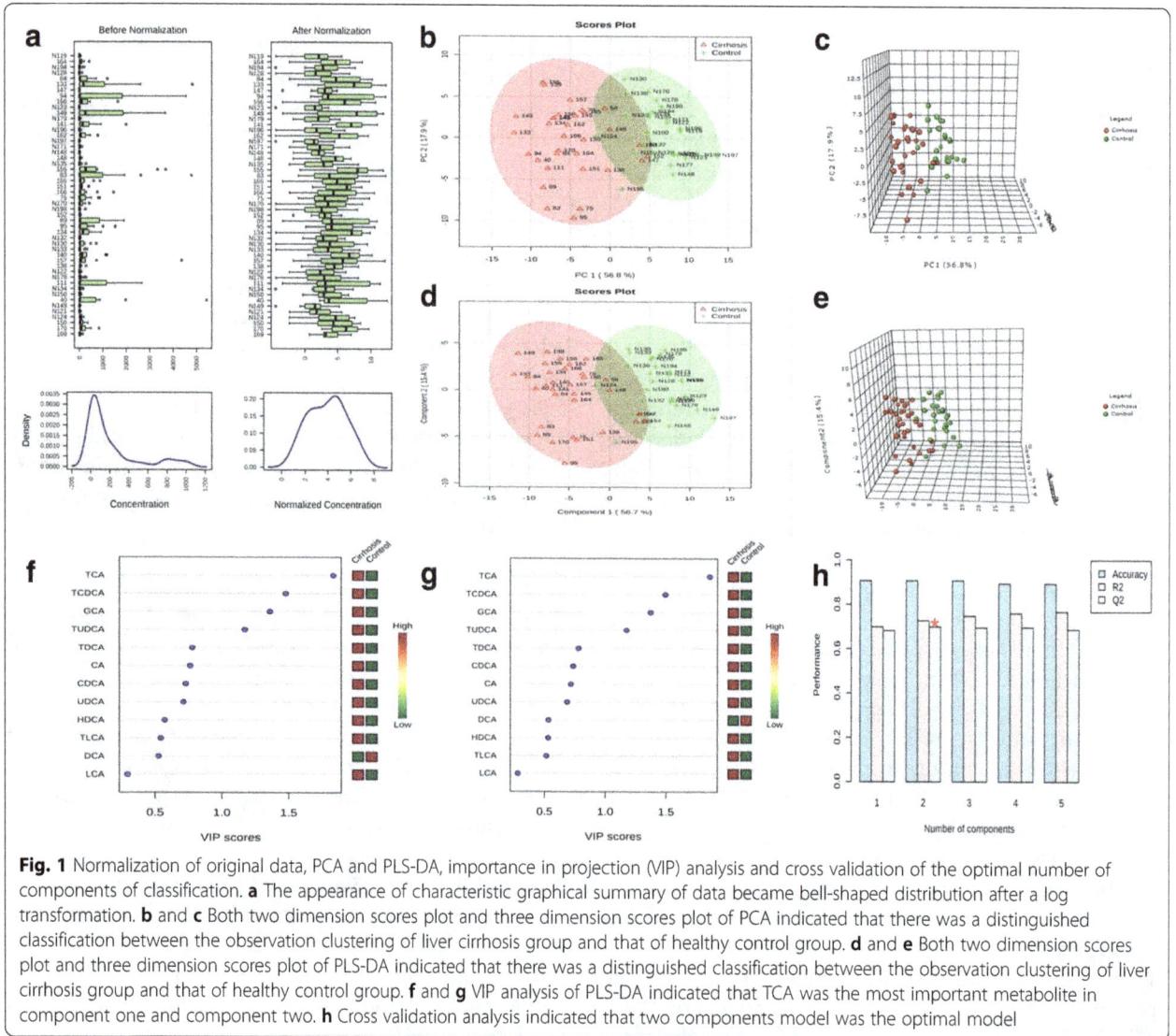

Fig. 1 Normalization of original data, PCA and PLS-DA, importance in projection (VIP) analysis and cross validation of the optimal number of components of classification. **a** The appearance of characteristic graphical summary of data became bell-shaped distribution after a log transformation. **b** and **c** Both two dimension scores plot and three dimension scores plot of PCA indicated that there was a distinguished classification between the observation clustering of liver cirrhosis group and that of healthy control group. **d** and **e** Both two dimension scores plot and three dimension scores plot of PLS-DA indicated that there was a distinguished classification between the observation clustering of liver cirrhosis group and that of healthy control group. **f** and **g** VIP analysis of PLS-DA indicated that TCA was the most important metabolite in component one and component two. **h** Cross validation analysis indicated that two components model was the optimal model

evaluated the effect of TCA on expression of TLR4 of LX-2 cells. Western blot showed that expression of TLR4 was increased by TCA treatment as compared with the control, and the effect was dose-dependent (Fig. 3d and e).

In order to mimic the interaction between hepatocytes and hepatic stellate cells in liver. We co-cultured LX-2 cells with HepG2 cells. Western blot showed that the effect of TCA on Collagen Type I and TLR4 expressions in co-culture group was more significant than that in mono-culture group (Fig. 3d and e).

Discussion

Cholestasis especially intra-hepatic cholestasis is very common in various liver diseases [14]. The mechanism of cholestasis including inflammatory damaging of biliary canaliculi and downregulation of critical bile acid transporters of hepatocytes [14–16]. As liver cirrhosis is the end stage of chronic liver diseases, cholestasis is also a

prominent manifestation of liver cirrhosis. Moreover, regenerative nodules surrounded by fibrous septa in liver cirrhosis can compress intrahepatic biliary trees to further aggravate cholestasis. Bile acid is an important component of bile and cholestasis can cause serum bile acid elevation [14]. So researchers postulate that bile acid might be associated with progression of liver cirrhosis, and have diagnostic value in classification of stages of liver cirrhosis.

A study conducted in 1986 showed that total serum-conjugated primary bile acids were more sensitive than conventional liver function test in evaluating prognosis of liver cirrhosis [17]. However, this study did not evaluate specific bile acid in diagnosis and prognosis of liver cirrhosis because of technology limitations. Recently, bile acid profiling method was used to study bile acid. One urinary metabolomic study showed that glycocholate 3-glucuronide, taurohyocholate, TCA, glycolithocholate 3-sulfate, and GUDCA were markedly elevated in hepatitis

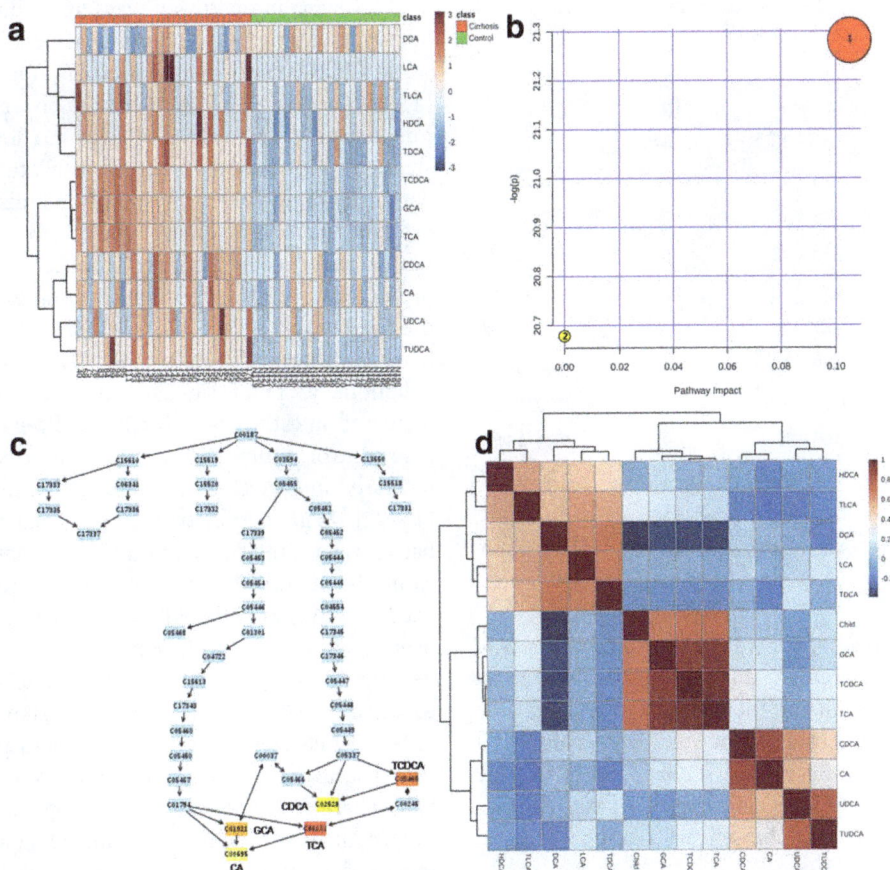

Fig. 2 Heatmap analysis, summary of pathway effect, compound impact on pathway and Spearman correlation. **a** Heatmap analysis indicated that TCA, TCDCA, TUDCA, GCA, UDCA, CDCA, CA, TLCA, TDCA, HDCA and LCA were increased in liver cirrhosis as compared with healthy controls. **b** Pathway analysis showed that primary bile acid biosynthesis was increased in liver cirrhosis. 1: bile acid biosynthesis. 2: taurine and hypotaurine metabolism. **c** Compound impact analysis implied that TCA impacted most in the increased primary bile acid biosynthesis in liver cirrhosis. **d** Spearman correlation analysis indicated that concentrations of TCA, GCA and TCDCA were significantly positively correlated with Child-Pugh classification (P < 0.0001). And concentrations of LCA, HDCA, CDCA, UDCA, CA, TLCA, TDCA and TUDCA were not correlated with Child-Pugh classification (P > 0.05)

B-induced liver cirrhosis compared with healthy controls [18]. Another metabolomic study revealed that TCA, TCDCA, GCA and GUDCA were the most elevated bile acids in serum of liver cirrhotic patients, and concentrations of these bile acids were positively correlated with Child–Pugh scores [6]. A recent metabolomic study further showed that TCA, TCDCA, GCDCA, GCA, GUDCA and CDCA in the serum of acute decompensated cirrhosis patients were significantly higher than those in the serum of patients with compensated cirrhosis, and bile acids could serve as maker for risk stratification of cirrhotic patients to develop new onset acute decompensation [7].

Our study indicated that TCA, TCDCA, TUDCA and GCA were the four most changed bile acids in liver cirrhosis, and TCA, TCDCA and GCA were positively correlated with Child-Pugh classification. Correspondingly, CA and DCA were the least changed bile acids, and were not correlated with Child-Pugh classification. The results of our study confirm the findings of previous studies. Moreover, when we observe results of the previous study and the present study, we find that TCA is the most changed bile acid in liver cirrhosis. Furthermore, previous studies did not conduct pathway analysis of bile acids. So we conducted a metabolomic pathway analysis of bile acid

Table 2 Fold change of bile acid in liver cirrhosis

	TCA	TCDCA	TUDCA	GCA	UDCA	CDCA	CA	TLCA	TDCA	HDCA	LCA	DCA
Fold Change(FC)	76.343	47.358	32.897	27.335	12.131	6.1778	5.714	4.9992	4.7731	3.4723	2.3062	1.1365
log2(FC)	6.2544	5.5655	5.0399	4.7727	3.6006	2.6271	2.5145	2.3217	2.2549	1.7959	1.2055	0.18464

Table 3 Comparison of concentration of twelve bile acids between liver cirrhosis and healthy control

	t	P	-log10(P)	FDR
TCA	10.11	2.51×10^{-14}	13.6	2.16×10^{-13}
TCDCA	10.013	3.59×10^{-14}	13.445	2.16×10^{-13}
GCA	9.7355	9.95×10^{-14}	13.002	3.98×10^{-13}
TUDCA	8.6658	5.45×10^{-12}	11.264	1.63×10^{-11}
TDCA	7.2181	1.38×10^{-9}	8.8608	3.31×10^{-09}
HDCA	4.69	1.75×10^{-5}	4.757	3.50×10^{-05}
LCA	4.2705	7.47×10^{-5}	4.1266	0.00012808
UDCA	3.4311	0.001125	2.9489	0.0016874
CDCA	3.2898	0.0017223	2.7639	0.0022964
TLCA	3.2346	0.0020289	2.6927	0.0024346
CA	3.0365	0.0036053	2.4431	0.003933
DCA	−2.3474	0.022403	1.6497	0.022403

FDR value is the false discovery rate adjusted P value

in our study, the results showed that primary bile acid biosynthesis was increased and TCA was the most important metabolite in the increased primary bile acid synthesis in liver cirrhosis. As one study revealed that fecal bile acids were decreased in liver cirrhosis, the attenuated feedback of bile acid enterohepatic circulation on primary bile acid biosynthesis might account for this phenomenon [19].

Although TCA is elevated in serum of liver cirrhotic patients, whether elevated TCA in liver cirrhosis is a promoting factor in progression of liver cirrhosis needs to be elucidated. So we conducted cell experiments to study the effect of TCA on hepatic stellate cell. Cell experiment showed that TCA increased proliferation of LX-2 cells and upregulated the expression of α-SMA and type I collagen of LX-2 cells, which implied that TCA was able to activate hepatic stellate cell to promote progression of liver cirrhosis. Moreover, the effect of TCA on hepatic stellate cell is dose-dependent, which accounts for the findings in the human metabolomic study that concentration of TCA is positively correlated with stages of liver cirrhosis. Moreover, the above effect of TCA on LX-2 cells was strengthened when LX-2 cells was co-cultured with HepG2 cells. These results support TCA as a promoting factor in liver cirrhosis, not just a manifestation of liver cirrhosis.

TLR4 signaling pathway plays an important role in the development of liver cirrhosis. Molecular epidemiology studies have revealed that polymorphisms of TLR4 gene (T399I and D299G) can affect the susceptibility of HCV infected patients to develop liver cirrhosis [20, 21]. Cell study also proves that hepatic stellate cell transfected with T399I and D299G mutations displays decreased cytokine and chemokine release and BAMBI downregulation in response to lipopolysaccharides (LPS) [22]. TLR4 promotes hepatic stellate cell activation by down-regulating the TGF-β pseudoreceptor BAMBI in order to render hepatic stellate cell sensitive to TGF-β signaling [12, 13]. Additionally, TLR4 signaling pathway orchestrates with increased intestinal permeability in liver cirrhosis. Various case control studies indicates that intestinal permeability is increased in liver cirrhosis compared with healthy controls [23–27]. With dysfunction of intestinal barrier, intestinal bacteria and LPS entering liver via portal vein system would be increased. LPS then activates hepatic stellate cell via TLR4. Activated hepatic stellate cell produces ECM in liver to remodel hepatic lobuli [28]. Moreover, activated hepatic stellate cells are recruited around sinusoidal vessels to increase intrahepatic vascular resistance to blood flow [29–31]. Activated hepatic stellate cell displaying decreased response to vasodilators also increases vascular resistance [32]. Therefore, TLR4 signaling in hepatic stellate cell plays important roles in both liver remodeling and portal hypertension development.

We evaluated the effect of TCA on expression of TLR4 of LX-2 cells. We found that TCA increased the expression of TLR4 of LX-2 cells and the effect was dose-dependent. Furthermore, in order to mimic the environment of hepatocyte and hepatic stellate cell interaction, LX-2 cells were co-cultured with HepG2 cells and the results showed that co-culture increased the effect of TCA on the expressions of TLR4 of LX-2 cells. Thus, TCA activates hepatic stellate cell via upregulating TLR4 signaling.

However, when evaluating the findings of our study we should be cautious. Our study has some limitations. First, we did not estimate the sample size in our metabolomic study, so the possibility of lack of power to come to a definite conclusion could not be ruled out. So future studies with large sample size are needed to validate the findings of our study. Second, our in vitro study only evaluated the effect of TCA on expression of TLR4 of

Table 4 Pathway analysis of twelve bile acids in liver cirrhosis compared with healthy volunteers

Pathway name	Hit	P	-log(P)	FDR	Impact
Primary bile acid biosynthesis	5	$5.72 \times 10-10$	21.281	$1.05 \times 10-9$	0.10527
Taurine and hypotaurine metabolism	1	$1.05 \times 10-9$	20.677	$1.05 \times 10-9$	0

Hit means the matched number of bile acid in metabolization pathway; The P value is calculated from the enrichment analysis; Impact value is calculate from pathway topography analysis; FDR value is the false discovery rate adjusted P value

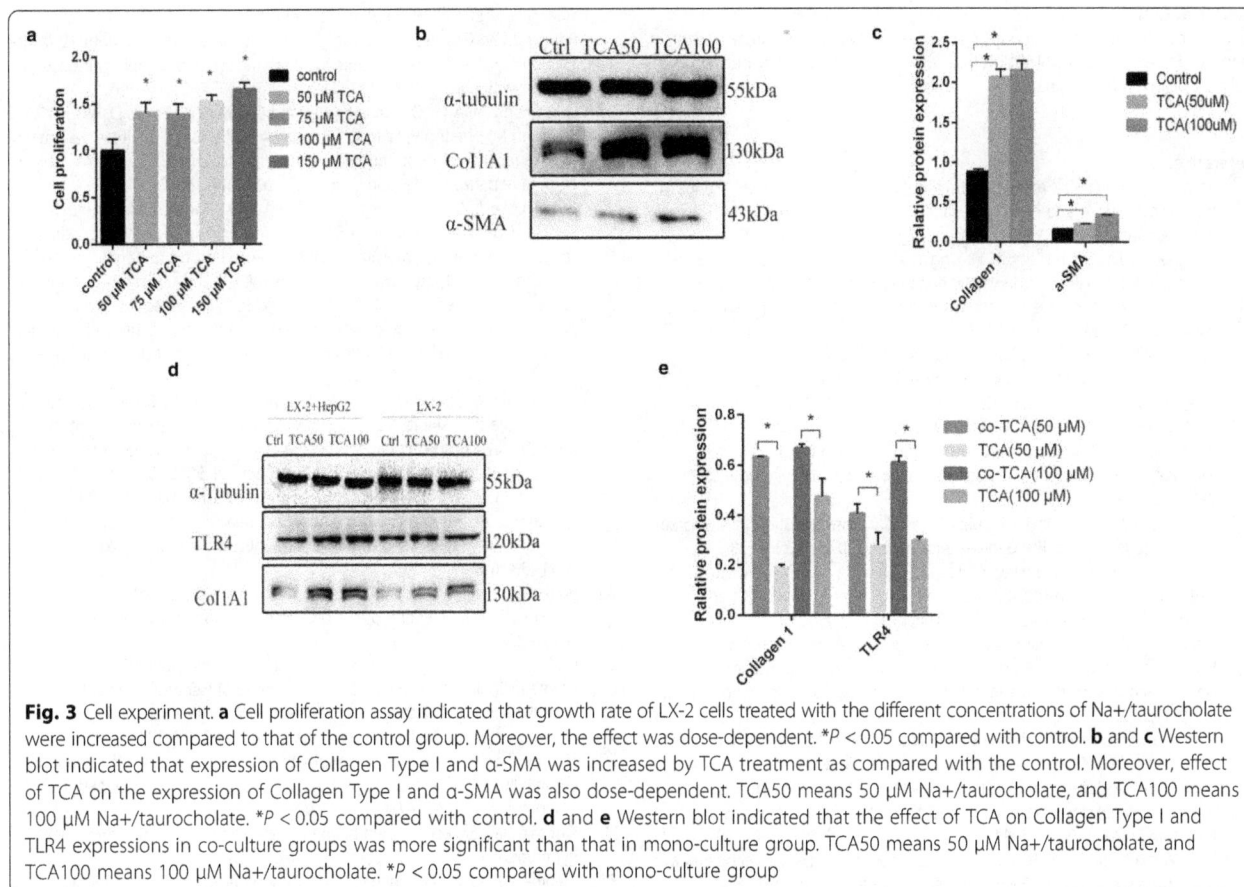

Fig. 3 Cell experiment. **a** Cell proliferation assay indicated that growth rate of LX-2 cells treated with the different concentrations of Na+/taurocholate were increased compared to that of the control group. Moreover, the effect was dose-dependent. *$P < 0.05$ compared with control. **b** and **c** Western blot indicated that expression of Collagen Type I and α-SMA was increased by TCA treatment as compared with the control. Moreover, effect of TCA on the expression of Collagen Type I and α-SMA was also dose-dependent. TCA50 means 50 μM Na+/taurocholate, and TCA100 means 100 μM Na+/taurocholate. *$P < 0.05$ compared with control. **d** and **e** Western blot indicated that the effect of TCA on Collagen Type I and TLR4 expressions in co-culture groups was more significant than that in mono-culture group. TCA50 means 50 μM Na+/taurocholate, and TCA100 means 100 μM Na+/taurocholate. *$P < 0.05$ compared with mono-culture group

LX-2 cells. Future studies can evaluate the detailed mechanism of TCA activating hepatic stellate cell via TLR4 signaling with transgenic animal studies.

Conclusion

The present study provides evidence of TCA as an active promoter in liver cirrhosis. Increased TCA concentration in cirrhosis is mainly due to increased bile acid biosynthesis. TCA is an active promoter of the progression of liver cirrhosis not just a bystander. The mechanisms of TCA promoting liver cirrhosis are likely through activating hepatic stellate cell via TLR4 pathways. TCA is a potential therapeutic target for the prevention and treatment of liver cirrhosis.

Abbreviations
AIH: Autoimmune hepatitis; ALD: Alcoholic liver disease; BAAT: Bile acid-CoA; BACS: Bile acyl-CoA synthetase; CA: Cholic acid; CDCA: Chenodeoxycholic acid; CYP: Cytochrome P450; DCA: Deoxycholic acid; DMEM: Dulbecco's Modified Eagle's Medium; ECM: Extracellular matrix; FBS: Fetal bovine serum; GCA: Glycocholic acid; GCDCA: Glycochenodeoxycholic acid; HBV: Hepatitis B virus; HDCA: Hyodeoxycholic acid; HSC: Hepatic stellate cell; LCA: Lithocholic acid; LSD: Least significant difference; MRM: Multiple reaction monitor; PBC: Primary biliary cholangitis; PBS: Phosphate buffered saline; PCA: Principal component analysis; PLS-DA: Partial least squares discriminant analysis; PSC: Primary sclerosing cholangitis; SD: Standard deviation; TCA: Taurocholic acid; TCDCA: Taurochenodeoxycholic acid; TDCA: Taurodeoxycholic acid;

TLCA: Taurolithocholic acid; TLR4: Toll-like receptor4; TTBS : Tris-buffered saline containing 0.05% Tween-20; TUDCA: Tauroursodeoxycholic acid; UDCA: Ursodeoxycholic acid; VIP : Importance in projection; α-SMA: Alpha smooth muscle actin

Funding
The present study was supported by the grants from the National Natural Science Foundation of China (No. 81670479) and Liaoning Provincial Research Program (No. 2016010223–301) .

Authors' contributions
Conceived and designed the experiments: ZJD. Performed the experiments: ZML and MH. Analyzed the data: ZML, ZFZ, MH, XPS, BJL, QYG and QSC. Wrote the paper: ZML, ZFZ and MH. All authors read and approved the final manuscript.

Consent for publication
Not applicable.

Competing interests
The authors declare that they have no competing interests.

Author details
[1]Second department of Gastroenterology, First Affiliated Hospital of Dalian Medical University, Dalian 116011, China. [2]The Sixth People's Hospital of Dalian, Dalian 116021, China.

References

1. Beste LA, Leipertz SL, Green PK, Dominitz JA, Ross D, Ioannou GN. Trends in burden of cirrhosis and hepatocellular carcinoma by underlying liver disease in US veterans, 2001-2013. Gastroenterology. 2015;149(6):1471–82.
2. Yonghao G, Jin X, Jun L, Pumei D, Ying Y, Xiuhong F, Yanyang Z, Wanshen G. An epidemiological serosurvey of hepatitis B virus shows evidence of declining prevalence due to hepatitis B vaccination in Central China. Int J Infect Dis. 2015;40:75–80.
3. Mokdad AA, Lopez AD, Shahraz S, Lozano R, Mokdad AH, Stanaway J, Murray CJ, Naghavi M. Liver cirrhosis mortality in 187 countries between 1980 and 2010: a systematic analysis. BMC Med. 2014;12:145.
4. Axelson M, Ellis E, Mörk B, Garmark K, Abrahamsson A, Björkhem I, Ericzon BG, Einarsson C. Bile acid synthesis in cultured human hepatocytes: support for an alternative biosynthetic pathway to cholic acid. Hepatology. 2000; 31(6):1305–12.
5. Jia W, Xie G, Jia W. Bile acid-microbiota crosstalk in gastrointestinal inflammation and carcinogenesis. Nat Rev Gastroenterol Hepatol. 2018;15(2):111–28.
6. Wang X, Xie G, Zhao A, Zheng X, Huang F, Wang Y, Yao C, Jia W, Liu P. Serum bile acids are associated with pathological progression of hepatitis B-induced cirrhosis. J Proteome Res. 2016;15(4):1126–34.
7. Horvatits T, Drolz A, Roedl K, Rutter K, Ferlitsch A, Fauler G, Trauner M, Fuhrmann V. Serum bile acids as marker for acute decompensation and acute-on-chronic liver failure in patients with non-cholestatic cirrhosis. Liver Int. 2017;37(2):224–31.
8. Ramm GA, Shepherd RW, Hoskins AC, Greco SA, Ney AD, Pereira TN, Bridle KR, Doecke JD, Meikle PJ, Turlin B, Lewindon PJ. Fibrogenesis in pediatric cholestatic liver disease: role of taurocholate and hepatocyte-derived monocyte chemotaxis protein-1 in hepatic stellate cell recruitment. Hepatology. 2009;49(2):533–44.
9. Xia J, Wishart DS. Using MetaboAnalyst 3.0 for comprehensive metabolomics data analysis. Curr Protoc Bioinformatics. 2016;55:14.10.1–14.10.91.
10. Chen Z, Zhu Y, Zhao Y, Ma X, Niu M, Wang J, Su H, Wang R, Li J, Liu L, Wei Z, Zhao Q, Chen H, Xiao X. Serum Metabolomic profiling in a rat model reveals protective function of Paeoniflorin against ANIT induced cholestasis. Phytother Res. 2016;30(4):654–62.
11. Maiers JL, Kostallari E, Mushref M, de Assuncao TM, Li H, Jalan-Sakrikar N, Huebert RC, Cao S, Malhi H, Shah VH. The unfolded protein response mediates fibrogenesis and collagen I secretion through regulating TANGO1 in mice. Hepatology. 2017;65(3):983–98.
12. Seki E, De Minicis S, Osterreicher CH, Kluwe J, Osawa Y, Brenner DA, Schwabe RF. TLR4 enhances TGF-beta signaling and hepatic fibrosis. Nat Med. 2007;13(11):1324–32.
13. Mencin A, Kluwe J, Schwabe RF. Toll-like receptors as targets in chronic liver diseases. Gut. 2009;58:704–20.
14. Jüngst C, Berg T, Cheng J, Green RM, Jia J, Mason AL, Lammert F. Intrahepatic cholestasis in common chronic liver diseases. Eur J Clin Investig. 2013;43(10):1069–83.
15. Zollner G, Fickert P, Zenz R, Fuchsbichler A, Stumptner C, Kenner L, Ferenci P, Stauber RE, Krejs GJ, Denk H, Zatloukal K, Trauner M. Hepatobiliary transporter expression in percutaneous liver biopsies of patients with cholestatic liver diseases. Hepatology. 2001;33:633–46.
16. Carey EJ, Ali AH, Lindor KD. Primary biliary cirrhosis. Lancet. 2015;386(10003): 1565–75.
17. Mannes GA, Thieme C, Stellaard F, Wang T, Sauerbruch T, Paumgartner G. Prognostic significance of serum bile acids in cirrhosis. Hepatology. 1986; 6(1):50–3.
18. Wang X, Wang X, Xie G, Zhou M, Yu H, Lin Y, Du G, Luo G, Jia W, Liu P. Urinary metabolite variation is associated with pathological progression of the post-hepatitis B cirrhosis patients. J Proteome Res. 2012;11(7):3838–47.
19. Kakiyama G, Muto A, Takei H, Nittono H, Murai T, Kurosawa T, Hofmann AF, Pandak WM, Bajaj JS. A simple and accurate HPLC method for fecal bile acid profile in healthy and cirrhotic subjects: validation by GC-MS and LC-MS. J Lipid Res. 2014;55(5):978–90.
20. Huang H, Shiffman ML, Friedman S, Venkatesh R, Bzowej N, Abar OT, Rowland CM, Catanese JJ, Leong DU, Sninsky JJ, Layden TJ, Wright TL, White T, Cheung RC. A 7 gene signature identifies the risk of developing cirrhosis in patients with chronic hepatitis C. Hepatology. 2007;46(2):297–306.
21. Li Y, Chang M, Abar O, Garcia V, Rowland C, Catanese J, Ross D, Broder S, Shiffman M, Cheung R, Wright T, Friedman SL, Sninsky J. Multiple variants in toll-like receptor 4 gene modulate risk of liver fibrosis in Caucasians with chronic hepatitis C infection. J Hepatol. 2009;51(4):750–7.
22. Guo J, Loke J, Zheng F, Hong F, Yea S, Fukata M, Tarocchi M, Abar OT, Huang H, Sninsky JJ, Friedman SL. Functional linkage of cirrhosis-predictive single nucleotide polymorphisms of toll-like receptor 4 to hepatic stellate cell responses. Hepatology. 2009;49(3):960–8.
23. Parlesak A, Schäfer C, Schütz T, Bode JC, Bode C. Increased intestinal permeability to macromolecules and endotoxemia in patients with chronic alcohol abuse in different stages of alcohol-induced liver disease. J Hepatol. 2000;32(5):742–7.
24. Scarpellini E, Valenza V, Gabrielli M, Lauritano EC, Perotti G, Merra G, Dal Lago A, Ojetti V, Ainora ME, Santoro M, Ghirlanda G, Gasbarrini A. Intestinal permeability in cirrhotic patients with and without spontaneous bacterial peritonitis: is the ring closed? Am J Gastroenterol. 2010;105(2):323–7.
25. Zuckerman MJ, Menzies IS, Ho H, Gregory GG, Casner NA, Crane RS, Hernandez JA. Assessment of intestinal permeability and absorption in cirrhotic patients with ascites using combined sugar probes. Dig Dis Sci. 2004;49(4):621–6.
26. Benjamin J, Singla V, Arora I, Sood S, Joshi YK. Intestinal permeability and complications in liver cirrhosis: a prospective cohort study. Hepatol Res. 2013;43(2):200–7.
27. Ersöz G, Aydin A, Erdem S, Yüksel D, Akarca U, Kumanlioglu K. Intestinal permeability in liver cirrhosis. Eur J Gastroenterol Hepatol. 1999;11(4):409–12.
28. Iwaisako K, Jiang C, Zhang M, et al. Origin of myofibroblasts in the fibrotic liver in mice. Proc Natl Acad Sci U S A. 2014;111:E3297–305.
29. Thabut D, Shah V. Intrahepatic angiogenesis and sinusoidal remodeling in chronic liver disease: new targets for the treatment of portal hypertension? J Hepatol. 2010;53:976–80.
30. Kim MY, Baik SK, Lee SS. Hemodynamic alterations in cirrhosis and portal hypertension. Korean J Hepatol. 2010;16:347–52.
31. Medina J, Arroyo AG, Sanchez-Madrid F, Moreno-Otero R. Angiogenesis in chronic inflammatory liver disease. Hepatology. 2004;39:1185–95.
32. Perri RE, Langer DA, Chatterjee S, Gibbons SJ, Gadgil J, Cao S, Farrugia G, Shah VH. Defects in cGMP-PKG pathway contribute to impaired NO-dependent responses in hepatic stellate cells upon activation. Am J Physiol Gastrointest Liver Physiol. 2006;290:G535–42.

10

Gall bladder wall thickening as non-invasive screening parameter for esophageal varices – a comparative endoscopic – sonographic study

Birgit Tsaknakis, Rawan Masri, Ahmad Amanzada, Golo Petzold, Volker Ellenrieder, Albrecht Neesse[*] and Steffen Kunsch

Abstract

Background: The mortality due to hemorrhage of esophageal varices (EV) is still high. The predominant cause for EV is liver cirrhosis, which has a high prevalence in Western Europe. Therefore, non-invasive screening markers for the presence of EV are of interest. Here, we aim to investigate whether non-inflammatory gall bladder wall thickening (GBWT) may serve as predictor for the presence of EV in comparison and combination with other non-invasive clinical and laboratory parameters.

Methods: One hundred ninety four patients were retrospectively enrolled in the study. Abdominal ultrasound, upper endoscopy and blood tests were evaluated. GBWT, spleen size and the presence of ascites were evaluated by ultrasound. Platelet count and Child-Pugh-score were also recorded. The study population was categorized in two groups: 122 patients without esophageal varices (non EV) compared to 72 patients with EV were analyzed by uni-and multivariate analysis.

Results: In the EV group 46% showed a non-inflammatory GBWT of ≥4 mm, compared to 12% in the non-EV group ($p < 0.01$). GBWT was significantly higher in EV patients compared to the non-EV group (mean: 4.4 mm vs. 2.8 mm, $p < 0.0001$), and multivariate analysis confirmed GBWT as independent predictor for EV ($p < 0.04$). The platelets/GBWT ratio (cut-off > 46.2) had a sensitivity and specificity of 78 and 86%, PPV 76% and NPV of 87%, and ROC analysis calculated the AUC of 0.864 (CI 0.809–0.919).

Conclusions: GBWT occurs significantly more often in patients with EV. However, because of the low sensitivity, combination with other non-invasive parameters such as platelet count is recommended.

Keywords: Esophageal varices, Gall bladder wall, Cirrhosis, Liver disease, Portal hypertension, Non-invasive parameter, Ultrasound parameter, Child-Pugh-score

Background

The prevalence of liver cirrhosis is estimated to be between 0.15 and 0.3% in European countries [1]. The main causes are alcohol abuse, infection with viral hepatitis B and C as well as autoimmune liver diseases [2]. A clinically relevant complication is the development of portal hypertension with all its clinical consequences such as ascites, spontaneous bacterial peritonitis and development of portosystemic collaterals. A progression rate of 12% has been reported for esophageal varices (EV) [3]. Although the mortality of variceal hemorrhage has declined in the last decades, it is still very high with a six-week-mortality of up to 37% [4], and a high recurrence rate after the first bleeding incident [5]. Although repeated endoscopic controls of patients with an advanced liver fibrosis or liver cirrhosis are justified, it is an invasive diagnostic procedure with its own risks, and it is not always widely available in countries with lower

* Correspondence: albrecht.neesse@med.uni-goettingen.de
Department Gastroenterology and Gastrointestinal Oncology, University Medical Centre Goettingen Georg-August-University, Robert-Koch-Str. 40, 37075 Goettingen, Germany

health care standards. Therefore, non-invasive predictors for portosystemic collaterals are of high interest. Notably, the venous blood is drained from the gall bladder in part via small vessels directly into the liver. An additional venous blood drain flows via small veins towards the cystic duct and then with vessels from the common bile duct terminating in the portal venous system [6].Therefore, the gall bladder should be directly affected by portal hypertension causing a thickened gall bladder wall due to impaired venous drainage. Here, we aim to determine whether non-inflammatory gall bladder wall thickness (GBWT) correlates with the presence of EV. To this end, we performed a retrospective endoscopic-ultrasonographic study correlating the presence of EV and GBWT with other non-invasive parameters for liver disease and portal hypertension.

Methods

In this study we retrospectively included all patients with chronic hepatic disease, who received an ultrasound of the abdomen either as an inpatient or outpatient in the Department of Gastroenterology and Gastrointestinal Oncology of the University Hospital of Goettingen between April 2015 and January 2016. Patients who had a cholecystectomy or complained of upper abdominal pain were excluded from the study. Gall stones and single gall bladder polyps without symptoms were no exclusion criteria. Of all patients who also had a documented upper endoscopy (median time interval 147 days), the following parameters were evaluated by ultrasound: The thickness of the gall bladder was measured twice after overnight fasting at two different locations and an average value was calculated. The spleen length was measured from a left lateral cross section. The diameter of the portal vein, the portal blood flow velocity and the liver size were measured. Ultrasound and endoscopy examinations were performed by experienced Gastroenterology trainees (> 3 years experience) and senior Gastroenterology consultants. The presence or absence of ascites was recorded. Additionally, clinical parameters such as the Child-Pugh-classification, laboratory results and upper endoscopic findings (presence of EV graded according the classification of Paquet) were obtained. Using the results of the cranio-caudal spleen diameter, gall bladder wall diameter and laboratory results, we calculated the ratio of platelet count to spleen diameter and the ratio of platelet count to gall bladder wall thickness. The statistical analysis was performed using the Mann Whitney U and Chi square test. Furthermore, variables with a P value < 0.1 from univariate analysis entered the multivariate binary logistic regression analysis and (receiver operating characteristic) ROC analysis was performed by SPSS Version 25 Mac OS. Since patient data were collected retrospectively and did not influence the diagnostic or therapeutic management of the patients, the ethic committee at the University Medical Centre Goettingen, Germany, was informed in written form about the study prior to data collection but did not request a separate ethical votum (24/7/15AN).

Results
Patient characteristics

A total of 194 patients were included in this study, of whom 84 were female and 110 were male. The average age of the patients at time of ultrasound examination was 57 years (range: 17–85 years). The main cause of hepatic disease was alcohol abuse ($n = 51$), followed by unknown cause of liver illness ($n = 38$) and viral hepatitis B and C ($n = 35$). The underlying liver diseases are summarized in Fig. 1. The patients were divided into two groups: 122 patients without EV (referred to as "non-EV" group) and 72 patients with EV in endoscopic diagnostic examination (referred to as "EV" group). Of those with EV 31 patients had 1° varices, 32 patients had 2° and further 9 patients had 3° varices. Interestingly, male patients were significantly more often represented in the EV group (73.6% EV group vs. 46.7% non-EV group; $p < 0.001$), potentially reflecting the high percentage (46%) of patients with alcohol abuse in the EV group. Histology of the liver was available in 53% of all patients ($n = 102$), and in those, cirrhosis was confirmed in 63% ($n = 22$) in the EV-group, and 19% ($n = 13$) in the non-EV group. As expected, hypertensive gastropathy, advanced Child Pugh Score and presence of ascites occurred significantly more frequently in the EV group. The patient characteristics disease severities are summarized in Table 1.

Ultrasonographic findings

In the EV group 46% of patients showed a non-inflammatory (absence of clinical and laboratory signs of acute cholecystitis) GBWT of ≥4 mm, compared to 12% in non-EV group ($p < 0.01$). GBWT was significantly higher in EV patients compared to the non-EV group (mean: 4.4 mm vs. 2.8 mm, $p < 0.0001$) Fig. 2a, b. The median of non-EV was lower with 2.5 mm than the median of 3.8 mm in the EV group. A more detailed analysis of the EV group revealed that there was no significant difference between first, second and third degree EV subgroups with an average thickness of 4.3 mm, 4.5 mm and 4.2 mm, respectively.

The spleen size as additional ultrasound parameter is also indicative for portal hypertension. In our cohort, the average spleen length was significantly higher in the EV group compared to the non-EV-group (138 mm vs. 113 mm; $p < 0,001$; Table 2). The portal vein diameter was also significantly higher in the EV group (12.4 mm vs. 11.6 mm; $p = 0.045$; Table 2). Further parameters

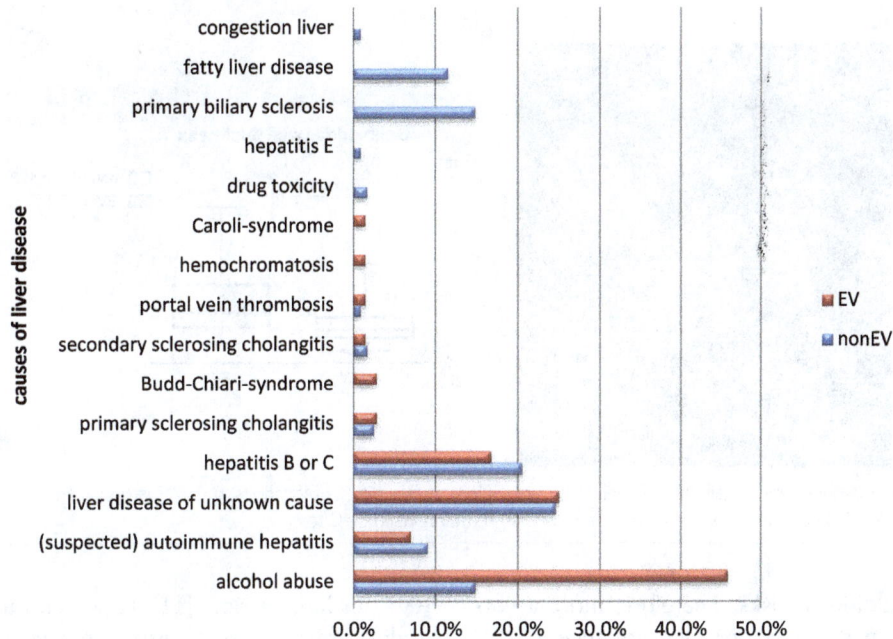

Fig. 1 Underlying liver diseases of study cohort (*n* = 194 patients)

measured by ultrasound such as average portal vein blood flow velocity, gall bladder length, and gall bladder diameter did not show any significant difference between the two groups (Table 2).

Biochemical analysis
The platelet count was significantly lower in the EV group (128.000/µl EV group vs. 227.000/µl non-EV group; *p*-value < 0.001; Table 2).

The average value of the INR differed significantly between the two groups with 1.09 ± 0.38 in the non-EV group and 1.39 ± 0.46 in the EV group (p-value < 0.0001). Sensitivity, specificity, positive and negative predictive value were calculated for single parameters regarding the presence of EV and showed sensitivities ranging between 40 and 70% (Table 3). In particular, the sensitivity of GBWT of ≥4 mm for the presence of EV was 46%, while

Table 1 Patient characteristics (comparison of group non-EV without esophageal varices and group EV with esophageal varices found by upper endoscopy)

Parameter	non-EV n = 120	EV n = 72	p-value
Male sex	47%	74%	< 0.001
Age (mean)	57 ± 14	57 ± 13	ns
Hypertensive gastropathy	14%	74%	< 0.0001
Child-Pugh-Classification A	92%	50%	< 0.0001
Child-Pugh-Classification B	3%	26%	< 0.0001
Child-Pugh-Classification C	5%	23%	< 0.001
presence of ascites	6%	44%	< 0.0001

the specificity was 89%. The positive predictive value was 70% and the negative predictive value 73%.

Using multivariate analysis by logistical regression including sex, Child-Pugh score, GBWT, liver size, spleen diameter, International Normalized Ratio (INR), platelet count, ascites and portal vein diameter, we show that GBWT, ascites, platelet count and spleen diameter are independent predictors of EV (Table 4).

However, platelet count/GBWT ratio (cut-off > 46.2) achieves a sensitivity of 78% and a specificity of 86%. The positive predictive value is 76% and the negative predictive value 87% (Table 5). Using our dataset, ROC analysis showed that the platelet count/GBWT ratio performed at a comparable level (area under the curve (AUC) 0.864 (confidence interval (CI) 0.809–0.919)) to the platelet count/spleen diameter ratio of 909 (AUC 0.841 (CI 0.782–0.901)) that was reported by Giannini et al. [7] (Fig. 3).

Discussion
Patients with compensated liver cirrhosis have a chance of up to 40% to develop EV [8]. To avoid hemorrhage from EV, it is recommended to perform an upper endoscopy as soon as there are signs for the presence of liver cirrhosis in patients [9, 10]. Therefore, many patients undergo upper endoscopy although they do not require treatment of EV (e.g. ligation) according to endoscopic classifications. While diagnostic gastroscopy itself is of low risk, low platelet counts as well as impaired coagulation parameters increase the risk of complications. Most patients prefer sedation during the procedure which is

A   B

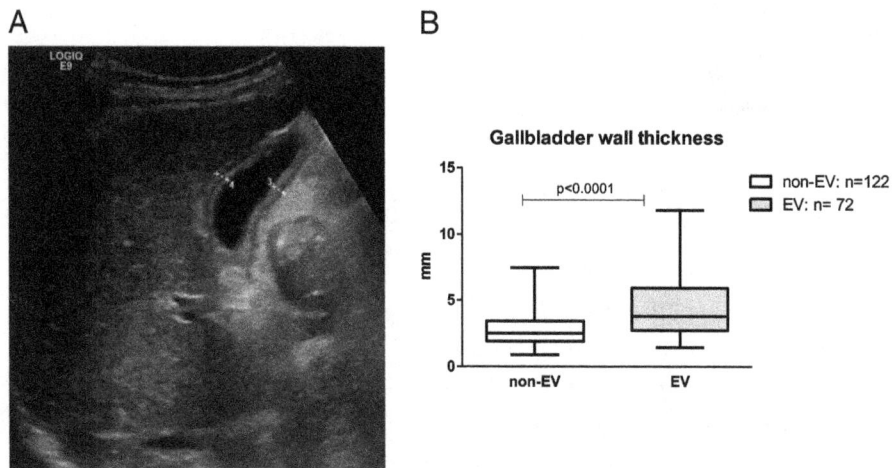

Fig. 2 a Sonographic measurement of gall bladder wall thickness (GBWT) at two different locations. **b** GBWT is significantly different in patients with esophageal varices (EV) compared to non-EV patients (*p* < 0.0001, Mann Whitney-U test)

associated with additional risks. Therefore, more accurate non-invasive parameters for the presence of EV could be a valuable and clinically relevant tool. We based our study on non-invasive, standard diagnostic tests, which are routinely performed in patients with chronic liver disease: ultrasound, clinical and laboratory results were evaluated in terms of prediction of EV.

Because of its portal-venous blood supply, we assumed that the GBWT may predict the presence of portal hypertension and EV. An interesting study by Maruyama et al. also reported a lower sensitivity of 62% regarding the detection of large esophageal varices using the platelet count to spleen diameter ratio in 229 cirrhosis patients. In this study, the authors showed that a diameter of the left gastric vein -as a non-variceal collateral- of more than 5.35 mm had a sensitivity of 90% and a specificity of 62% for presence of large esophageal varices. Its sonographic detection was associated with a sensitivity of 84% for any esophageal varices and a sensitivity of

100% for large varices [11]. However, further prospective studies are required to assess the value of portal vein velocity as non-invasive parameter for the presence of esophageal varices.

A small Chinese study showed a correlation between portal vein velocity and GBWT supporting the hypothesis that GBWT could also predict the presence of EV [12]. From a pathophysiological point of view, GBWT may be a microcirculatory driven event caused by impaired portalvenous outflow before significant changes in portal vein velocity occur. However, the development of GBWT may also be caused by other factors such as the serum-ascites albumin gradient (SAAG) [13].

Several studies have investigated non-invasive parameters as predictors for the presence of EV. A platelet count to spleen diameter ratio of 909 and less was associated with EV [7]. The enlarged spleen is caused by portal hypertension and low platelets were also associated with a lowered thrombopoetin serum level due to reduced liver

Table 2 Sonographic, clinical and laboratory findings in patients without esophageal varices (non-EV = 122) and endoscopically confirmed varices (EV = 72)

Parameter	non-EV *n* = 120	EV *n* = 72	*p*-value
Gall bladder wall thickness	2.8 ± 1.2 mm	4.4 ± 2.1 mm	**< 0.0001**
Gall bladder length	61.6 ± 17.6 mm	61.1 ± 21.8 mm	0.867
Gall bladder diameter	25.0 ± 8.6 mm	27.1 ± 10.0 mm	0.128
Liver size in MCL	13.8 ± 2.1 cm	14.7 ± 2.6 cm	**0.015**
Spleen diameter	112.9 ± 23.9 mm	138.0 ± 28.2 mm	**< 0.0001**
Portal vein diameter	11.6 ± 2.1 mm	12.4 ± 2.9 mm	**0.045**
Portal vein velocity	18.0 ± 3.9 cm/s	18.0 ± 5.8 cm/s	0.968
INR	1.09 ± 0.38	1.39 ± 0.46	**< 0.0001**
Platelet count	226.6 ± 85.9 × 1.000/µl	128.1 ± 99.2 × 1.000/µl	**< 0.0001**

INR International ratio; *MCL* Medioclavicular line
Significant are all values <0.05

Table 3 Sensitivity, specificity, positive and negative predictive value for the presence of esophageal varices using gall bladder wall thickness (GBWT) ≥4 mm, spleen length (≥130 mm), ascites, thrombocytes (< 160.000/µl) and Child-Pugh classification

Parameter	GBWT (≥4 mm)	Spleen (≥130 mm)	Thrombocytes (< 160.000/µl)	Ascites	Child-Pugh B or C
Sensitivity	46%	62%	69%	44%	50%
Specificity	89%	81%	78%	94%	92%
Positive predictive value	70%	67%	64%	82%	78%
Negative predictive value	73%	78%	81%	74%	76%

function [14]. Chen performed a meta-analysis to confirm the usefulness of this ratio and calculated a summative sensitivity of the ratio of 84% with a specificity of 78% to predict EV. The sensitivity of this ratio was also influenced by etiology of the liver disease with a sensitivity of 92% in viral liver cirrhosis [15]. Using the platelet count to spleen diameter ratio as previously described [7], the sensitivity was somewhat lower with our dataset. The reasons might be the greater variety of causes for liver disease in our cohort than in previous evaluations. Another non-invasive method is the use of computed tomography (CT) imaging with a sensitivity of 90% and a specificity of 72% for the detection of EV [16]. The higher sensitivity is traded against higher costs, exposure to irradiation, and the use of contrast agents. Other non-invasive measurements such as liver stiffness measurements are promising but further studies need to be performed. Meta-analysis of data so far collected by using transient elastography (FibroScan®) showed lower prognostic values for liver stiffness [17]. A meta-analysis of studies using different modes of elastography techniques to measure spleen stiffness showed heterogeneous results to detect EV [18]. The sensitivity of liver stiffness was 84% in predicting any varices, compared to 78% using the stiffness of the spleen as parameter. The specificity of the spleen stiffness was higher when compared to liver stiffness (76% versus 62%) [18] [16]. The use of capsule endoscopy to detect EV is also discussed in the literature [19] but high costs and its semi-invasive nature need to be kept in mind. Because of those limitations of the aforementioned non-invasive methods, the use of GBWT could represent a novel and feasible clinical marker for the detection of EV.

Alcantara previously published a cut-off value of 4.35 mm for a thickened gall bladder wall and found a sensitivity of 60% and a specificity of 90% regarding the presence of EV in pediatric patients [20]. The sensitivity was higher than in our study, although a higher value was used as cut-off. Other reasons for this difference might be the different patient cohorts, since de Alcantara based his study on data from children with various causes of cirrhosis such as biliary atresia and auto-immune hepatitis [20]. In our study we used data from adult patients with chronic liver disease and common causes for cirrhosis in Western Europe, but lack of histological confirmation in almost half of them. The cut-off-value of 4 mm was arbitrarily set for univariate analysis and seems reasonable since a lower value could be measured in individuals that did not fast overnight with a higher rate of falsely positive cases. A higher cut-off value would lower sensitivity.

In addition, a lowered velocity within the portal vein seems reasonable in the presence of portal hypertension and esophageal varices, but existing data are still conflicting. An Indian study of sonographic parameters predicting esophageal varices in 56 patients showed a significant difference of mean portal vein velocity. In presence of esophageal varices the mean velocity was 14.77 cm/s and in absence of varices 17.66 cm/s [21]. However, Li et al. did not report a significant difference in portal vein velocity between patients with and without esophageal varices. The mean velocity was 15.3 cm/s in healthy individuals, 14.2 cm/s in patients with first degree varices, 13.1 cm/s in second degree varices and 12.0 cm/s in third degree varices [22]. In our study there

Table 4 Results of logistic regression analysis for prediction esophageal varices

Logistic regression for prediction esophageal varices						
	B	S.E.	df	p	OR = Exp(B)	95% CI for OR
GBWT	−0.323	0.155	1	0.037	0.724	0.534–0.977
Spleen diameter	−0.023	0.009	1	0.007	0.977	0.961–0.994
Platelet count	0.009	0.003	1	0.001	1.009	1.004–1.015
Ascites	1.674	0.717	1	0.019	5.336	1.310–21.731

B Regression coefficient; *S.E.* Standard error; *df* Degree of freedom; *OR* Odds ratio; *GBWT* Gall bladder wall thickness

Table 5 Sensitivity, specificity, positive and negative predictive value and area under the curve (AUC) for the presence of EV using the combination of platelet count/GBWT ratio (> 46.2), and platelet count/spleen diameter 909 as described by Giannini et al. [7]

Parameters	Platelet count/GBWT (> 46.2)	Th/Spleen (< 909)
Sensitivity	78%	63%
Specificity	86%	87%
Positive predictive value	76%	75%
Negative predictive value	87%	80%
Area under the curve	0.864 (CI 0.809–0.919)	0.841 (CI 0.782–0.901)

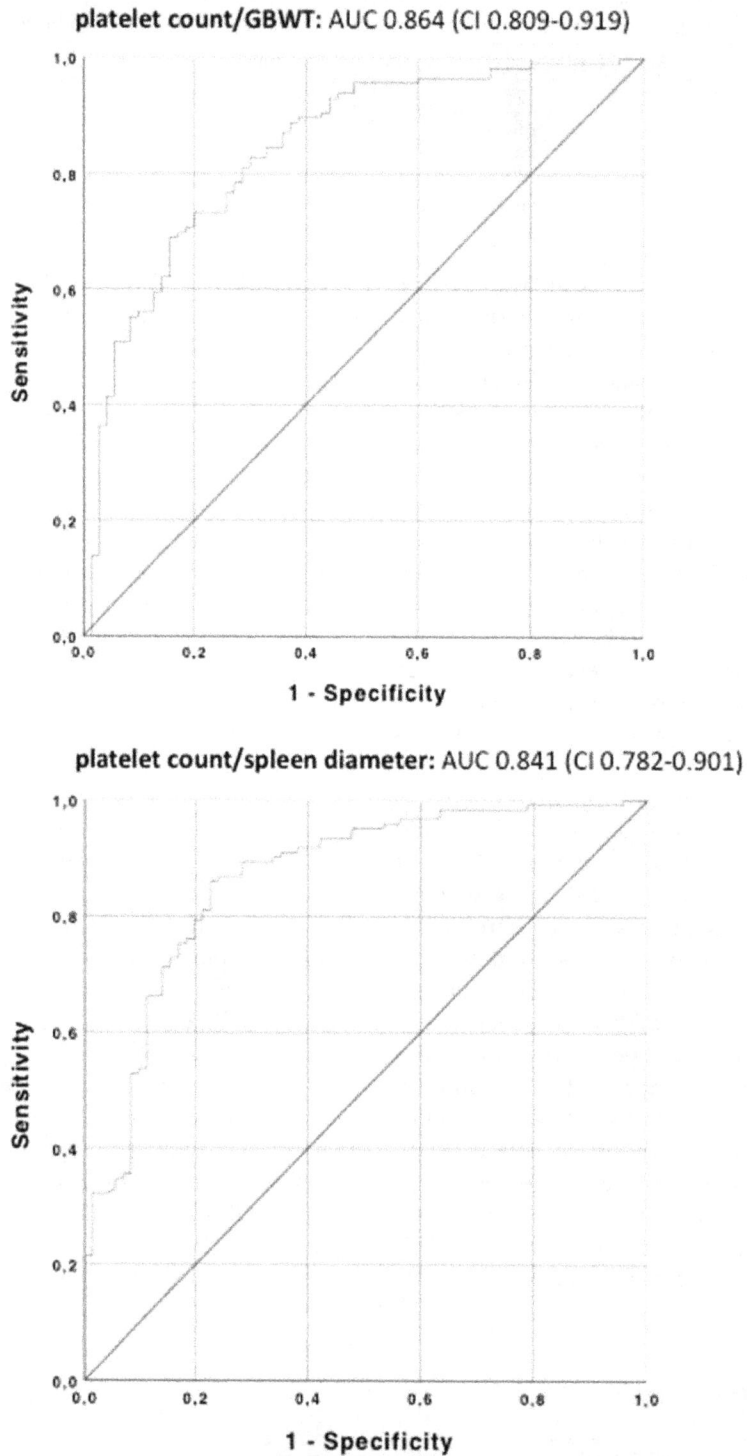

Fig. 3 Receiver operating characteristic (ROC) analysis and area under the curve (AUC) Top platelet count/GBWT ratio. Bottom platelet count/spleen diameter ratio

was no difference in average portal vein velocity with 18.0 cm/s in both groups.

Our study has several limitations. First, ultrasonography and endoscopy were not always performed within a few days and may have biased results in case of rapidly changing endoscopy or ultrasonography findings. Furthermore, retrospective data collection could not establish a clear cause for chronic liver disease in almost 20% of patients.

Secondly, although performed by experienced Gastro-enterology trainees and consultants, GBWT measurements were performed by only one examiner, and inter-observer variability could thus not be accounted for. Third, we could not detect significant differences between small and large EV most likely due to the relatively low number of 3° EVs ($n = 9$) in the EV cohort.

Conclusions

To conclude, GBWT may improve the non-invasive monitoring of liver disease patients to assess the risk for the presence of EV. However, a distinction between different severity grades of EV was not possible with the cut-off values used in our study. To improve upon the predictive value of GBWT, the combination with additional non-invasive parameters such as the platelet count is recommended.

Abbreviations
AUCa: Area under the curve; CI: Confidence interval; EV: Esophageal varices; GBWT: Gall bladder wall thickening; INR: International normalized ratio; ROC: Receiver operating characteristic

Authors' contributions
AN and SK initiated the study. BT and RM collected the data for this study. BT, AA and GP analyzed and interpreted the patient data. AN, SK and VE were major contributors in writing the manuscript. All authors read and approved the final manuscript.

Consent for publication
Not applicable.

Competing interests
The authors declare that they have no competing interests.

References
1. Blachier M, Leleu H, Peck-Radosavljevic M, Valla D-C, Roudot-Thoraval F. The burden of liver disease in Europe: a review of available epidemiological data. J Hepatol. 2013;58:593–608.
2. Fleming KM, Aithal GP, Card TR, West J. All-cause mortality in people with cirrhosis compared with the general population: a population-based cohort study. Liver Int Off J Int Assoc Study Liver. 2012;32:79–84.
3. Merli M, Nicolini G, Angeloni S, Rinaldi V, De Santis A, Merkel C, et al. Incidence and natural history of small esophageal varices in cirrhotic patients. J Hepatol. 2003;38:266–72.
4. Hsieh Y-C, Lee K-C, Chen P-H, Su C-W, Hou M-C, Lin H-C. Acute kidney injury predicts mortality in cirrhotic patients with gastric variceal bleeding. J Gastroenterol Hepatol. 2017;32:1859-66.
5. de Franchis R, Primignani M. Natural history of portal hypertension in patients with cirrhosis. Clin Liver Dis. 2001;5:645–63.
6. Way LW, Pellegrini CA, editors. Surgery of the gallbladder and bile ducts. Philadelphia: Saunders; 1987.
7. Giannini E, Botta F, Borro P, Risso D, Romagnoli P, Fasoli A, et al. Platelet count/spleen diameter ratio: proposal and validation of a non-invasive parameter to predict the presence of oesophageal varices in patients with liver cirrhosis. Gut. 2003;52:1200–5.
8. Pagliaro, et al. In: Bosch J, Groszmann RJ, editors. Portal Hypertens Pathophysiol Treat Portal hypertension in cirrhosis: natural history. Oxford: Blackwell Science; 1992. p. 72–92.
9. Denzer U, Beilenhoff U, Eickhoff A, Faiss S, Hüttl P, In der Smitten S, et al. S2k guideline: quality requirements for gastrointestinal endoscopy, AWMF registry no. 021-022. Z Gastroenterol. 2015;53:E1–227.
10. Sarin SK, Lahoti D, Saxena SP, Murthy NS, Makwana UK. Prevalence, classification and natural history of gastric varices: a long-term follow-up study in 568 portal hypertension patients. Hepatol Baltim Md. 1992;16:1343–9.
11. Maruyama H, Kobayashi K, Kiyono S, Ogasawara S, Ooka Y, Suzuki E, et al. Left gastric vein-based noninvasive test for esophageal varices: a same-day comparison of portal hemodynamic assessment with endoscopic appearance. Clin Transl Gastroenterol. 2018;9:154.
12. Li C, Yang Z, Ma E, Liu Y. Analysis of the correlation between the degree of GBWT and hemodynamic changes of portal vein system. Sheng Wu Yi Xue Gong Cheng Xue Za Zhi J Biomed Eng Shengwu Yixue Gongchengxue Zazhi. 2010;27:583–5. 625
13. Colli A, Cocciolo M, Buccino G, Parravicini R, Martinez E, Rinaldi G, et al. Thickening of the gallbladder wall in ascites. J Clin Ultrasound. 1991;19:357–9.
14. Giannini E, Botta F, Borro P, Malfatti F, Fumagalli A, Testa E, et al. Relationship between thrombopoietin serum levels and liver function in patients with chronic liver disease related to hepatitis C virus infection. Am J Gastroenterol. 2003;98:2516–20.
15. Chen R, Deng H, Ding X, Xie C, Wang W, Shen Q. Platelet count to spleen diameter ratio for the diagnosis of gastroesophageal varices in liver cirrhosis: a systematic review and meta-analysis. Gastroenterol Res Pract. 2017;2017:7407506.
16. Tseng Y-J, Zeng X-Q, Chen J, Li N, Xu P-J, Chen S-Y. Computed tomography in evaluating gastroesophageal varices in patients with portal hypertension: a meta-analysis. Dig Liver Dis Off J Ital Soc Gastroenterol Ital Assoc Study Liver. 2016;48:695–702.
17. Pu K, Shi J-H, Wang X, Tang Q, Wang X-J, Tang K-L, et al. Diagnostic accuracy of transient elastography (FibroScan) in detection of esophageal varices in patients with cirrhosis: a meta-analysis. World J Gastroenterol. 2017;23:345–56.
18. Singh S, Eaton JE, Murad MH, Tanaka H, Iijima H, Talwalkar JA. Accuracy of spleen stiffness measurement in detection of esophageal varices in patients with chronic liver disease: systematic review and meta-analysis. Clin Gastroenterol Hepatol Off Clin Pract J Am Gastroenterol Assoc. 2014;12:935–945.e4.
19. Colli A, Gana JC, Turner D, Yap J, Adams-Webber T, Ling SC, et al. Capsule endoscopy for the diagnosis of oesophageal varices in people with chronic liver disease or portal vein thrombosis. Cochrane Database Syst Rev. 2014;10:CD008760.
20. de Alcantara RV, Yamada RM, Cardoso SR, de Fátima M, Servidoni CP, Hessel G. Ultrasonographic predictors of esophageal varices. J Pediatr Gastroenterol Nutr. 2013;57:700–3.
21. Chakrabarti R, Sen D, Khanna V. Is non-invasive diagnosis of esophageal varices in patients with compensated hepatic cirrhosis possible by duplex Doppler ultrasonography? Indian J Gastroenterol Off J Indian Soc Gastroenterol. 2016;35:60–6.
22. Li F-H, Hao J, Xia J-G, Li H-L, Fang H. Hemodynamic analysis of esophageal varices in patients with liver cirrhosis using color Doppler ultrasound. World J Gastroenterol. 2005;11:4560–5.

11

Tolvaptan treatment improves survival of cirrhotic patients with ascites and hyponatremia

Shuzhen Wang[1], Xin Zhang[1], Tao Han[2], Wen Xie[3], Yonggang Li[4], Hong Ma[5], Roman Liebe[6], Honglei Weng[6] and Hui-Guo Ding[1]*

Abstract

Background: Although tolvaptan treatment improves hyponatremia, only few studies have investigated whether tolvaptan actually benefits the survival of cirrhotic patients. This study evaluated the impact of tolvaptan on six-month survival of decompensated cirrhotic patients with and without hyponatremia.

Methods: Two hundred forty-nine decompensated cirrhotic patients with or without hyponatremia were enrolled in a multicenter cohort study. Patients were divided into two groups according to receiving either tolvaptan or placebo treatment for 7-day. Subsequently, the patients were followed up for 6 months.

Results: Two hundred thirty patients, including 98 with hyponatremia (tolvaptan vs. placebo: 69 vs. 29) finished the study. Tolvaptan did not alter serum sodium levels and survival outcome of decompensated cirrhotic patients without hyponatremia. However, tolvaptan treatment remarkably improved serum sodium levels and six-month survival in patients with hyponatremia. Following tolvaptan treatment, serum sodium levels were restored to normal in 63.8% of patients, whereas in patients receiving placebo, only 36.2% showed the same effect ($P < 0.05$). Compared to a six-month survival rate of 68.97% in patients receiving placebo, the survival rate in tolvapatan-treated patients was 89.94% ($P < 0.05$). Furthermore, six-month survival rate in the tolvaptan-treated hyponatremia patients with resolved serum sodium was 81.32%, whereas the survival in those with unresolved serum sodium was only 24% ($P < 0.05$).

Conclusions: Tolvaptan improves short term survival in most decompensated cirrhotic hyponatremia patients with resolved serum sodium.

Keywords: Ascites, Hyponatremia, Liver cirrhosis, Survival, Tolvaptan

Background

Cirrhotic patients with ascites and hyponatremia have a poor quality of life and high mortality [1]. One-year survival rate in these patients is less than 60% [2]. Development of ascites with or without hyponatremia is associated with multiple pathophysiological alteration, i.e. renal water and

* Correspondence: dinghuiguo@medmail.com.cn; dinghuiguo@ccmu.edu.cn
[1]Department of Gastroenterology and Hepatology, Beijing You'an Hospital, Affiliated with Capital Medical University, Fengtai District, Beijing 100069, China
Full list of author information is available at the end of the article

sodium retention, hyperdynamic cardiovascular dysfunction secondary to arterial splanchnic vasodilation, activation of the renin-aldosterone system, and increased aldosterone and vasopressin levels in the peripheral circulation [3, 4].

Classic diuretics such as furosemide and aldosterone antagonists spironolactone improve water retention and edema, but exacerbate hyponatremia in cirrhotic patients [5]. Distinct from the classic diuretics, tolvaptan, a highly selective vasopressin V2 antagonist, effectively improves levels of serum sodium by increasing the excretion of electrolyte-free water without altering total level of electrolyte excretion [6]. Previous clinical studies showed that tolvaptan improved serum sodium levels in cirrhotic patients with ascites [6–8]. However, few studies to date have assessed whether tolvaptan treatment improves the survival of cirrhotic patients when hyponatremia is resolved [9]. The current cohort study addresses this question by following up cirrhotic patients for six months after tolvaptan treatment. The factors that influenced the efficacy of tolvaptan in liver cirrhotic patients with ascites are also analyzed.

Methods
Patients
The prospective cohort enrolled 249 cirrhotic patients with ascites from three clinical trials, which were conducted in five medical centers between 2008 and 2012 (Fig. 1). The patients enrolled in three clinical trials were divided into two groups according to receiving tolvaptan (7.5 mg/day to 15 mg/day) or placebo for 7 days. The followings were a brief clinical trial descriptions. The first clinical trial performed from May 5, 2008 to July 7, 2009 was a multicenter, randomized (1:1), double-blind, placebo-controlled, which was designed to evaluate the efficacy and safety of the tolvaptan in patients with non-hypovolemic, and non-acute hyponatremia (ClinicalTrials.gov ID:NCT00664014). Cirrhotic patients with hyponatremia, defined as serum sodium< 135 mmol/L, were hospitalized to receive drug administration. They received 15 mg/day tolvaptan or placebo for the first 4 days. After 4 days, the dose was increased to 30 mg/day and 60 mg/day in the patients whose

serum sodium levels did not respond. The remaining patients remained on the same dosage as on days 1–4 until the 7th day.. The second clinical trial, which was performed from 2009 to 2010, was a multicenter, open-label, double-blinded, and placebo-controlled design (ClinicalTrials.gov ID:NCT01349335) [10]. The aim of the trial was to evaluate the effect of tolvaptan in cirrhotic patients with ascites. The patients enrolled in this trial had insufficient response to combination diuretics treatment (furosemide ≥40 mg/day and spironolactone ≥20 mg/day; or furosemide ≥20 mg/day and spironolactone ≥40 mg/day). Patients were randomly assigned to three groups (1:1:1) receiving placebo, tolvaptan 15 mg/day and tolvaptan 30 mg/day for 7 days, respectively. The third clinical trial, which was performed between October 5, 2010 and January 20, 2012, was a multicenter randomized, double-blind, and placebo-controlled study (ClinicalTrials.gov ID:NCT01349348). This trial evaluated the efficacy and safety of tolvaptan in cirrhotic patients with ascites. Patients who had insufficient response to combination therapies of diuretics were treated with tolvaptan 7.5 mg/day, tolvaptan 15 mg/day or placebo (1:2:1) for 7 days, respectively. Patients were followed up for 6 months after treatment. The endpoints of the study were (1) survival of patients and (2) resolved serum sodium levels. Normal serum sodium was defined as serum sodium concentration between 135 and 155 mmol/L. Mild, moderate and severe hyponatremia were considered when levels of serum sodium between 130 and 135 mmol/L, 125 and

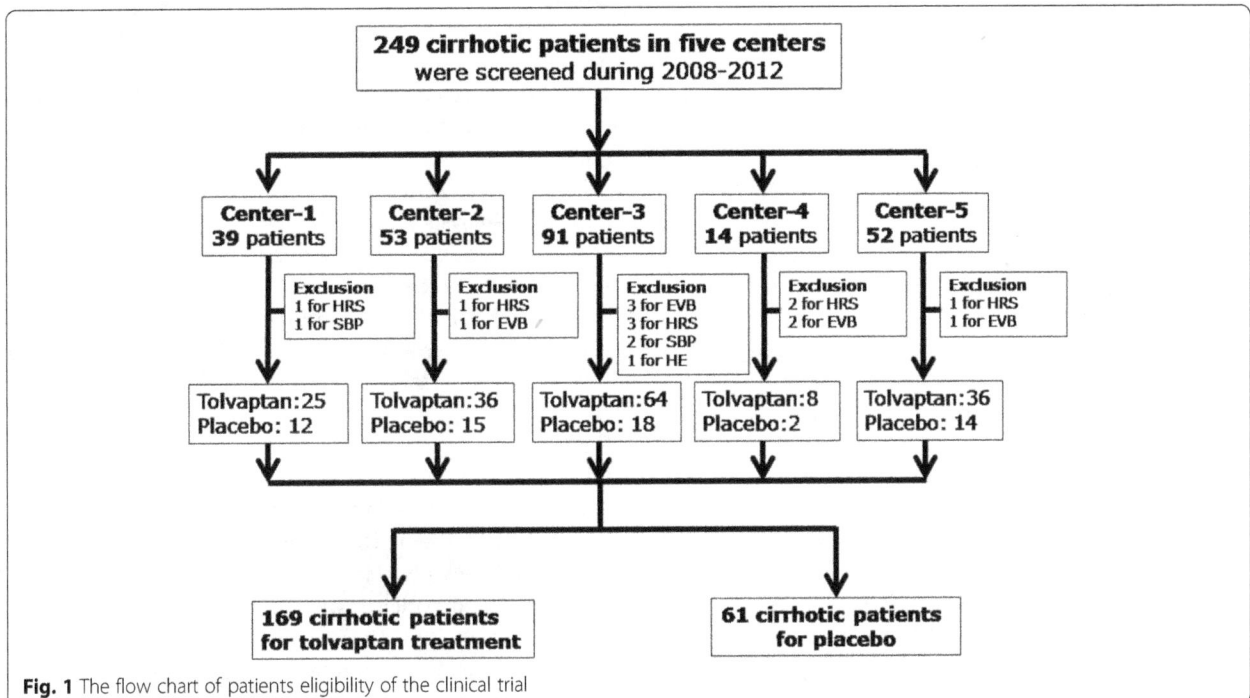

Fig. 1 The flow chart of patients eligibility of the clinical trial

130 mmol/L, and less than 125 mmol/L, respectively (Table 1). "Resolved serum sodium" was defined as a patient with hyponatremia before treatment restoring levels of serum sodium to between 135 and 155 mmol/L after treatment.

Decompensated cirrhotic patients were enrolled according to the following criteria: (1) aged between 18 and 75 years, (2) definite history of cirrhosis, (3) signs and symptoms of decompensated cirrhosis, such as splenomegaly, hypersplenism, variceal bleeding, ascites, and hepatic encephalopathy, (4) confirmed cirrhosis by image measurements, i.e. B-ultrasound scanning (LOGIQ9; GE

Table 1 The baseline characteristics of the patients enrolled in this study

Index	Tolvaptan (n = 169)	Placebo (n = 61)	P value
Age (mean ± SD)	54.6 ± 8.58	51.6 ± 10.71	0.03
Gender (F/M)	33/136	12/49	0.98
Etiology of cirrhosis (n,%)			
Hepatitis B	102 (60.3)	41 (67.3)	0.03
Hepatitis C	9 (5.3)	3 (4.9)	
Alcohol liver disease	33 (19.5)	11 (18.0)	
PBC	2 (1.2)	0 (0)	
Mixed[a]	13 (7.7)	5 (8.2)	
Cryptogenic	4 (2.4)	0 (0)	
Others[b]	6 (3.6)	1 (1.6)	
Child-Pugh grade (n, %)			
A (5–6)	2 (1.2)	1 (1.6)	0.36
B (7–9)	113 (66.8)	45 (73.8)	
C (10–15)	54 (32.0)	15 (24.6)	
Edema of lower limbs (n, %)			
No	123 (72.8)	43 (70.5)	0.86
Yes	46 (27.2)	18 (29.5)	
Serum sodium (mmol/L)			0.56
Median	135.8	135.0	
(Min, Max)	(117.2, 146.3)	(124.8, 142.7)	
Normal serum sodium (n, %) (≥ 135 and < 150 mmol/L)	100 (59.2)	32 (52.5)	
Mild hyponatremia (n, %) (≥ 130 and < 135 mmol/L)	44 (26.0)	21 (34.4)	
Middle hyponatremia (n, %) (≥ 125 and < 130 mmol/L)	19 (11.2)	7 (11.5)	
Severe hyponatremia (n, %) (< 125 mmol/L)	6 (3.6)	1 (1.6)	
Serum potassium (mmol/L)	4.2 ± 0.5	4.1 ± 0.7	0.98
Serum urea nitrogen (mmol/L)	5.3 ± 0.8	5.6 ± 0.8	0.93

[a]Mixed etiology: Hepatitis B + alcoholic hepatitis, hepatitis B + primary biliary cirrhosis (PBC), hepatitis C + alcoholic hepatitis, alcoholic hepatitis+ PBC. PBC:primary biliary cirrhosis
[b]Other etiology: 3 drug-induced hepatitis, 2 cardiac disease, 2 autoimmune liver disease

Company, Fairfield, United States) and computerized tomography (CT; GE HISPEED DXI; GE Company) and (5) consenting to follow-up for six months.

Patients with the following diseases were excluded: (1) type I hepatorenal syndrome, (2) nervous system diseases such as Alzheimer's disease, Parkinson's disease, multiple sclerosis, epilepsy, Guillain-Barré syndrome, etc., (3) poorly controlled diabetes (fasting glucose > 220 mg/dL), (4) heart failure with ascites, (5) anuria (urine volume < 100 mL/day), (6) dysuresia, (7) hepatic encephalopathy ≥ Grade II, (8) hepatocellular carcinoma, (9) chronic liver failure, (10) cerebrovascular accident within 30 days prior to the study medication, and (11) history of cerebral infarction or stroke.

The study protocol was performed in compliance with the Declaration of Helsinki and approved by the Ethics Committees of Beijing Youan Hospital affiliated to Capital Medical University. Signed informed consent was obtained from each patient for using samples, materials and publication.

Clinical and laboratory data

Symptoms, signs, and adverse events were recorded. Serum markers for hepatitis B and C viruses were detected by electrochemiluminescence immunoassay (Roche E170 modular immunoassay analyzer, Roche Diagnostics, Mannheim, Germany). Serum sodium and potassium levels, liver and renal function, including serum alanine aminotransferase (ALT), aspartate aminotransferase (AST), total bilirubin (TBIL), albumin, creatinine, and urea nitrogen, were measured with an automatic biochemical analyzer (AU5400, Olympus Company, Tokyo, Japan).

Safety

Patients were routinely monitored throughout the study. Any occurrences of adverse events and deaths were recorded.

Statistical analysis

Student's t test, χ2, and Fisher's exact test were used to test the intergroup difference according to the types of variables. The Kaplan–Meier estimator and log-rank test were used to calculate the survival rate. A P value less than 0.05 (two-way) was considered statistically significant.

Results
Study patients

After 6-month of follow-up, 230 patients finished the study. Among them, 169 patients were treated with tolvaptan and 61 with placebo. The baseline characteristics of the enrolled patients were shown in Table 1. Except for age and etiology, there were no differences of demographic and clinical parameters, i.e. gender, Child-Pugh grades, edema, levels of serum sodium, potassium and urea nitrogen, between the two groups of patients at the baseline of the clinical study. The mean age of patients treated with tolvaptan and with placebo were 54 and 51 years, respectively ($P < 0.05$). The major etiology in both groups was chronic hepatitis B infection (60.3% vs. 67.3%, $P < 0.05$).

Tolvaptan does not impact serum sodium levels of cirrhotic patients without hyponatremia

First we investigated whether tolvaptan impacted serum sodium levels in cirrhotic patients without hyponatremia. This clinical study enrolled 132 cirrhotic patients with normal serum sodium levels. Among these, 100 patients received tolvaptan treatment and 32 placebo (Table 1). The dynamic alteration of serum sodium levels in cirrhotic patients treated with tolvaptan or placebo were shown in Table 2. Tolvaptan treatment for 7 days increased mean values of serum sodium from 138.15 ± 2.58 mmol/L to 139.83 ± 3.32 mmol/L ($P < 0.05$). In the period of follow-up levels of serum sodium in these patients decreased compared to those at the baseline ($P < 0.05$), however, the concentrations of serum sodium during the follow-up still remained within the normal range: 136.88 ± 5.09 mmol/L after 3 months and 136.97 ± 6.92 mmol/L after 6 months. Placebo treatment for 7 days did not alter serum sodium levels of cirrhotic patients: 138.60 ± 2.24 mmol/L vs. 138.23 ± 2.16 mmol/L ($P > 0.05$). During the follow-up, levels of serum sodium in these patients reduced to 136.97 ± 4.18 mmol/L at 3 months and 133.18 ± 9.31 mmol/L ($P > 0.05$).

Tolvaptan improves serum sodium levels of cirrhotic patients with hyponatremia

Next, we assessed the effect of tolvaptan on cirrhotic patients with hyponatremia. In this study, 69 cirrhotic patients (44 with mild, 19 with moderate and 16 with severe hyponatremia) received tolvaptan treatment while 29 (21 with mild, 7 with moderate and 1 with severe hyponatremia) were treated with placebo.

Tolvaptan treatment for 7 days significantly improved levels of serum sodium of cirrhotic patients with hyponatremia (Table 2). Thirty-two patients (72.7%) with mild, 10 (52.6%) with moderate and 2 (33.3%) with severe hyponatremia restored serum sodium levels to normal levels. The mean value of serum sodium in mild, moderate and severe hyponatremia patients with tolvaptan treatment for 7 days increased from 132.98 ± 1.31, 127.35 ± 1.17 and 120.87 ± 3.33 mmol/L to 136.59 ± 3.51, 132.29 ± 2.87 and 126.50 ± 6.61 mmol/L, respectively ($P < 0.01$ for all). Three months after tolvaptan treatment, levels of serum sodium in patients with mild, moderate and severe hyponatremia remained at 133.78 ± 4.13, 132.24 ± 5.71 and 131.10 ± 6.15 mmol/L, respectively ($P < 0.01$). At the end of follow-up, levels of serum sodium

in 23 patients with mild hyponatremia had decreased to 131.96 ± 5.29 mmol/L ($P < 0.01$,). However, 10 patients with moderate and 2 with severe hyponatremia kept at 129.81 ± 7.02 and 132.30 mmol/L, higher than the baseline levels ($P < 0.01$).

Placebo treatment did not alter levels of serum sodium in patients with hyponatremia (Table 2). One patient with severe hyponatremia died 2 days after hospitalization. The mean values of serum sodium in patients with mild and moderate hyponatremia before and after placebo treatment were 131.96 ± 1.44 vs. 131.06 ± 4.65 mmol/L and 127.94 ± 0.92 vs. 129.20 ± 10.32 mmol/L, respectively ($P > 0.05$). Only 9 patients with mild and 2 patients with moderate hyponatremia in this group finished follow-up. The mean value of serum sodium in patients with mild hyponatremia was 134.50 ± 6.20 mmol/L ($P > 0.05$ compared to the baseline).

Tolvaptan improves six-month survival of cirrhotic patients with hyponatremia

Next, we examined the six-month survival of cirrhotic patients. First we analyzed the impact of tolvaptan treatment on survival of cirrhotic patients without hyponatremia. Although tolvaptan-treated patients showed higher six-month survival rate than placebo-treated ones, the difference was not statistically significant ($P > 0.05$, Fig. 2a). The differences in three or six-month survival rates of cirrhotic patients with hyponatremia between tolvaptan treated patients and control patients were not statistically significant either ($P > 0.05$, Fig. 2b). Compared to patients receiving placebo, however, three or six-month survival rates in the hyponatremia patients receiving tolvaptan increased from 75.87% (22/29) and 68.97% (19/29) to 91.31% (63/69) and 89.94%, respectively.

In hyponatremia patients receiving tolvaptan, survival depended on the serum sodium responded to tolvaptan treament or not. The three or six-month survival rates in hyponatremia patients with restored normal serum sodium (tolvaptan responders) reached 86.36% (38/44) and 81.32% (36/44), whereas in those with unrestored serum sodium levels (non-responders) were a mere 40% (10/25) and 24% (6/25) ($P < 0.05$).

Notably, even in the hyponatremia patients receiving placebo, survival of the patients depended on restoring serum sodium levels to normal during follow-up. The six-month survival rate of patients with restored serum sodium levels (62.5%) was significantly higher than of those without (28.7%), $P < 0.01$. The Kaplan–Meier survival curves shown that the survival of patients with resolved serum sodium was significantly higher than of those unresolved serum sodium either tolvaptan or placebo treatment (Fig. 2c).

Safety assessment

No side-effects were detected during treatment and follow-up of this study. Monitoring liver function did

Table 2 Dynamic alteration of serum sodium levels in cirrhotic patients treated with tolvaptan or placebo

	Tolvaptan (n = 169)					Placebo (n = 61)					
	0 day	4 days	7 days	3 months	6 months	0 day	4 days	7 days	3 months	6 months	
Normal sodium, mmol/L (n)	138.15 ± 2.58 (100)	140.28 ± 3.07 (95)	139.83 ± 3.32* (95)	136.88 ± 5.09* (56)	136.97 ± 6.92* (49)	138.60 ± 2.24 (32)	138.52 ± 2.39 (29)	138.23 ± 2.16 (24)	136.97 ± 4.18 (14)	133.18 ± 9.31 (11)	
Mild hyponatremia, mmol/L (n)	132.98 ± 1.31 (44)	138.02 ± 3.11** (44)	136.59 ± 3.51** (41)	133.78 ± 4.13** (33)	131.96 ± 5.29** (23)	131.96 ± 1.44 (21)	131.34 ± 3.03 (13)	131.06 ± 4.65 (13)	129.45 ± 6.66 (11)	134.50 ± 6.20 (9)	
Middle hyponatremis, mmol/L (n)	127.35 ± 1.17 (19)	131.50 ± 2.85** (18)	132.29 ± 2.87** (18)	132.24 ± 5.71** (11)	129.81 ± 7.02** (10)	127.94 ± 0.92 (7)	130.30 ± 3.82 (5)	129.20 ± 10.32 (3)	134.30 (2)	139.30 (2)	
Severe hyponatremia, mmol/L (n)	120.87 ± 3.33 (6)	126.87 ± 7.05** (6)	126.50 ± 6.61** (5)	131.10 ± 6.15** (3)	132.30 (2)	124.80 (1)	ND	ND	ND	ND	

Compared with 0 day, *P > 0.05, **P < 0.01

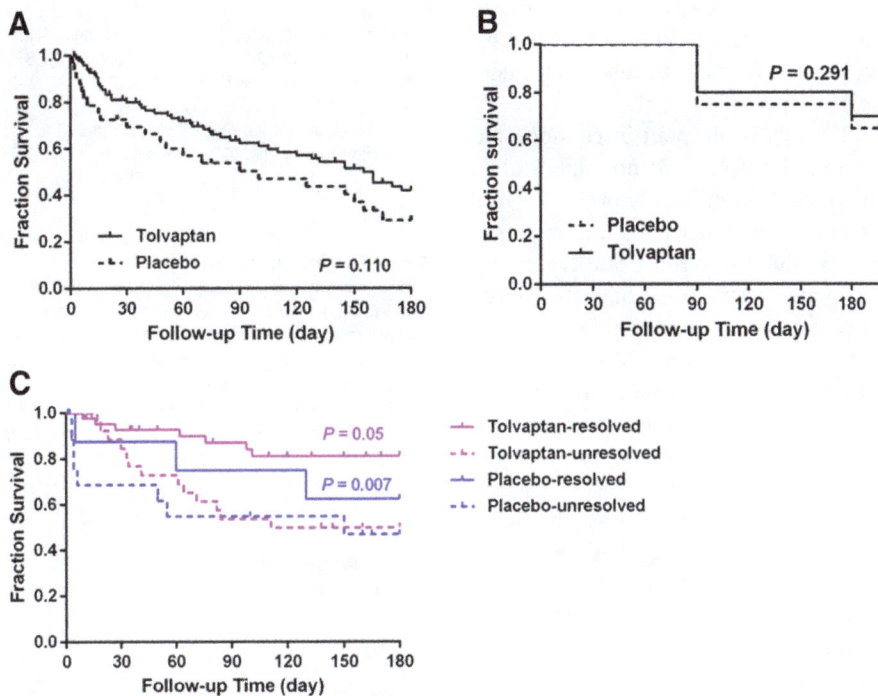

Fig. 2 Six-month survival of cirrhotic patients with ascites who received tolvaptan or placebo treatment. The Kaplan–Meier survival curves was not statistically significant difference in patients without hyponatremia between tolvaptan and placebo treatment ($P > 0.05$, **a**), also in cirrhotic patients with hyponatremia($P > 0.05$, **b**).However, the survival of patients with resolved serum sodium was significantly higher than of those unresolved serum sodium either tolvaptan or placebo treatment($P < 0.01$, **c**)

not detect any tolvaptan-associated alterations in serum ALT and TBIL levels (data not shown).

Discussions

Hyponatremia is tightly associated with cirrhotic complications, including hepatic encephalopathy, refractory ascites, renal failure, spontaneous bacterial peritonitis, and hepatic hydrothorax, and concomitant high mortality [11]. Tolvaptan is a recently FDA approved drug used to treat hyponatremia in cirrhotic patients. Given only several clinical trials of tolvaptan have been published to date [11–16], including for treatment of liver cirrhotic patients with refractory ascites [17], the safety and efficacy of this drug in cirrhotic patients are not clarified yet. It is unknown to date whether tolvaptan treatment improves the survival of cirrhotic patients. It is also not clear whether tolvaptan has similar or different efficacy in cirrhotic patients with different degree of hyponatremia. A single-center retrospective study in Japan included 95 cirrhotic patients who received tolvaptan for ascites treatment [9]. Among patients with hyponatremia (serum sodium level < 135 mEq/L), 60.0% achieved a normal level after 1 week treatment, and the survival rate was significantly higher in patients with a normalized serum sodium level.

In this prospective cohort study, which comprised 249 cirrhotic patients with ascites from three clinical trials

and five medical centers, we investigated the impact of tolvaptan on six-month mortality of cirrhotic patients with different levels of serum sodium. We found that low dosage of tolvaptan (7.5 mg/day or 15 mg/day) treatment for 7 days significantly improved six-month survival of decompensated cirrhotic patient with hyponatremia. Compared to placebo-treated patients whose six-month survival rate was 68.97%, 89.94% of decompensated cirrhotic patients with hyponatremia survived after tolvaptan treatment. Survival in tolvaptan-treated patients was determined by whether they responded to tolvapatan or not. Hyponatremic patients who restored normal levels of serum sodium after tolvaptan treatment (tolvaptan responders) demonstrated a six-month survival rate of 89.31%, whereas those with refractory hyponatremia (non-responders) only had a 24% survival rate. The baseline serum sodium levels were closely associated with the efficacy of tolvaptan. Compared to the impressive benefit of tolvaptan on cirrhotic patients with mild and moderate hyponatremia whose six-month survival rate was more than 50%, the drug seems to have limited effects on cirrhotic patients with severe hyponatremia. Among 6 patients with severe hyponatremia, only 2 patients survived and maintained normal serum sodium levels 6 months after tolvaptan treatment. The result is consistent with two previous studies [18, 19]. It is unknown why severe hyponatremia in cirrhotic patients is difficult to treat with tolvaptan. The existence of an adaptive renal response to chronic hyponatremia, which results in a diminished response to a selective antagonist such as tolvaptan, might be an explanation [20].

In contrast to its efficacy of tolvaptan in cirrhotic patients with hyponatremia, tolvaptan did not significantly alter serum sodium concentration and improve survival in cirrhotic patients without hyponatremia. Interestingly, placebo-treated patients who recovered from hyponatremia had significantly higher survival outcome than those who didn't. These results argue a crucial role of restoring hyponatremia for cirrhosis recovery. More than 80% hyponatremic patients who did not respond to tolvaptan treatment died of hepatorenal syndrome (data not shown). Therefore, it is very important to predict the therapeutic response to tolvaptan in clinical practice. Several recent clinical studies showed that serum BUN/ Cr ratio ≥ 17.5, urine Na/K ratio < 3.09, and decreased urinary aquaporin 2 levels were predictive of being non-responsiveness to tolvaptan [21–23]. It is not totally clear why a short tolvaptan administration can improve survival in cirrhotic patients. Based on current knowledge, hyponatremia is the most important factors affecting the prognosis of patients with cirrhosis and ascites [2, 11]. Resolved hyponatremia may directly reduce the risk of hepatic encephalopathy, hepatorenal syndrome and spontaneous peritonitis in decompensated cirrhotic patients, which may directly improve survival in patients who respond to tolvaptan treatment [9]. This might partially explain why the survival is significantly improved in resolved hyponatremia patients following tolvaptan treatment.

Considering the safety of patients, this clinical trial adopted low dosages of tolvaptan. These dosages are safe. No tolvaptan-associated side effects were reported in this study. Notably, whether increasing dosage can improve the efficacy of tolvaptan and thus increase response rate or survival rates in responders should be further investigated in the future clinical studies.

Conclusions
Taken together, we found that the six-month survival may be improved in cirrhotic patients with hyponatremia after tolvaptan short administration, particularly in tolvaptan responders. Severity of hyponatremia in cirrhotic patients impacts the response of tovalptan. The underlying mechanisms should be further investigated.

Abbreviations
ALT: Alanine aminotransferase; AST: Aspartate aminotransferase; TBIL: Total bilirubin

Acknowledgements
The authors would like to acknowledge Mrs.Zhang wei for statistical analysis assistance of the Beijing Otsuka Pharmaceutical Co., Ltd., China.

Funding
This study was supported by the Beijing Natural Science Foundation-Beijing Municipal Committee of Education (KZ201810025037), the State Key Projects Specialized on Infectious Diseases(2017ZX10203202–004, 2017ZX10201201–008), Beijing Municipal Administration of Hospitals Clinical Medicine Development of special funding (ZYLX201610), and Beijing Municipal Administration of Hospitals'Ascent Plan (DFL20151602).

Authors' contributions
Conception and design: WSZ, ZX and DHG, Analysis and interpretation of data: WSZ,WHL and DHG. Drafting the manuscript: WSZ,LR and DHG. Patients' care, follow-up and acquisition of data: ZX,HT, XW, LYG, and MH. Revising the manuscript and language polishing: WHL, LR and DHG. All authors read and approved the final manuscript. All authors agreed to be accountable for all aspects of the work in ensuring that questions related to the accuracy or integrity of any part of the work are appropriately investigated and resolved.

Consent for publication
Not applicable.

Competing interests
The authors have no competing interest.

Author details
[1]Department of Gastroenterology and Hepatology, Beijing You'an Hospital, Affiliated with Capital Medical University, Fengtai District, Beijing 100069, China. [2]Department of Gastroenterology, Tianjin Third Central Hospital, Tianjin, China. [3]Department of Hepatology, Beijing Ditan Hospital, Affiliated with Capital Medical University, Beijing, China. [4]Department of Hepatology, PLA 302 Hospital, Beijing, China. [5]Liver Diseases Center, Beijing Friendship Hospital, Affiliated with Capital Medical University, Beijing, China. [6]Department of Medicine II, Section Molecular Hepatology, Medical Faculty Mannheim, Heidelberg University, Mannheim, Germany.

References
1. Moore CM, Van Thiel DH. Cirrhotic ascites review: pathophysiology, diagnosis and management. World J Hepatol. 2013;5:251–63.
2. Yu C, SharmaN SS. Hyponatremia: clinical associations, prognosis, and treatment in cirrhosis. ExpClin Transplant. 2013;11:3–11.
3. Gordon FD. Ascites. Clin Liver Dis. 2012;16:285–99.
4. Runyon BA, AASLD. Introduction to the revised American Association for the Study of Liver Diseases Practice Guideline management of adult patients with ascites due to cirrhosis, 2012. Hepatology. 2013;57:1651–3.
5. Leiva JG, Salgado JM, Estradas J, Torre A, Uribe M. Pathophysiology of ascites and dilutional hyponatremia: contemporary use of aquaretic agents. Ann Hepatol. 2007;6:214–21.
6. Josiassen RC, Curtis J, Filmyer DM, Audino B, Skuban N, Shaughnessy RA. Tolvaptan: a new tool for the effective treatment of hyponatremia in psychotic disorders. Expert Opin Pharmacother. 2010;11:637–48.
7. Sakaida I, Kawazoe S, Kajimura K, Saito T, Okuse C, Takaguchi K, et al. Tolvaptan for improvement of hepatic edema: a phase 3, multicenter, randomized, double-blind, placebo-controlled trial. Hepatol Res. 2014;44:73–82.
8. Berl T, Quittnat-Pelletier F, Verbalis JG, Schrier RW, Bichet DG, Ouyang J, et al. Oral tolvaptan is safe and effective in chronic hyponatremia. J Am SocNephrol. 2010;21:705–12.
9. Kogiso T, Kobayashi M, Yamamoto K, Ikarashi Y, Kodama K, Taniai M, et al. The outcome of cirrhotic patients with ascites is improved by the

normalization of the serum sodium level by tolvaptan. Intern Med. 2017;56: 2993–3001.

10. Wang YF, Tang JT, Han T, Ding HG, Ye WJ, Wang MR, et al. Tolvaptan in Chinese cirrhotic patients with ascites: a randomized, placebo-controlled phase 2 trial. J Dig Dis. 2018;19:144–54.

11. Umemura T, Shibata S, Sekiguchi T, Kitabatake H, Nozawa Y, Okuhara S, et al. Serum sodium concentration is associated with increased risk of mortality in patients with compensated liver cirrhosis. Hepatol Res. 2015;45: 739–44.

12. Cárdenas A, Ginès P, Marotta P, et al. The safety and efficacy of tolvaptan, an oral vasopressin antagonist in the treatment of hyponatremia in cirrhosis. J Hepatol. 2012;56:571–8.

13. Yan L, Xie F, Lu J, Ni Q, Shi C, Tang C, Yang J. The treatment of vasopressin V2-receptor antagonists in cirrhosis patients with ascites: a meta-analysis of randomized controlled trials. BMC Gastroenterol. 2015;15:65.

14. Kogiso T, Tokushige K, Hashimoto E, Ikarashi Y, Kodama K, Taniai M, et al. Safety and efficacy of long-term tolvaptan therapy for decompensated liver cirrhosis. Hepatol Res. 2016;46:E194–200.

15. Zhang X, Wang SZ, Zheng JF, Zhao WM, Li P, Fan CL, et al. Clinical efficacy of tolvaptan for treatment of refractory ascites in liver cirrhosis patients. World J Gastroenterol. 2014;20:11400–5.

16. Akiyama S, Ikeda K, Sezaki H, Fukushima T, Sorin Y, Kawamura Y, et al. Therapeutic effects of short- and intermediate-term tolvaptan administration for refractory ascites in patients with advanced liver cirrhosis. Hepatol Res. 2015;45:1062–70.

17. Wang SZ, Ding HG. New therapeutic paradigm and concepts for patients with cirrhotic refractory ascites. Zhonghua Gan Zang Bing Za Zhi. 2017;25: 249–53.

18. Pose E, Solà E, Piano S, Gola E, Graupera I, Guevara M, et al. Limited efficacy of Tolvaptan in patients with cirrhosis and severe Hyponatremia: real-life experience. Am J Med. 2017;130:372–5.

19. Ahluwalia V, Heuman DM, Feldman G, Wade JB, Thacker LR, Gavis E, et al. Correction of hyponatraemia improves cognition, quality of life, and brain oedema in cirrhosis. J Hepatol. 2015;62:75–82.

20. Esteva-Font C, Baccaro ME, Fernández-Llama P, Sans L, Guevara M, Ars E, et al. Aquaporin-1 and aquaporin-2 urinary excretion in cirrhosis: relationship with ascites and hepatorenal syndrome. Hepatology. 2006;44: 1555–63.

21. Nakai M, Ogawa K, Takeda R, Ohara M, Kawagishi N, Izumi T, et al. Increased serum C-reactive protein and decreased urinary aquaporin 2 levels are predictive of the efficacy of tolvaptan in patients with liver cirrhosis. Hepatol Res. 2018;48:E311–9.

22. Komiyama Y, Kurosaki M, Nakanishi H, Takahashi Y, Itakura J, Yasui Y, et al. Prediction of diuretic response to tolvaptan by a simple, readily available spot urine Na/K ratio. PLoS One. 2017;12:e0174649.

23. Kawaratani H, Fukui H, Moriya K, Noguchi R, Namisaki T, Uejima M, et al. Predictive parameter of tolvaptan effectiveness in cirrhotic ascites. Hepatol Res. 2017;47:854–61.

12

Apatinib affect VEGF-mediated cell proliferation, migration, invasion via blocking VEGFR2/RAF/MEK/ERK and PI3K/AKT pathways in cholangiocarcinoma cell

Manping Huang[1], Bin Huang[1], Guowen Li[1] and Sainan Zeng[2*]

Abstract

Background: Cholangiocarcinoma (CCA) is a form of cancer that easily aggress to contiguous structures. Vascular endothelial growth factor (VEGF) and VEGF receptor 2 (VEGFR2) are increased in majority species of cancers and suppress tumor progression by blocking VEGF/VEGFR2. Apatinib is a highly selective VEGFR2 antagonist which has inhibitive effect on antiapoptotic and cell growth in CCA. While, the effect of apatinib cell migration and invasion in CCA is still unknown.

Methods: CCA cell lines QBC939 and TFK-1 were transfected with siKDR to establish the KDR function loss cell model, and recombined human VEGF (rhVEGF) protein was added into the culture medium to enhance the VEGF expression. RT-qPCR and western bloting were used to detect the mRNA and protein expression levels of VEGFR2 to investigate whether it was effectively repressed or activated with rhVEGF or apatinib treatment. Then, MTT, wound healing assay, and transwell matrix assay were applied to measure the effect of apatinib and rhVEGF on cell viability, migration and invasion, respectively.

Results: The mRNA and protein expressions of VEGFR2 were significantly reduced with KDR RNAi in both QBC939 and TFK-1 cells, and rhVEGF treatment increased these expression levels ($p < 0.05$). Apatinib dramatically suppressed VEGF-mediated cell migration and invasion at the concentration of 100 nM treatment and significantly decreased the expression of metastasis-associated protein such as Slug, snail and MMP9. Moreover, all of these inhibiting effects of apatinib depended on the VEGFR2 existence. In addition, VEGFR2/RAF/MEK/ERK and PI3K/AKT signal pathways were enhanced by the introduction of rhVEGF, but were dramatically suppressed after the apatinib treatment.

Conclusion: Apatinib inhibit VEGF-mediated cell migration and invasion in CCA cell lines via inhibiting the VEGFR2/RAF/MEK/ERK and PI3K/AKT pathways. It will be a potentially effective targeted drug for CCA.

Keywords: Cholangiocarcinoma, Apatinib, VEGF, KDR (VEGFR2), RAF/MEK/ERK pathway, PI3K/AKT pathway

Background

Cholangiocarcinoma(CCA), also known as bile duct cancer, is a form of cancer that originates in the epithelial cells of bile ducts, along intrahepatic and extrahepatic biliary tree, that is defined as intrahepatic, peri-hilar and distal CCA [4, 22]. Due to the high aggressive ability, CCA could easily infiltrate into adjacent organs such like liver, hepatic artery and portal vein [29]. The infiltration patterns of CCA were distributed in lymph, vascular infiltration site, and lymph node metastases, which is a basic feature of CCA [6, 12].

Vascular endothelial growth factor (VEGF), originally known as vascular permeability factor (VPF), is a signal protein produced by epithelial cells [23]. It has been identified as a key player in neovascularization and cell proliferation in a variety of cancers, including the fatal biliary CCA [5, 21]. Clinical data shows VEGF was significantly

* Correspondence: zengsainan1121@163.com
[2]Infection Controlling Center, The Third Xiangya Hospital of Central South University, Tongzipo Road, Yuelu District, Changsha 410013, People's Republic of China
Full list of author information is available at the end of the article

increased in the biopsy samples of CCA [2, 18, 26]. Furthermore, there is evidences that blocking VEGF/VEGFR2 pathway can effectively inhibit the proliferation, migration, invasion, survival and adhesion ability of hepatocellular carcinoma, hyperplastic cholangiocyte and non-small cell lung cancer [14, 32].

Apatinib, a tyrosine kinase inhibitor that selectively inhibits the vascular endothelial growth factor receptor-2 (VEGFR2, also known as KDR), could significantly inhibit intracellular VEGF signaling [28]. Benefiting from the blocking effect of VEGF pathway, apatinib play a prominent role in inhibiting tumor cells anti-apoptosis, cells proliferation in vitro and repressing the growth of xenograft tumor in vivo [19, 20]. In additon, apatinib reveals inhibition effect on migration and invasion in KIF5B-RET driven tumors therapy [13]. However, up to now there are currently few studies on the impact of CCA migration and invasion. In this study, we investigated the role of apatinib in CCA migration and invasion via the QBC939 and TFK-1 cell line. Moreover, we also explored the potential mechanism that the inhibition effect of apatinib may via VEGFR2/RAF/MEK/ERK and PI3K/AKT pathways.

Methods

Cell culture and transfection

Human CCA cell lines QBC939 and TFK-1 were purchased from Suer Biological Inc. (Shanghai, China). QBC939 cells were cultured in Dulbecco's Modified Eagle Medium (DMEM, Sigma-Aldrich, St. Louis, MO, USA) and TFK-1 cells were cultured in RPMI-1640 medium (Gibco-BRL, Gaithersburg, MD), both supplemented with 10% heat-inactivated fetal bovine serum (Gibco; Thermo Fisher Scientific, Inc., Waltham, MA, USA), and incubated at 37 °C with 5% CO_2.

Cells were sub-cultured to 6-well plates until the confluence reached 80%. The final concentration 50 mM siKDR and siControl (labeled with a fluorescent, synthesize by Gene Pharma, Suzhou, China) were diluted in serum-free MEM, and gently mixed with Lipofectamine 2000 (6 μl/well, Sigma-Aldrich, St. Louis, MO, USA) following 5 min stand, respectively. Before added this mixture to cells, another 20 min stand at room temperature is needed. The transfected cells incubated at 37 °C with 5% CO_2 for 8 h, and then change the medium into McCoy's 5A medium containing 10% FBS without antibiotics. 24 h post transfection, the transfection efficiency was checked by fluorescence detection.

RT-qPCR

VEGFR2 mRNA levels from two group cells were tested by RT-qPCR. The first group cells were transfected with siKDR and siControl for 24 h. Cells in the second group was treated with 0, 20, 50, 100, and 200 ng/ml recombinant human VEGF (rhVEGF, PeproTech, 100–20-2)

for 2 h. Cells were subsequently homogenized and centrifuged (12,000 x g, 10 min, 4 °C) using TRIzol reagent (Sigma-Aldrich, St. Louis, MO, USA) for total RNA extraction. RNA purity and concentration were determined by Nano-Drop (Thermo Scientific).

1 mg total RNA was reverse transcribed into cDNA using GoScript™ RT system (Promega, Madison, WI, USA). qPCR was performed in triplicate as: 95 °C for 30 s, 40 cycles of 95 °C for 5 s, 58 °C for 10 s and 72 °C for 30 s, subsequently analyze melting curve. GAPDH was used as the reference gene. Primers (forward, reverse) were: VEGFR2 5'-GGAC TCTCTCTGCCTACCTCAC-3', 5'-GGCTCTTTCGCT TACTGTTCTG-3', GAPDH 5'-AGAAGGCTGGGGCT CATTTG-3', reverse 5'-AGGGGCCATCCACAGTCTT C-3'. The relative fold change of VEGFR2 was calculated by $2^{-\Delta\Delta Ct}$ method.

MTT assay

After QBC939 cells and TFK-1 cells were cultured to 96-well plates (1×10^5 cells/well) overnight, three conditions of drug treatment were set: (1) cells treated with 0, 10, 100, 1000 and 10,000 nM apatinib (MCE, HY13342) for 24 h; (2) cells treated with 0, 20, 50, 100 and 200 ng/ml rhVEGF for 2 h; (3) cells treated with 100 ng/ml rhVEGF for 2 h following treated with 10, 100, 1000 and 10,000 nM apatinib for 24 h And then cells were cultured for another 24 h, 10 mg/ml MTT was added and incubated for further 4 h. After that, cells were centrifuged at 1,000×g for 5 min at room temperature, removed supernatant, and added 100 μl DMSO to each well for 30 min to dissolve the formazan product. The optical density (OD) was measured at 492 nm by a microplate reader (FLx800; BioTek, Winooski, VT, USA). The relative cell viability was normalized with control group using optical density values.

Wound healing assay

Cells were cultured to 6-well plates (2×10^5 cells/well) until about 100% confluence. 100 nM apatinib or 100 ng/ml rhVEGF + 100 nM apatinib were added into medium and cultured 24 h. 200 μl pipette tip was used to create a wound gap on cell monolayer, and Olympus IX71 microscope (Olympus Corporation, Tokyo, Japan) at 100 times magnification was used for imaging immediately. Migration was then observed 24 h post wound scratched. Image-Pro Plus software (Media Cybernetics, Inc., Rockville, MD, USA) was used to calculated the relative migration distant% as: [(The relative distance recorded at 0 h - the relative distance recorded at 24 h)/the relative distance recorded at 0 h] × 100.

Transwell matrix assay

Control and siKDR transfected cells (1×10^4 cells/well) were incubated into the top chamber of matrigel coated polyethylene terephthalate membrane (50 μl/well, Corning,

Corning, USA), and 100 nM apatinib or 100 ng/ml rhVEGF were added into the upper chamber,. After culturing for 24 h, cells in the upper chamber were removed gentlyand the invaded cells left at the bottom of chamber were fixed with 4% paraformaldehyde for 30 min and then stained with 0.1% crystal violet for 30 min. Following by counting under an optical microscope (Olympus Corporation, Tokyo, Japan) at a magnification of 200.

Western blotting

After cells treated with/without 100 ng/ml rhVEGF, 100 nM apatinib or 100 ng/ml rhVEGF + 100 nM apatinib, cells were lysed using lysis buffer (Cell Signaling Technology, Danvers, USA) to extract total protein. Protein lysates were separated by 10% SDS-PAGE, followed by transfer to nitrocellulose membranes. The membrane was then blocked with 5% milk diluted in PBS at room temperature for 1 h, followed by incubated with 1:1000 VEGFR2 antibody (ab10972, Abcam, Cambridge, MA, USA),1:5000 p-VEGFR2 (ab38473, Abcam), 1:2000 p-MEK (2338, CST), 1:1000 MEK (4694, CST), 1:2000 p-ERK1/2 (4370, CST), 1:1000 ERK (4695, CST), 1:2000 slug (ab51772, Abcam), 1:3000 Snail (ab53519, Abcam), 1:2500 MMP9 (ab38898, Abcam), 1:1500 P-AKT (ab81283, Abcam), 1:1500 AKT (ab179463, Abcam) and 1:5000 GAPDH antibody (ab8245, Abcam) overnight at 4 °C separately. Once primary antibodies were washed, membrane was incubated with goat anti-rabbit horseradish peroxidase-labeled secondary antibody (Sangon Biotech, Shanghai, China). Protein bands were detected by incubating the membrane with Western Bright enhanced chemiluminescence working solution (Advansta, Menlo Park, CA, USA). The film (Kodak XBT-1, Carestream, Xiamen, China) was scanned with Bio-rad Gel Doc XR+ (BIO-RAD, Shanghai, China).

Statistical analyses

Statistical analysis was conducted with the Social Sciences software version 17.0. Quantitative data were presented as mean ± SD. The two-tailed Student's t test was applied to analyze statistical differences between two groups. For multiple comparisons, the one-way ANOVA was used to analyze the difference. $p < 0.05$ was considered to be statistically significant. Each test data was repeated at least three times.

Results

RNA interference reduced VEGFR2 mRNA and protein levels in QBC939 and TFK-1 cells

q-PCR and western blotting were performed to investigate the mRNA and protein levels of VEGFR2 in si-KDR or si-Control transfected QBC939 and TFK-1 cells. VEGFR2 mRNA level reduced significantly, showed five and two times lower in siKDR group compared to siControl group in QBC939and TFK-1 cells, respectively ($p < 0.01$; Fig. 1a). Similarly, the protein level also reduced about 2-fold which caused by siKDR (Fig. 1b-c). Both q-PCR and western blotting results suggested KDR interference significantly reduced VEGFR2 expression in both mRNA and protein levels.

VEGF activated VEGFR2 and promoted proliferation in QBC939 and TFK-1 cells

After 2 h treatment of 0, 20, 50, 100, or 200 ng/ml rhVEGF, VEGFR2 mRNA and protein level were detected by q-PCR and western blotting. Results showedVEGFR2 mRNA level elevated along the increasing concentration of rhVEGF treatment and reached peak value at 100 ng/ml, which was about 5-fold compared to control group (Fig. 2a). Moreover, VEGFR2 mRNA level kept stable when rhVEGF concentration higher than 100 ng/ml (Fig. 2a). Similarly, the intensity of VEGFR2 protein bands appeared stronger continuously accompany the increasing concentration of rhVEGF treatment and reached strongest at 100 ng/ml rhVEGF (Fig. 2b). These data showed 100 ng/ml rhVEGF is the most suitable concentration for activating VEGFR2.

Following that, MTT assay was performed to show that 100 ng/ml rhVEGF had a significant greater (1.4-fold) enhancement of relative cell viability compared to control ($p < 0.05$; Fig. 2c), suggested that rhVEGF promoted cell viability in QBC939 and TFK-1 cells effectively. In addition, we analyzed the protein level of VEGFR2 by western blot, and found rhVEGF caused a significant increase of VEGFR2 while siKDR caused a significant reduction. However, 100 ng/ml rhVEGF did not significantly reverse the decrease of VEGFR2 in the KDR knockout group ($p < 0.01$; Fig. 2d).

Apatinib inhibites the migration and invasion of QBC939 and TFK-1 cells

There were no changes of relative cell viability on both QBC939 and TFK-1 cells with 10 and 100 nM apatinib treatment, but 1,000 and 10,000 nM apatinib caused a greatly reduction of relative cell viability compared to control group, suggested 1,000 nM and higher concentration of apatinib could cause cytotoxicity on CCA cells (Fig. 3a). However, we found 100 nM apatinib was enough for CCA cell lines QBC939 and TFK-1 to cause migation and invasion inhibition ($p < 0.01$; Fig. 3b, and $p < 0.05$, $p < 0.01$, respectively; Fig. 3c), Furthermore, metastatic marker Slug, snail and MMP9 protein levels in the cells treated with or without 100 nM apatinib were detected by western blot. Result showed that apatinib could significantly inhibit the protein expression of Slug, snail and MMP9 (Fig. 3d). All these data suggested that apatinib has the effection on inhibiting cell migration and invasion of CCA.

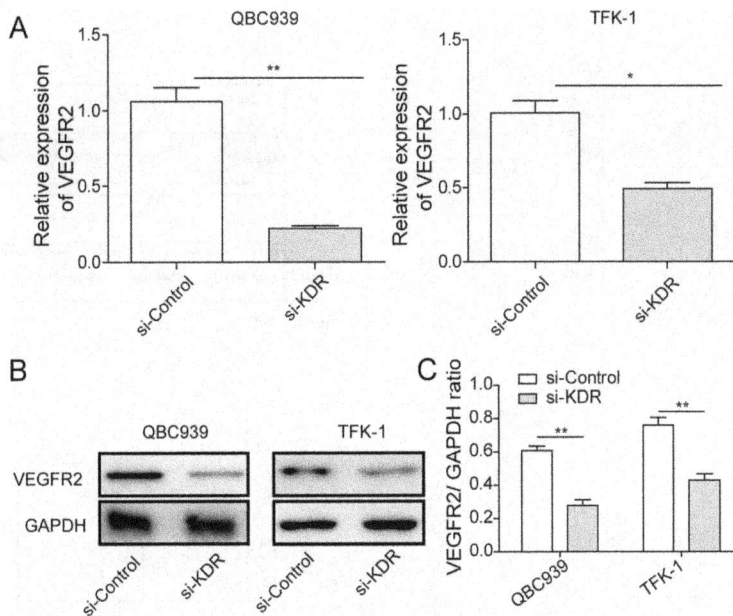

Fig. 1 VEGFR2 expression in QBC939 and TFK-1 cells transfected with siKDR or siControl. **a** Cells were transfected with 50 nM siKDR or siControl for 48 h. qRT-PCR was performed to evaluate the mRNA level of VEGFR2 Data shown are means ± SD ($n = 3$). **$P < 0.01$ and * $P < 0.05$ in QBC939 and TFK-1 cells versus si-Control group, respectively. **b** Protein expression of VEGFR2 in transfected QBC939 and TFK-1 cells were also detected by western-blotting. GAPDH was detected as reference. **c** Densitometric analysis of the autoradiographic plaques of these proteins is shown on the Fig. 1b. Data shown are means ± SD ($n = 3$). **$P < 0.01$ in QBC939 and TFK-1 cells versus si-Control group

Apatinib played an essential role on VEGF-mediated migration and invasion in QBC939 and TFK-1 cells

The effect of apatinib on VEGF-mediated cell viability was determined by MTT assay, that total 6 groups were set using increased concentration of apatinib from 0 nM to 10,000 nM with 100 ng/ml rhVEGF. 100 ng/ml rhVEGF significantly increased relative cell viability about 26%compared to control group ($p < 0.05$, $p < 0.01$, respectively Fig. 4a, b). In addition to this, 10 nM and 100 nM apatinib reverses the viability caused by 100 ng/ml VEGF to the normal rate ($p < 0.05$). But 1,000 nM and the higher concentration showed cytotoxicity in both QBC939 and TFK-1 cells (Fig. 4a, b).

Followed that, wound healing was performed to detect the effect of apatinib (100 nM) on VEGF-mediated QBC939 and TFK-1 cell migration. On siControl group, the wound width significantly reduced 24 h post rhVEGF treatment), while, apatinib treatment suppressed this reduction effectively ($p < 0.001$; Fig. 4c, d). However, on siKDR group, rhVEGF and apatinib treatment showed no significant differenceon wound width as a cause of VEGFR2 knock-down (Fig. 4c, d). These data revealed rhVEGF facilitates QBC939 and TFK-1 cell migration, and apatinib can reverse thiseffect in a VEGFR2 dependent manner.Next, transwell assays were conducted to assess the invasion ability of rhVEGF-induced cells with or without apatinib. On siControl group, rhVEGF significantly promoted the invasion of QBC939 and TFK-1 cells ($p < 0.01$; Fig. 5a), but this invasion was

totally suppressed by apatinib ($p < 0.01$; Fig. 5a). However, cells in the rhVEGF and apatinib treating groups had little difference of invasion ability when KDR expression is disturbed (Fig. 5a). Protein levels of metastatic marker slug, snail, MMP9 were also detected, in siControl group, 100 ng/ml rhVEGF significantly promoted the protein expression of slug, snail and MMP9, but 100 nM apatinib dramatically reverse this elevation effect. On the contrary, the protein levels of Slug, snail and MMP9 were stable with rhVEGF and apatinib treatment in the siKDR group (Fig. 5b). These results would reveal that effect of apatinib on AAC cell invasion relying on the presence of VEGFR2.

Apatinib suppresses VEGF/VEGFR2-mediated signaling through the RAF/MEK/ERK and AKT signaling pathways

Western blotting was performed on siControl and siKDR transfection cells which treated 100 ng/ml rhVEGF with/without 100 nM apatinib, to determine the signaling pathway related to VEGF and its receptor VEGFR2. The expression of p-VEGFR2, VEGR2, RAF, p-MEK, MEK, p-ERK1/2, ERK1/2, p-AKT and AKT were examined, since RAF, MEK and ERK1/2 are the downstream pathway molecules of VEGFR2. Treatment with rhVEGF significantly increased the phosphorylation and total protein of VEGFR2, RAF, phosphorylated MEK, ERK1/2 and AKT protein expression level in siControl group, but had little influence on total protein level of MEK ERK1/2 and AKT

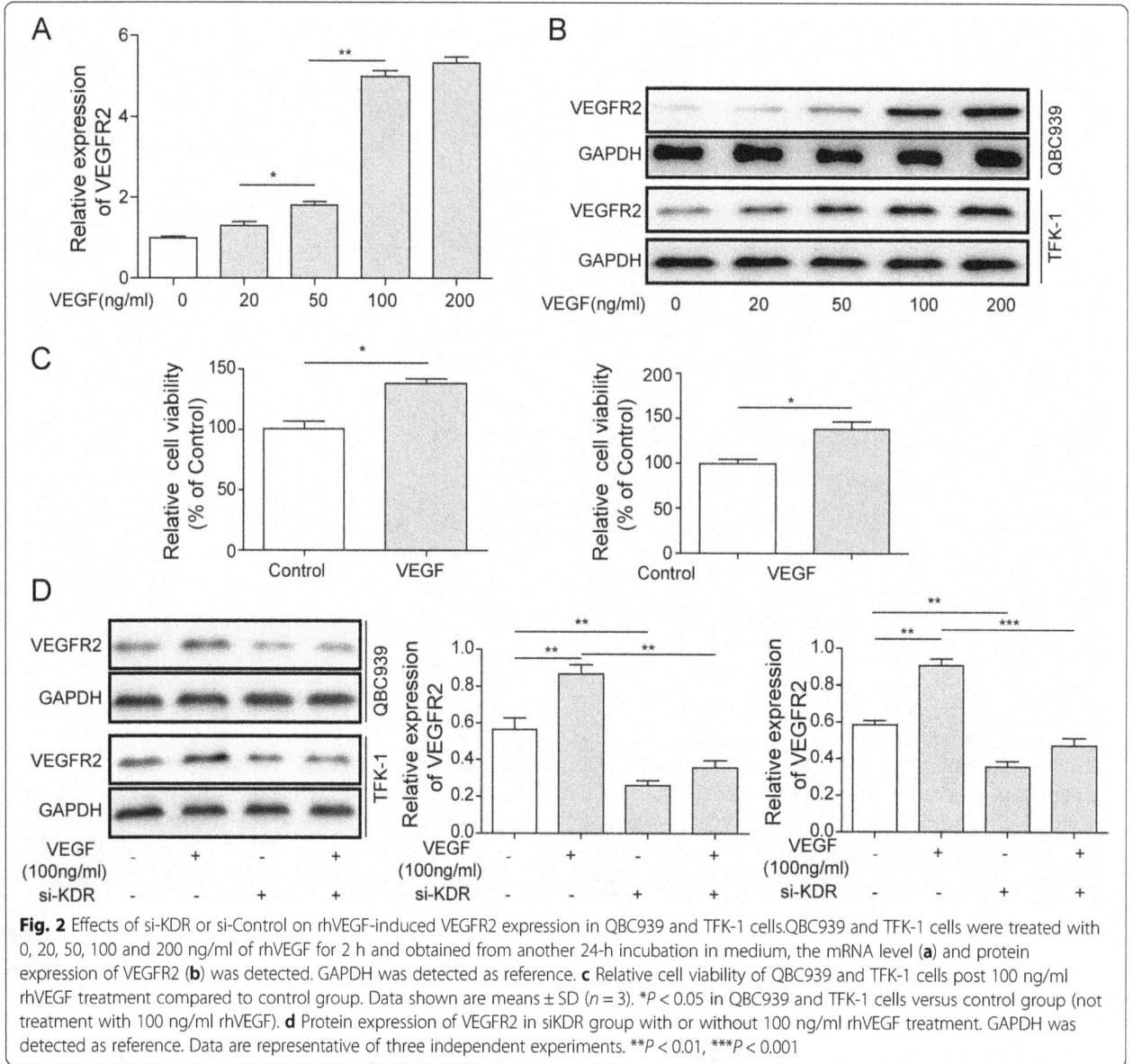

Fig. 2 Effects of si-KDR or si-Control on rhVEGF-induced VEGFR2 expression in QBC939 and TFK-1 cells.QBC939 and TFK-1 cells were treated with 0, 20, 50, 100 and 200 ng/ml of rhVEGF for 2 h and obtained from another 24-h incubation in medium, the mRNA level (**a**) and protein expression of VEGFR2 (**b**) was detected. GAPDH was detected as reference. **c** Relative cell viability of QBC939 and TFK-1 cells post 100 ng/ml rhVEGF treatment compared to control group. Data shown are means ± SD (*n* = 3). *P < 0.05 in QBC939 and TFK-1 cells versus control group (not treatment with 100 ng/ml rhVEGF). **d** Protein expression of VEGFR2 in siKDR group with or without 100 ng/ml rhVEGF treatment. GAPDH was detected as reference. Data are representative of three independent experiments. **P < 0.01, ***P < 0.001

(Fig. 6a, b). After blocking VEGFR2 by apatinib, the phosphorylation and total protein level of VEGFR2, phosphorylated MEK and ERK1/2 were reverse to basal level (Fig. 6a, b). On the contrary, both rhVEGF and apatinib treatments had no influence on phosphorylation and total protein level of MEK and ERK1/2 in siKDR group (Fig. 6a, b). Phosphorylation and total protein level of VEGFR2, RAF and phosphorylated AKT were expressed very weak in siKDR group, and this weak expression were stable with or without rhVEGF and apatinib treatment (Fig. 6a, b).

Discussion

VEGF exerts its biological effects by combining and activating its receptors, which known as VEGFR2 [8, 27]. Publications reveal VEGF plays key role in CCA as the

high expression level was detected in the patients' tumor tissues [1, 15]. Hence, as the antagonist of VEGFR2, apatinib has the potential to become an effective targeted medicine of CCA [16, 19, 20]. In this study, we firstly confirmed the role of VEGF in QBC939 and TFK-1 cells, and then comfirmed the inhibition functions of apatinib in migration and invasion of these two CCA cell lines. Finally, we analyzed the potential signaling pathways Raf/MEk/ERK and PI3K/AKT that might be influenced by apatinib.

Publication reported VEGF could regulate kinds of cancer cells growth through binding to VEGFR [10]. Results in our study showed that exogenous rhVEGF activated the VEGFR2 expression and promoted the cell viability both in QBC939 and TFK-1 cells. It was consistent with publications that blocking VEGF/VEGFR2

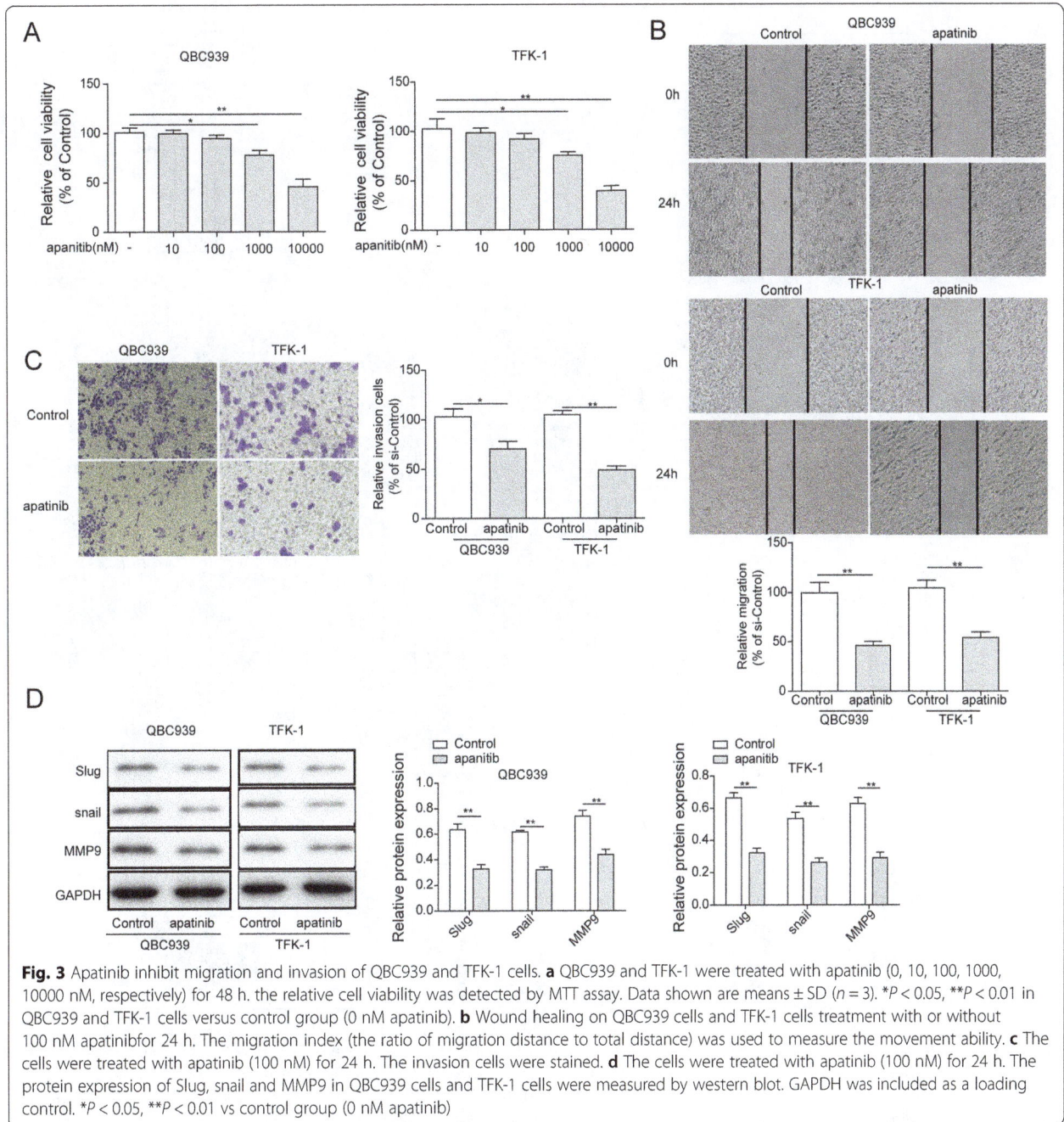

Fig. 3 Apatinib inhibit migration and invasion of QBC939 and TFK-1 cells. **a** QBC939 and TFK-1 were treated with apatinib (0, 10, 100, 1000, 10000 nM, respectively) for 48 h. the relative cell viability was detected by MTT assay. Data shown are means ± SD (n = 3). *P < 0.05, **P < 0.01 in QBC939 and TFK-1 cells versus control group (0 nM apatinib). **b** Wound healing on QBC939 cells and TFK-1 cells treatment with or without 100 nM apatinibfor 24 h. The migration index (the ratio of migration distance to total distance) was used to measure the movement ability. **c** The cells were treated with apatinib (100 nM) for 24 h. The invasion cells were stained. **d** The cells were treated with apatinib (100 nM) for 24 h. The protein expression of Slug, snail and MMP9 in QBC939 cells and TFK-1 cells were measured by western blot. GAPDH was included as a loading control. *P < 0.05, **P < 0.01 vs control group (0 nM apatinib)

pathway have inhibition effect on the growth of cancer cells [7, 14, 32]. Moreover, one paper revealed the role of VEGF in promoting cell growth and inducing the cell apoptosis in CCA [19, 20]. However, whether VEGF was an necessity for tumor migration or invasion in CCA remains unknown.

As the antagonist of VEGFR2, the biological functions of apatinib towards cell migration and invasion in CCA cell lines were performed in this study, and the results provide a first ever comprehensive elucidation of apatinib in anti-CCA progress. We found that it significantly

inhibited cell migration and invasion. Moreover, apatinib significantly decreased the expression of metastatic marker such like Slug, snail, and MMP9 in the CCA cell lines. It was consistent with the previous research in lung adenocarcinomas, which found apatinib inhibits cellular invasion and migration by fusion kinase KIF5B-RET via suppressing RET/Src signaling pathway [13]. In addition, it was report intracellular autocrine VEGF signaling promotes EBDC cell proliferation, which can be inhibited by apatinib [19, 20]. And we also found that exogenous rhVEGF significantly promoted migration and invasion in QBC939 and TFK-1

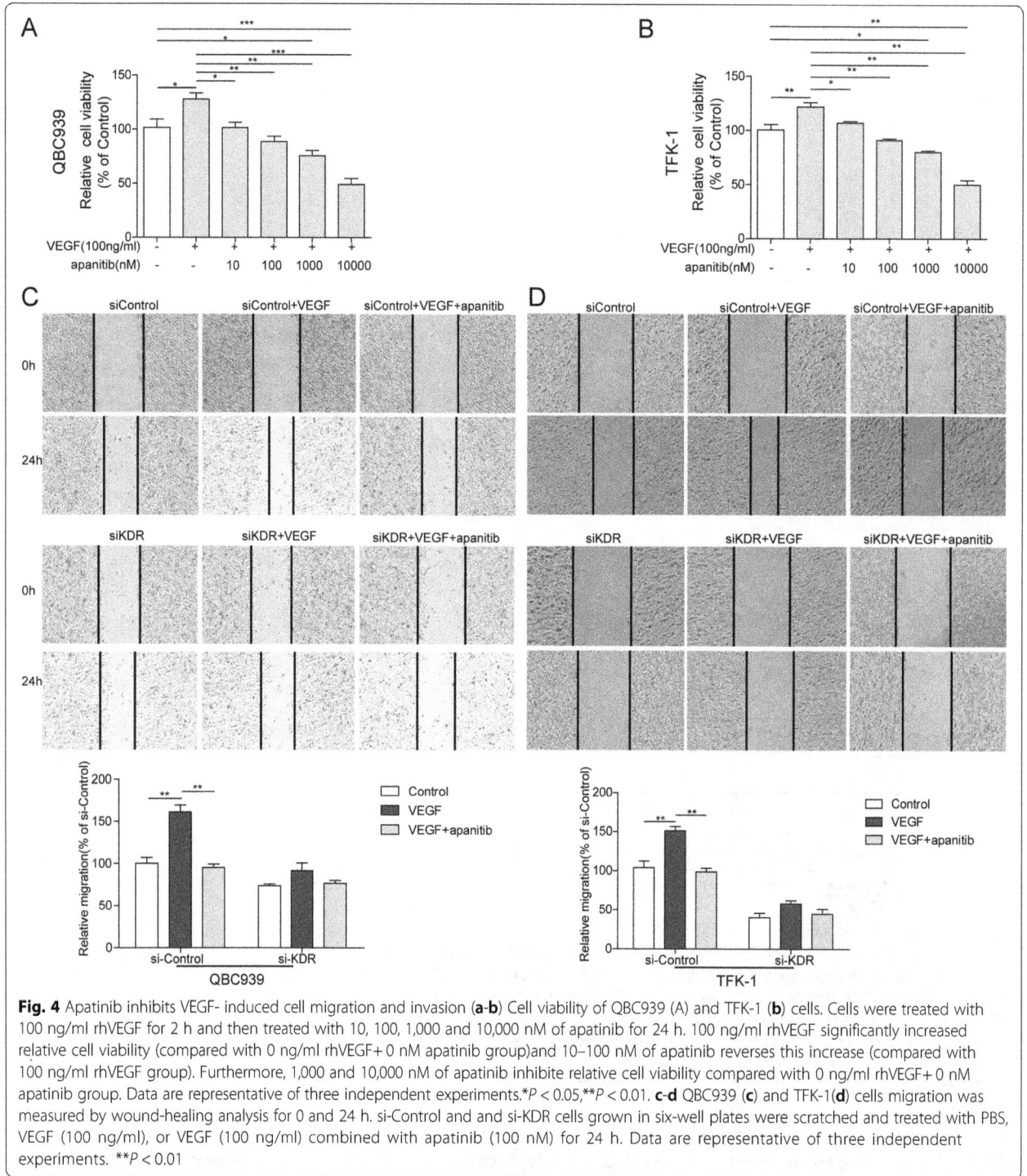

Fig. 4 Apatinib inhibits VEGF- induced cell migration and invasion (**a-b**) Cell viability of QBC939 (A) and TFK-1 (**b**) cells. Cells were treated with 100 ng/ml rhVEGF for 2 h and then treated with 10, 100, 1,000 and 10,000 nM of apatinib for 24 h. 100 ng/ml rhVEGF significantly increased relative cell viability (compared with 0 ng/ml rhVEGF+ 0 nM apatinib group)and 10–100 nM of apatinib reverses this increase (compared with 100 ng/ml rhVEGF group). Furthermore, 1,000 and 10,000 nM of apatinib inhibite relative cell viability compared with 0 ng/ml rhVEGF+ 0 nM apatinib group. Data are representative of three independent experiments.*$P < 0.05$,**$P < 0.01$. **c-d** QBC939 (**c**) and TFK-1(**d**) cells migration was measured by wound-healing analysis for 0 and 24 h. si-Control and and si-KDR cells grown in six-well plates were scratched and treated with PBS, VEGF (100 ng/ml), or VEGF (100 ng/ml) combined with apatinib (100 nM) for 24 h. Data are representative of three independent experiments. **$P < 0.01$

cells, whereas apatinib could reverse these effects. Combine our data and references mentioned above, it exposes the essential role of apatinib in anti-tumour effect, and the apatinib induced inhibition of cell migration and invasion in CCA.

RAF/MEK/ERK pathway has been linked in endothelial cell proliferation [17] and VEGF mediated cell survival [3, 11]. To investigate the possible mechanism of

how apatinib works on CCA cells. We found exogenous rhVEGF markedly elevated phosphorylation and total of VEGFR2 protein, and the major downstream targets: phosphorylation of RAF, MEK and ERK1/2, but did not affect the levels of total MEK and ERK1/2. On the contrary, apatinibprominently inhibited this promotion. These results disclosed apatinib could efficiently inhibit the activation of VEGFR2/RAF/MEK/ERK1/2 signal transduction

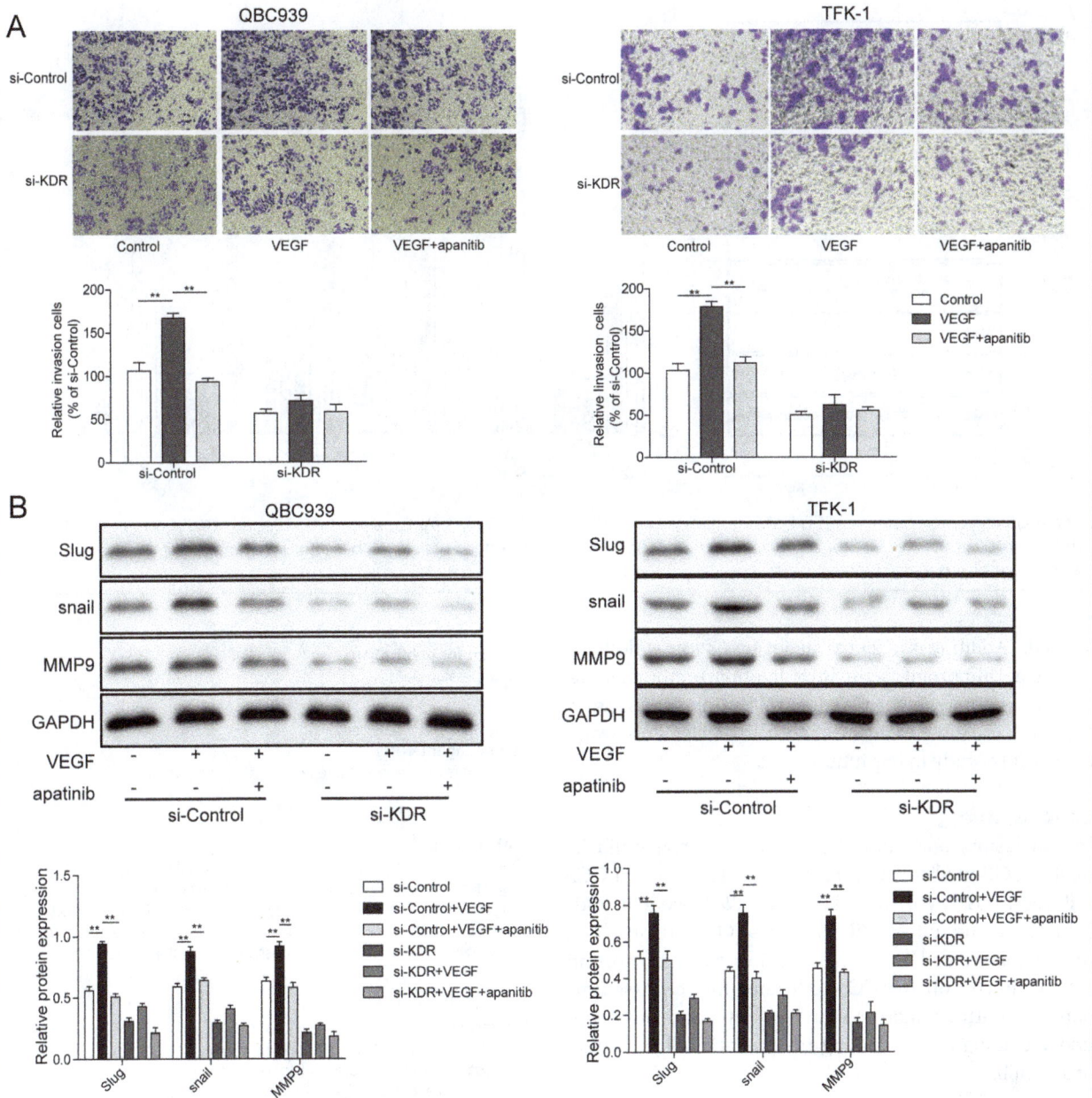

Fig. 5 Apatinib inhibits VEGF- induced cell invasion. **a** Representative images of transwell (up) and quantification of invasion cell number (bottom). si-Control and and si-KDR cells grown in six-well plates were scratched and treated with PBS, VEGF (100 ng/ml), or VEGF (100 ng/ml) combined with apatinib (100 nM) for 24 h. Data are representative of three independent experiments. **P < 0.01. **b** Protein expression of Slug, snail and MMP9 in si-Control and si-KDR cells when treated with 100 ng/ml rhVEGF or 100 ng/ml rhVEGF + 100 nM apatinib for 24 h. GAPDH was detected as reference. **P < 0.01

which was induced by VEGF, Besides, we also checked the PI3K/AKT pathway, which was identified as a VEGF related signaling pathway [9, 19, 20, 31]. Same results were gained such like the detection of RAF/MEK/ERK1/2 pathway, which provided another molecular mechanism of apatinib acted on CCA cells. These results are supported by several studies that the anti-apoptosis effect of VEGF closely related to PI3K/AKT/mTOR signaling pathway [9, 19, 20, 31]. Previous studies has revealed that both VEGF/

MEK/ERK and PI3K/AKT pathways play key role in developing CCA [9, 24, 25, 30]. Here, we found that apatinib could reverse the rhVEGF induced cell migration and invasion by blocking these two pathways. Combined with our data and references we have mentioned above, apatinib has an important role in CCA migration and invasion, and apatinib exerts excellent anti-tumor function in CCA cell lines. However, whether apatinib could perform the same antitumor function of CCA in vivo still needs to be

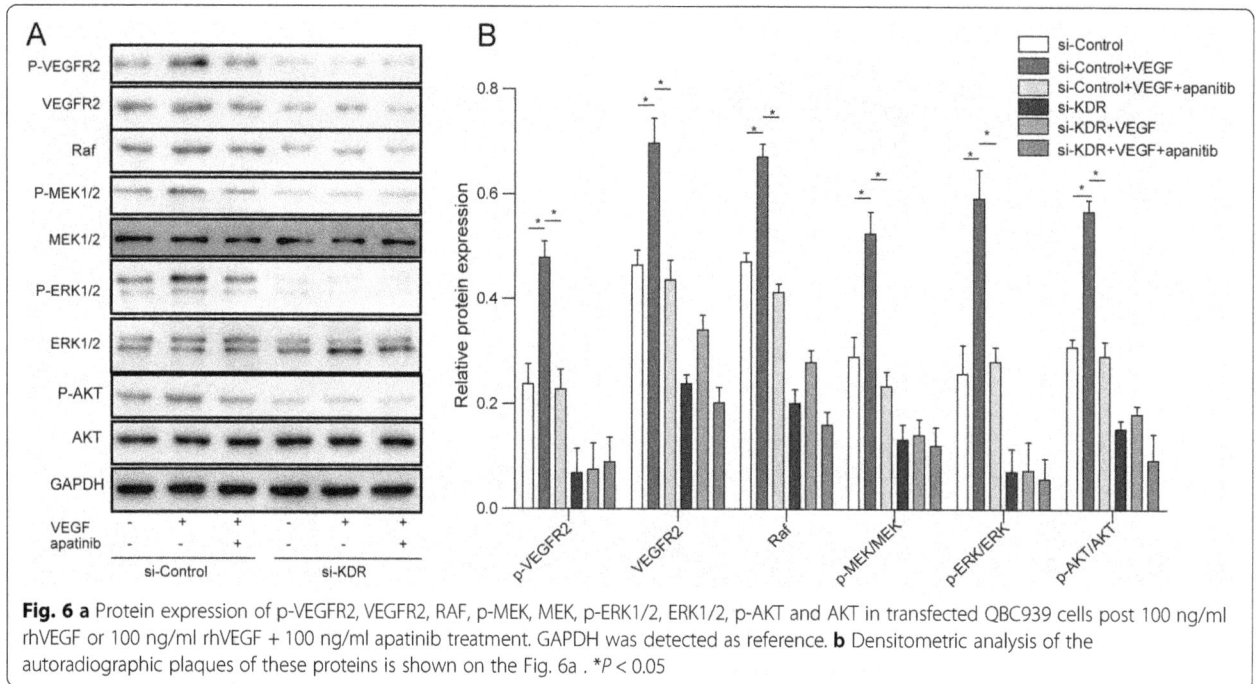

Fig. 6 a Protein expression of p-VEGFR2, VEGFR2, RAF, p-MEK, MEK, p-ERK1/2, ERK1/2, p-AKT and AKT in transfected QBC939 cells post 100 ng/ml rhVEGF or 100 ng/ml rhVEGF + 100 ng/ml apatinib treatment. GAPDH was detected as reference. **b** Densitometric analysis of the autoradiographic plaques of these proteins is shown on the Fig. 6a . *$P < 0.05$

studied. Additionally, since angiogenesis of endothelial cells is an important factor in promoting tumor metastasis, and apatinib might play key role in angiogenesis via VEGFR2 as it expressed in endothelial cells. This would be worth to study in our future work.

Conclusions

In conclusion, our study demonstrates that apatinib inhibits VEGF-mediated cell migration and invasion of CCA cell lines, possibly by blocking VEGFR2-dependent RAF/MEK/ERK and PI3K/AKT pathways. Our article shows the migration and invasion inhibition effect of apatinib acting directly on the CCA cell lines for the first time, hoping to attract more researchers' attention on deeper understanding and evaluating the potential clinical utility of apatinib.

Abbreviations
CCA: Cholangiocarcinoma; KDR: Kinase insert domain receptor, also known as VEGFR2; rhVEGF: Recombined human VEGF; siKDR: Small interference KDR; VEGF: Vascular endothelial growth factor; VEGFR2: VEGF receptor 2

Acknowledgements
This work was supported by the Joint Project of Natural Science Foundation of Hunan Province and Department of Science and Technology of Hunan Province and Commission of Health and Family Planning of Hunan Province [No.2018JJ6029].

Authors' contributions
HMP designed the study, prepared and edited the manuscript. HB performed experimental studies and acquired data. LGW analysed data and did literature research. ZSN designed the study and reviewed the manuscript. All authors have read and approved the manuscript.

Consent for publication
Not applicable.

Competing interests
The authors declare that there are no competing interests.

Author details
[1]Department of Intervention, Hunan Cancer Hospital & The Affiliated Cancer Hospital of Xiangya School of Medicine, Central SouthUniversity, No.283 , Tongzipo Road, Changsha 410013, People's Republic of China. [2]Infection Controlling Center, The Third Xiangya Hospital of Central South University, Tongzipo Road, Yuelu District, Changsha 410013, People's Republic of China.

References
1. Abdel-Razik A, ElMahdy Y, Hanafy EE, Elhelaly R, Elzehery R, Tawfik AM, Eldars W. Insulin-like growth Factor-1 and vascular endothelial growth factor in malignant and benign biliary obstructions. Am J Med Sci. 2016;351(3): 259–64.
2. Amo Y, Masuzawa M, Hamada Y, Katsuoka K. Serum concentrations of vascular endothelial growth factor-D in angiosarcoma patients. Br J Dermatol. 2004;150(1):160–1.
3. Berra E, Milanini J, Richard DE, Le GM, Viñals F, Gothié E, Roux D, Pagès G, Pouysségur J. Signaling angiogenesis via p42/p44 MAP kinase and hypoxia. Biochem Pharmacol. 2000;60(8):1171.
4. Callea F, Sergi C, Fabbretti G, Brisigotti M, Cozzutto C, Medicina D. Precancerous lesions of the biliary tree. J Surg Oncol. 2010;53(S3):131–3.
5. Chatterjee S, Heukamp LC, Siobal M, Schottle J, Wieczorek C, Peifer M, Frasca D, Koker M, Konig K, Meder L, Rauh D, Buettner R, Wolf J, Brekken RA, Neumaier B, Christofori G, Thomas RK, Ullrich RT. Tumor VEGF:VEGFR2 autocrine feed-forward loop triggers angiogenesis in lung cancer. J Clin Invest. 2013;123(4):1732–40.
6. Deoliveira ML, Cunningham SC, Cameron JL, Kamangar F, Winter JM, Lillemoe KD, Choti MA, Yeo CJ, Schulick RD. Cholangiocarcinoma: thirty-one-year experience with 564 patients at a single institution. Ann Surg. 2007;245(5):755–62.

7. Gaudio E, Barbaro B, Alvaro D, Glaser S, Francis H, Ueno Y, Meininger CJ, Franchitto A, Onori P, Marzioni M, Taffetani S, Fava G, Stoica G, Venter J, Reichenbach R, De Morrow S, Summers R, Alpini G. Vascular endothelial growth factor stimulates rat cholangiocyte proliferation via an autocrine mechanism. Gastroenterology. 2006;130(4):1270.

8. Eremina V, Quaggin SE. The role of VEGF-A in glomerular development and function. Curr Opin Nephrol Hypertens. 2004;13(1):9–15.

9. Ewald F, Norz D, Grottke A, Hofmann BT, Nashan B, Jucker M. Dual inhibition of PI3K-AKT-mTOR- and RAF-MEK-ERK-signaling is synergistic in cholangiocarcinoma and reverses acquired resistance to MEK-inhibitors. Investig New Drugs. 2014;32(6):1144–54.

10. Ferrara N, Gerber HP, Lecouter J. The biology of VEGF and its receptors. Nat Med. 2003;9(6):669.

11. Gupta K, Kshirsagar S, Li W, Gui L, Ramakrishnan S, Gupta P, Law PY, Hebbel RP. VEGF prevents apoptosis of human microvascular endothelial cells via opposing effects on MAPK/ERK and SAPK/JNK signaling. Exp Cell Res. 1999;247(2):495.

12. Li YY, Li H, Lv P, Liu G, Li XR, Tian BN, Chen DJ. Prognostic value of cirrhosis for intrahepatic cholangiocarcinoma after surgical treatment. J Gastrointest Surg. 2011;15(4):608–13.

13. Lin C, Wang S, Xie W, Zheng R, Gan Y, Chang J. Apatinib inhibits cellular invasion and migration by fusion kinase KIF5B-RET via suppressing RET/Src signaling pathway. Oncotarget. 2016;7(37):59236–44.

14. Liu Y, Qiao Y, Hu C, Liu L, Zhou L, Liu B, Chen H, Jiang X. VEGFR2 inhibition by RNA interference affects cell proliferation, migration, invasion, and response to radiation in Calu-1 cells. Clinical & translational oncology. 2016;18(2):212–9.

15. Lv L, Wei M, Lin P, Chen Z, Gong P, Quan Z, Tang Z. Integrated mRNA and lncRNA expression profiling for exploring metastatic biomarkers of human intrahepatic cholangiocarcinoma. Am J Cancer Res. 2017;7(3):688–99.

16. Ma FC, Yu Q, Zeng ZM, He RQ, Mo CH, Zhong JC, Ma J, Feng ZB, Chen G, Hu XH. Progression-free survival of up to 8 months of an advanced intrahepatic cholangiocarcinoma patient treated with apatinib: a case report. Onco Targets Ther. 2017;10:5237–42.

17. Meadows KN, Bryant P, Pumiglia K. Vascular endothelial growth factor induction of the angiogenic phenotype requires Ras activation. J Biol Chem. 2001;276(52):49289–98.

18. Park BK, Paik YH, Park JY, Park KH, Bang S, Park SW, Chung JB, Park YN, Song SY. The clinicopathologic significance of the expression of vascular endothelial growth factor-C in intrahepatic cholangiocarcinoma. Am J Clin Oncol. 2006;29(2):138.

19. Peng H, Zhang Q, Li J, Zhang N, Hua Y, Xu L, Deng Y, Lai J, Peng Z, Peng B, Chen M, Peng S, Kuang M. Apatinib inhibits VEGF signaling and promotes apoptosis in intrahepatic cholangiocarcinoma. Oncotarget. 2016b;7(13):17220–9.

20. Peng S, Zhang Y, Peng H, Ke Z, Xu L, Su T, Tsung A, Tohme S, Huang H, Zhang Q, Lencioni R, Zeng Z, Peng B, Chen M, Kuang M. Intracellular autocrine VEGF signaling promotes EBDC cell proliferation, which can be inhibited by Apatinib. Cancer Lett. 2016d;373(2):193–202.

21. Ramirez-Merino N, Aix SP, Cortes-Funes H. Chemotherapy for cholangiocarcinoma: an update. World J Gastrointest Oncol. 2013;5(7):171–6.

22. Rizvi S, Gores GJ. Pathogenesis, diagnosis, and management of cholangiocarcinoma. Gastroenterology. 2013;145(6):1215–29.

23. Senger DR, Galli SJ, Dvorak AM, Perruzzi CA, Harvey VS, Dvorak HF. Tumor cells secrete a vascular permeability factor that promotes accumulation of ascites fluid. Science. 1983;219(4587):983–5.

24. Shroff RT, Yarchoan M, O'Connor A, Gallagher D, Zahurak ML, Rosner G, Ohaji C, Sartorius-Mergenthaler S, Subbiah V, Zinner R, Azad NS. The oral VEGF receptor tyrosine kinase inhibitor pazopanib in combination with the MEK inhibitor trametinib in advanced cholangiocarcinoma. Br J Cancer. 2017;116(11):1402–7.

25. Simone V, Brunetti O, Lupo L, Testini M, Maiorano E, Simone M, Longo V, Rolfo C, Peeters M, Scarpa A, Azzariti A, Russo A, Ribatti D, Silvestris N. Targeting angiogenesis in biliary tract cancers: an open option. Int J Mol Sci. 2017;18(2).

26. Tang D, Nagano H, Yamamoto H, Wada H, Nakamura M, Kondo M, Ota H, Yoshioka S, Kato H, Damdinsuren B. Angiogenesis in cholangiocellular carcinoma: expression of vascular endothelial growth factor, angiopoietin-1/2, thrombospondin-1 and clinicopathological significance. Oncol Rep. 2006;15(3):525–32.

27. Terman BI, Dougher-Vermazen M, Carrion ME, Dimitrov D, Armellino DC, Gospodarowicz D, Bohlen P. Identification of the KDR tyrosine kinase as a receptor for vascular endothelial cell growth factor. Biochem Biophys Res Commun. 1992;187(3):1579–86.

28. Tian S, Quan H, Xie C, Guo H, Lu F, Xu Y, Li J, Lou L. YN968D1 is a novel and selective inhibitor of vascular endothelial growth factor receptor-2 tyrosine kinase with potent activity in vitro and in vivo. Cancer Sci. 2011;102(7):1374–80.

29. Tsuzuki T, Ogata Y, Iida S, Nakanishi I, Takenaka Y, Yoshii H. Carcinoma of the bifurcation of the hepatic ducts. Arch Surg. 1983;118(10):1147.

30. Wiedmann MW, Mossner J. Molecular targeted therapy of biliary tract cancer--results of the first clinical studies. Curr Drug Targets. 2010;11(7):834–50.

31. Xu D, Ma Y, Zhao B, Li S, Zhang Y, Pan S, Wu Y, Wang J, Wang D, Pan H, Liu L, Jiang H. Thymoquinone induces G2/M arrest, inactivates PI3K/Akt and nuclear factor-kappaB pathways in human cholangiocarcinomas both in vitro and in vivo. Oncol Rep. 2014;31(5):2063–70.

32. Zhang L, Wang JN, Tang JM, Kong X, Yang JY, Zheng F, Guo LY, Huang YZ, Zhang L, Tian L. VEGF is essential for the growth and migration of human hepatocellular carcinoma cells. Mol Biol Rep. 2012;39(5):5085–93.

13

Stapleless laparoscopic left lateral sectionectomy for hepatocellular carcinoma: reappraisal of the Louisville statement by a young liver surgeon

Chao-Wei Lee[1,2,3] (iD), Hsin-I Tsai[3,4], Hao-Tsai Cheng[2,3,5], Wei-Ting Chen[5], Heng-Yuan Hsu[1], Chien-Chih Chiu[6], Yi-Ping Liu[1], Tsung-Han Wu[1], Ming-Chin Yu[1,2,7*], Wei-Chen Lee[1] and Miin-Fu Chen[1,2]

Abstract

Background: Laparoscopic liver resection has been regarded as the standard treatment for liver tumors located at the left lateral liver sector. However, few studies have reported the results of laparoscopic left lateral sectionectomy (LLS) for HCC, not to mention the feasibility of this emerging technique for the less experienced liver surgeons. The current study would reappraise the Louisville statement by examining the outcome of LLS performed by a young liver surgeon.

Methods: We retrospectively reviewed two separate groups of patients who underwent open or laparoscopic left lateral sectionectomies at Chung Gung Memorial Hospital, Linkou. All laparoscopic hepatectomies were performed by the index young surgeon following a stepwise stapleless LLS. The surgical results and oncological outcomes of laparoscopic vs. open hepatectomies (LH and OH, respectively) with the surgical indication of HCC at left lateral liver sector were further compared and analyzed.

Results: 18 of 29 patients in the laparoscopic group and 75 patients in the conventional open group had primary HCC. The demographic data was essentially the same for the two groups. Statistical analysis revealed that the LH group had smaller tumor size, higher blood transfusion requirement, longer duration of inflow control and parenchymal transection, and longer operation time. However, no significant difference was observed in terms of complication rate, mortality rate, and hospital stay between the two groups. After adjusting for tumor size, LH and OH showed no statistical difference in the amount of blood transfusion, operation time and patient survival.

Conclusions: This study demonstrated that stapleless LLS is a safe and feasible procedure for less experienced liver surgeons to resect HCC located at the left lateral liver sector. This stepwise stapleless LSS can not only achieve surgical results comparable to OH but also can provide a platform for liver surgeons to apply laparoscopic technique before conducting more complicated liver resections.

Keywords: Laparoscopic hepatectomy, Liver resection, Left lateral sectionectomy, Hepatocellular carcinoma, Hepatoma, Stapleless, Louisville statement, Laparoscopic surgery, Hepatectomy, Young surgeon

* Correspondence: mingchin2000@gmail.com
[1]Department of Surgery, Linkou Chang Gung Memorial Hospital, No.5, Fuxing St, Guishan Dist, Taoyuan City 33305, Taiwan, Republic of China
[2]College of Medicine, Chang Gung University, Guishan, Taoyuan, Taiwan, Republic of China
Full list of author information is available at the end of the article

Background

Laparoscopic surgery has been proven to be an effective surgical approach in many abdominal diseases, including acute cholecystitis, colon cancer, and gastroesophageal reflux disesase [1–3]. With improvements in surgical techniques and laparoscopic instruments, laparoscopic surgery has also shown promising results in major abdominal operations in recent decades. Laparoscopic liver resection, for example, has been shown to be a feasible and safe technique for hepatic tumors with surgical results comparable to conventional open hepatectomy [4, 5]. However, because the liver is a highly vascular solid organ, the resection of liver tumors still carries substantial risk of morbidity, especially in patients with liver cirrhosis [6]. In an attempt to guide liver surgeons worldwide, the first International Consensus Conference on Laparoscopic Liver Resections was thus convened and a statement formulated. In this so-called "Louisville Statement", laparoscopic liver resection was considered a standard practice for liver tumors located in the left lateral liver sector [7]. Hence, laparoscopic left lateral sectionectomy (LLS) was to be performed by surgeons who had developed sufficient laparoscopic techniques. However, due to lack of strong evidence in case of hepatocellular carcinoma (HCC), this recommendation was not strongly supported by the second International Consensus Conference on Laparoscopic Liver Resections [8]. The fact that HCC may arise in the context of liver cirrhosis while most of the series published so far were based on evidence from colorectal liver metastasis or benign liver lesions leaves the status of laparoscopic liver resection for HCC undetermined.

A recent study published by a Hong Kong group demonstrated their long-term outcome for HCC. In their study, laparoscopic left lateral sectionectomy resulted in survival outcome comparable to the conventional open approach [9]. Their promising result was exhilarating. However, the operating surgeons in that study were all well-known and experienced liver surgeons. Their excellent results were not unexpected. The surgical outcome of less experienced surgeons or surgeons with lower case volumes, on the other hand, remains unknown. To further address this issue, we conducted the current study and aim to reappraise the Louisville statement by examining the outcome of LLS performed by a young liver surgeon.

Methods

Patients

From 2009 to 2017, records of patients who underwent standard left lateral sectionectomy at Chang Gung Memorial Hospital, Linkou, Taiwan, were retrospectively reviewed. Only patients who had histologically proven primary HCC were included in the final comparative study. The conventional open hepatectomies were performed by experienced liver surgeons in the same surgical department. Laparoscopic left lateral sectionectomy, on the other hand, was conducted by a young surgeon who had a special interest in the laparoscopic procedures. The index young surgeon had received a 5-year postgraduate training as a surgical resident at Linkou Chang Gung Memorial Hospital. The surgeon received, in addition to trainings in conventional open hepatobiliary surgeries, comprehensive training in fundamental laparoscopic procedures including laparoscopic cholecystectomy (LC) and laparoscopic appendectomy (LA) during his last two years of residency. Since the index surgeon had become a board-certified gastrointestinal surgeon in 2012, the LLS also started from 2012. Moreover, because the instruments required by laparoscopic liver resections were not reimbursed by health insurance in Taiwan, only patients who were able to afford the cost were assigned to the LLS group.

With the approval of the Institutional Review Boards of Chang Gung Memorial Hospital (CGMH IRB No: 201701574B0 and No: 201600359B0), the recruited patients' clinicopathological data were retrieved from the prospectively collected database. Patients who did not have detailed preoperative/intraoperative clinical records, or who did not have regular postoperative out-patient follow-up were excluded from our study. The tumor staging of the current study was based on the AJCC TNM staging system for HCC [10].

Preoperative diagnosis of HCC was established by characteristic features on imaging by either triphasic computed tomography (CT), magnetic resonance imaging (MRI), hepatic arteriography, and/or a serum α-fetoprotein (AFP) level greater than 200 ng/ml. Resection criteria were constant over the entire study period, including a lack of cancerous thrombi in the main trunk of the portal vein, no distant metastasis to other organs, a technically operable main tumor in the preoperative evaluation, and a adequate liver functional reserve. Liver function was routinely assessed preoperatively by Child–Pugh classification and indocyanine green retention test. A previous study identified an indocyanine green retention at 15 min (ICG-15) of less than 14% as the safety limit for major hepatic resection [11]. In our institute, an ICG-15 $\leq$ 10% was the prerequisite for major hepatic resection.

For LLS, the patients were placed in the reversed Trendelenburg position. Most procedures were performed by two surgeons, with the index operating surgeon standing on the right side of the patient and assistant surgeon on the left. The video laparoscope was introduced via a 12 mm vertical incision at the supraumbilical region. Another 12 mm working port was created at the right subcostal area in line with the falciform ligament. Two more 5 mm assistant ports were introduced at the lateral aspect of the right subcostal area, and at about the left mid-clavicular line in the left subcostal area, respectively. The peritoneal cavity was inspected to confirm the absence of metastatic disease. Laparoscopic ultrasound was introduced via the 12 mm working port to locate the primary tumor, search for possible additional tumors at bilateral lobes, identify the location and patency of major vascular structures, and define the transection line. After ultrasonic evaluation, the round ligament and falciform ligament were divided by energy device. The energy devices used for tissue dissection or liver parenchymal transection were usually Harmonic scalpels (EthiconTM) or Thunderbeat dissectors (OlympusTM). During liver parenchymal transection, the central venous pressure was maintained as low as possible (around 5 mmHg) and pneumopeirtoneum was kept at 15 mmHg to reduce venous bleeding from the transected surface. The liver parenchyma was transected along the lateral border of the falciform ligament, and the portal pedicles supplying segment 3 and 2, small hepatic veins, and left hepatic vein were identified and ligated individually by double HEM-O-LOK (Teleflex). In the current study, no vascular staplers were employed for liver parenchymal transection. Upon completion of liver transection, the transected surface was meticulously examined for bleeding or bile leakge. Electrocauterization, hemoclips, or suture were applied whenever necessary. The resected specimen was delivered through a transverse incision created at the suprapubic area. A Jackson-Pratt drain was routinely placed at the left subphrenic space for postoperative drainage.

For conventional open left lateral sectionectomy, an upper midline and right subcostal incision was usually made. Intraoperative exploration by both manual palpation and ultrasonography was performed to define the extent of the tumor(s), the texture of liver parenchyma, any invasion of the portal or hepatic veins, and the size of future liver remnant. A low central venous pressure was maintained to reduce venous bleeding as for the laparoscopic approach. For either LLS or conventional open surgery, inflow control with Pringle's maneuver was predetermined and applied according to individual surgeon's discretion. Parenchymal transection was performed using either crush clamp technique or Cavitron ultrasonic surgical aspirator (CUSA) based on surgeon's preference. Hemostasis was achieved and bile leakage meticulously repaired in each operation.

Patients were cared for and monitored postoperatively according to a protocolized approach published previously [6]. All patients received blood exams and triphasic CT study one to two months after the operation. Out-patient follow-up with serial lab tests and image study was arranged every 2–3 months after hospital discharge.

Definition

Operation duration was defined as the time interval elapsed from anesthesia induction to extubation. Major surgical complications comprised grade III and IV surgical complications as described previously [6, 12]. Thirty-day mortality was defined as the occurrence of death within 30 days after the operation, and in-hospital mortality was defined as death during the same hospital stay. Recurrence was defined as the appearance of characteristic image findings during regular postoperative radiologic examinations. Early recurrence was defined as recurrence within two years of the initial curative operation [13]. Disease-free survival (DFS) was calculated from the date of surgery to the date of the first documented clinical disease recurrence. Overall survival (OS) was defined as the time elapsed from the date of surgery to either the date of death or the date of the last contact. Cases with surgical mortality, defined as death within one month of surgery, were excluded from the survival analyses.

Statistical analysis

The statistical analysis was performed with IBM SPSS Statistics 21 (IBM Corporation, Software Group, Somers, NY, USA). Fisher's exact test or Pearson's $\chi 2$ test was used to analyze categorical data. Student's t test was used to analyze continuous variables. Kaplan-Meier analysis and log-rank test were used to determine and compare the OS and DFS. Statistical significance was defined as P values < 0.05 in two-sided tests.

Results

From 2012 to 2017, a total of twenty-nine LLS were performed by the index surgeon. The demographic data of these patients receiving LLS is summarized in Table 1. Almost half of the patients were older than 60 years old. The most common etiology was HCC (18 patients, LH group), followed by hepatic hemangioma, hepatic cysts, focal nodular hyperplasia (FNH), cholelithiasis, and amebic liver abscess. The size of the tumors was mostly less than 5 cm in diameter. Twenty-five patients (86.2%) received purely laparoscopic surgery, 3 had (10.3%) robotic surgery, and 1 (3.4%) underwent hybrid operation. No conversion laparotomy was encountered. Inflow control was employed in only 5 patients (17.2%). Surgical complication rate was 13.8%. For comparison, a further 75 patients who underwent conventional open left lateral sectionectomy for their primary HCC (OH group) from 2009 to 2017 were included for subsequent analysis.

Table 1 Demographic data of patients receiving laparoscopic left lateral sectionectomy by a single surgeon (n = 29)

Variables	(%)	Variables	(%)
Age ≦60 years	15 (51.7)	OP method	
Male gender	17 (58.6)	Pure laparoscopic	25 (86.2)
Disease entity		Hybrid	1 (3.4)
Hepatocellular carcinoma	18 (62.1)	Pure robotic	3 (10.3)
Hemangioma	5 (17.2)	Conversion laparotomy	0 (0)
Liver cysts	3 (10.3)	Inflow control	
Focal nodular hyperplasia	1 (3.4)	Pringle's maneuver	5 (17.2)
Cholelithiasis	1 (3.4)	No inflow control	24 (82.8)
Amebic liver abscess	1 (3.4)	Duration of operation (hour) [a] (range)	4.63 ± 1.81 (2.3–10.4)
Tumor size (cm) (range 1.0–12.6 cm)		Duration of parenchymal transection [a] (minute) (range)	90.81 ± 52.78 (35–300)
≤ 2	5 (17.2)	Blood loss [a] (ml) (range)	179.53 ± 161.9 (20–600)
2–5	17 (58.6)	Complication (Yes)	4 (13.8)
> 5	7 (24.1)	Grade II/III/V	4 / 0 / 0

[a] Mean ± standard deviation

Table 2 Comparison of clinical characteristics between laparoscopic stapleless left lateral sectionectomy (LH) and open left lateral sectionectomy (OH) for hepatocellular carcinoma

Categorical variables	LH group [a] (n = 18)	OH group (n = 75)	p value
Age (> 65 years (%))	9 (50.0)	27 (36.0)	0.293
Gender (Male(%) / Female(%))	13(72.2) / 5(27.8)	56(74.7) / 19(25.3)	1.000
Diabetes Mellitus (Yes (%))	6 (33.3)	18 (24.0)	0.549
Hypertension (Yes (%))	7 (38.9)	23 (37.7)	1.000
ESRD[b] (Yes (%))	0 (0)	3 (4.0)	1.000
Smoking (Yes (%))	4 (22.2)	13 (17.3)	0.735
Alcohol (Yes (%))	7 (38.9)	14 (18.7)	0.112
HBV surface antigen (Positive (%))	10 (55.6)	36 (48.0)	0.608
Hepatitis C virus (Positive (%))	7 (38.9)	27 (36.0)	1.000
Child-Pugh Classification (A(%) / B(%))	18(100) / 0(0)	72(97.3) / 2(2.7)	1.000
Symptoms (Yes (%))	0 (0)	19 (25.3)	0.019
ICG-15 (> 10% (%))	8 (44.4)	23 (31.9)	0.407
Preoperative α-fetoprotein (> 15 ng/mL (%))	8 (44.4)	33 (44.0)	1.000

Continuous variables [c]	LH group [a] (n = 18)	OH group (n = 75)	p value
Age (years)	60.2 ± 3.24	61.4 ± 1.32	0.707
BMI (kg/m²)	25.7 ± 1.00	25.3 ± 0.42	0.704
ICG-15 (%)	10.4 ± 1.90	10.5 ± 1.25	0.970
Hemoglobin (g/dL)	13.3 ± 0.51	13.3 ± 0.25	0.998
Albumin (g/dL)	4.0 ± 0.11	4.1 ± 0.06	0.423
Bilirubin total (mg/dL)	0.54 ± 0.06	0.72 ± 0.05	0.122
Preoperative α-fetoprotein (ng/mL)	1496.4 ± 1356.6	1147.4 ± 42.5	0.748

[a] include laparoscopic and robotic left lateral sectionectomy
[b] end-stage renal disease
[c] mean ± standard error of mean

As for HCC per se, the LH group and OH group shared similar clinical characteristics (Table 2). The rate of comorbid illness was comparable between the two groups. Hepatitis B virus (HBV) infection accounted for about 50% of cases, while around 35% of patients had chronic hepatitis C virus (HCV) infection. The BMI was 25.7 kg/m² for the LH group and 25.3 kg/m² for the OH group. In both groups, the vast majority of patients were Child-Pugh A. However, one-fourth of patients in the OH group were symptomatic upon presentation, in contrast to 0% in the LH group (p = 0.019). The median follow-up time was 35.8 months for the LH group and 37.1 months for the OH group.

As for surgical variables, the LH group had significantly lower rate of inflow control when compared to the OH group (27.8% vs. 63.8%, p = 0.008). However, higher blood transfusion requirement, longer duration of inflow control and parenchymal transection, and longer operation time were observed in the LH group. No significant difference was found in terms of complication rate, mortality rate, and hospital stay. The early recurrence rate was also comparable between the two groups (Table 3).

The pathological characteristics are summarized in Table 4. The tumor size in the LH group was significantly smaller than that in the OH group (mean tumor size: 3.2 cm vs. 4.9 cm, p = 0.011). The OH group had a slightly higher rate of tumor rupture when compared to the LH group (17.3% vs. 0%, p = 0.066). Negative resection margin was achieved in every patient in the LH group and in all but one patient in the OH group. In addition to 100% R0 resection rate, more than 60% of the LH group had their safety margin larger than 1 cm in width. Histologically-proven liver cirrhosis was present in 44 and 58% of the LH and OH groups, respectively. The other pathological parameters were essentially the same between the two groups.

The oncological survival outcome has been illustrated in Fig. 1a-b. The mean disease-free survival (DFS) was 49.25 ± 6.29 months for the LH group and 39.24 ± 3.67 months for the OH group (P = 0.110). The mean overall survival (OS) was 60.73 ± 2.70 months for the LH group and 61.58 ± 2.61 months for the OH group (P = 0.400). Laparoscopic surgery can achieve satisfactory oncological outcome when compared to conventional open surgery.

Table 3 Comparison of surgical variables and outcome between laparoscopic stapleless left lateral sectionectomy (LH) and open left lateral sectionectomy (OH) for hepatocellular carcinoma

Categorical variables	LH group [a] (n = 18)	OH group (n = 75)	p value
Inflow control (Yes (%))	5 (27.8)	44 (63.8)	0.008
Blood transfusion (Yes(%))	3 (16.7)	1 (1.4)	0.023
Complications (Yes (%))	6 (33.3)	22 (29.3)	0.778
Major complications [b] (Yes (%))	0 (0)	9 (12)	0.198
Thirty-day mortality (Yes (%))	0 (0)	0 (0)	N.A.
In-hospital mortality (Yes (%))	0 (0)	1 (1.3)	1.000
Early recurrence [c](Yes (%))	3 (16.7)	30 (40.0)	0.098

Continuous variables [d]	LH group [a] (n = 18)	OH group (n = 75)	p value
Operative duration (minutes)	287.0 ± 28.91	221.4 ± 8.00	0.041
Blood loss (ml)	217.2 ± 45.00	239.8 ± 40.58	0.794
Duration of inflow control [e] (minutes)	85.6 ± 8.04	35.0 ± 3.16	< 0.001
Duration of parenchymal transection (minutes)	96.7 ± 15.98	53.8 ± 3.80	0.018
Post-OP hospital stay (days) (range)	8.44 ± 0.54 (5–15)	9.7 ± 0.50 (6–29)	0.238

[a]include laparoscopic and robotic left lateral sectionectomy
[b]major surgical complications include grade III-IV surgical complications
[c]recurrence within two years after the index operation
[d]mean ± standard error of mean
[e]mean duration among those who had inflow control

Table 4 Comparison of pathologic characteristics between laparoscopic stapleless left lateral sectionectomy (LH) and open left lateral sectionectomy (OH) for hepatocellular carcinoma

Variables	LH group [a] (n = 18)	OH group (n = 75)	p value
Tumor size (cm)[b]	3.2 ± 0.50	4.9 ± 0.41	0.011
Tumor size (> 5 cm (%))	2 (11.1)	26 (34.7)	0.083
Encapsulation (Yes (%))	16 (88.9)	64 (85.3)	1.000
Capsular invasion (Yes (%))	12 (66.7)	45 (60.8)	0.789
Tumor rupture (Yes (%))	0 (0)	13 (17.3)	0.066
Vascular invasion (Yes (%))	5 (27.8)	20 (26.7)	1.000
Daughter nodules (Yes (%))	2 (11.1)	9 (12.0)	1.000
Resection margin (Negative (%))	18 (100)	74 (98.7)	1.000
Safety margin (≥1 cm (%))	11 (61.1)	35 (46.7)	0.304
Edmonson and Steiner grade (III and IV (%))	6 (35.3)	27 (37.0)	1.000
Cirrhosis (Yes (%))	8 (44.4)	44 (58.7)	0.302
T stage			
T1 (%)	11 (61.1)	37 (52.9)	0.631
T2 (%)	4 (22.2)	15 (21.4)	
T3a/T3b (%)	0/4 (0/5.7)	1/2 (1.4/11.1)	
T4 (%)	1 (5.6)	13 (18.6)	

[a]include laparoscopic and robotic left lateral sectionectomy
[b]mean ± standard error of mean

For more matched analysis, patients with HCC less than 5 cm in diameter were included for subgroup analysis. The clinical backgrounds were comparable between the two groups and are summarized in Table 5. After adjusting for tumor size, the LH group still had lower rate of inflow control than the OH group. However, the rate of blood transfusion became similar when smaller tumors were concerned. In addition, despite longer duration of inflow control and parenchymal transection, the total operative duration was comparable between the two groups. There were still no significant differences found in terms of complication rate, mortality rate, hospital stay, or early recurrence rate (Table 6). The pathological variables in the adjusted cohort are summarized in Table 7. Like the original cohort, more than 60% of the LH group had their safety margin larger than 1 cm in width. The other pathological characteristics remain similar between the two groups. The oncological outcome has been illustrated in Fig. 1c-d. The mean DFS was 45.80 ± 5.99 months for the LH group and 42.46 ± 4.36 months for the OH group (P = 0.266). The mean OS was 60.02 ± 3.32 months for the LH group and 62.51 ± 2.43 months for the OH group (P = 0.962).

Laparoscopic hepatectomy can achieve comparable oncological outcome when compared to conventional open surgery, especially for smaller HCC.

The influence of liver cirrhosis on laparoscopic hepatectomy was investigated and is summarized in Table 8. There was no significant differences found in terms of rate of inflow control, blood transfusion, complications, mortality, or early recurrence between cirrhotic and non-cirrhotic groups. The duration of parenchymal transection and total operative duration were also comparable between the two groups. However, the cirrhotic group tended to have more operative blood loss and longer postoperative hospital stay than the non-cirrhotic group.

Discussion

HCC is the most common primary malignancy of the liver and causes more than 8000 deaths each year in Taiwan [14, 15]. With improvements in patient selection, surgical instruments, operative techniques, and postoperative care, the mortality rate of curative surgical resection has improved dramatically in recent decades [16–19]. According to a recent study, the 30-day mortality rate was only 1.8% and the in-hospital mortality rate was 2.9% after hepatectomy for HCC [6, 20]. Minimally invasive liver resection was thus developed

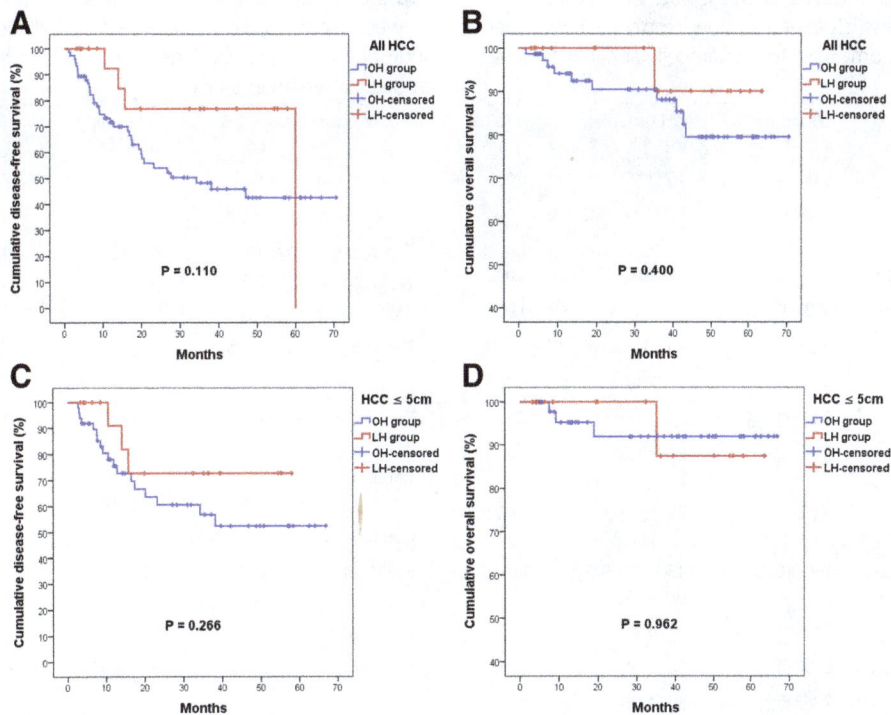

Fig. 1 Kaplan–Meier disease-free survival (DFS) curves and overall survival (OS) curves for hepatocellular carcinoma treated by LH or OH. (**a** and **b**, all HCC) The mean DFS was 49.25 months for the LH group and 39.24 months for the OH group ($P = 0.110$). The mean OS was 60.73 months for the LH group and 61.58 months for the OH group ($P = 0.400$). Laparoscopic liver resection for HCC located at left lateral liver sector can achieve satisfactory oncological outcome when compared to the conventional open surgery. (**c** and **d**, HCC less than 5 cm in diameter). The mean DFS was 45.80 months for the LH group and 42.46 months for the OH group ($P = 0.266$). The mean OS was 60.02 months for the LH group and 62.51 months for the OH group ($P = 0.962$). Laparoscopic hepatectomy can achieve comparable oncological outcome when compared to the conventional open surgery, especially for smaller HCC

in the late 1990s after significant improvements in surgical outcome [21]. It has received worldwide acknowledgement and more and more liver surgeons have started to perform laparoscopic liver resections during the last decade. According to a review article in 2009, as many as 2804 minimally invasive liver resections were conducted for either benign or malignant liver diseases in the early twenty-first century [5]. Due to this widespread acceptance, the First World Consensus Conference on Laparoscopic Liver Surgery suggested laparoscopic liver resection become standard practice for lesions located at the left lateral liver sector [7]. This statement has encouraged liver surgeons to devote themselves to conducting laparoscopic left lateral sectionectomy. Nevertheless, this recommendation failed to gain full support from the juries at the Second International Consensus Conference on Laparoscopic Liver Resection. The fact that most of the evidence presented for LLS were from series of colorectal liver metastasis rendered this recommendation less convincing [8]. For this reason, many studies have since been conducted to investigate the result of LLS for HCC. In these series, LLS has been shown to have surgical

morbidity and mortality rates comparable to the open approach [9, 22–24]. Nevertheless, most studies failed to compare the long-term oncological outcome between laparoscopic approach and conventional open approach. In addition, since most studies were obtained from operations performed by experienced and authorative liver surgeons, their results may not be fully applicable to the "real world" scenario. Our study, in which all of the LLS was performed by a single young surgeon, may be the first one in the English literature to provide strong evidence for beginners or hospitals with lower case volumes to perform this operation for HCC.

In the current study, we demonstrated that for HCC located in the left lateral liver sector, laparoscopic liver resection provided results comparable to the conventional open approach in terms of blood loss, surgical complication rate, mortality rate, and early recurrence rate. The total operative duration was also similar between the two approaches when smaller tumors were concerned. Moreover, the presence of liver cirrhosis did not affect the results of laparoscopic liver resection, in that the amount of blood products transfused, surgical

Table 5 Comparison of clinical characteristics between laparoscopic stapleless left lateral sectionectomy (LH) and open left lateral sectionectomy (OH) for hepatocellular carcinoma less than 5 cm

Categorical variables	LH group [a] (n = 16)	OH group (n = 49)	p value
Age (> 65 years (%))	8 (50.0)	15 (30.6)	0.229
Gender (Male(%) / Female(%))	12(75.0) / 4(25.0)	35(71.4) / 14(28.6)	1.000
Diabetes Mellitus (Yes (%))	5 (31.3)	15 (30.6)	1.000
Hypertension (Yes (%))	5 (31.3)	14 (33.3)	1.000
ESRD[b] (Yes (%))	0 (0)	1 (2.0)	1.000
Smoking (Yes (%))	4 (25.0)	10 (20.4)	0.732
Alcohol (Yes (%))	7 (43.8)	13 (26.5)	0.223
HBV surface antigen (Positive (%))	8 (50.0)	24 (49.0)	1.000
Hepatitis C virus (Positive (%))	9 (56.3)	29 (59.2)	1.000
Child-Pugh Classification (A(%) / B(%))	16(100) / 0(0)	48(100) / 0(0)	N.A.
Symptoms (Yes (%))	0 (0)	9 (18.4)	0.098
ICG-15 (> 10% (%))	8 (50.0)	16 (34.8)	0.374
Preoperative α-fetoprotein (> 15 ng/mL (%))	7 (43.8)	24 (49.0)	0.779
Continuous variables [c]	LH group [a] (n = 16)	OH group (n = 49)	p value
Age (years)	60.1 ± 3.61	61.1 ± 1.33	0.790
BMI (kg/m^2)	25.8 ± 1.10	25.5 ± 0.55	0.837
ICG-15 (%)	11.0 ± 2.09	9.78 ± 1.04	0.575
Hemoglobin (g/dL)	13.6 ± 0.52	13.5 ± 0.30	0.963
Albumin (g/dL)	4.1 ± 0.12	4.2 ± 0.05	0.101
Bilirubin total (mg/dL)	0.56 ± 0.07	0.60 ± 0.04	0.655
Preoperative α-fetoprotein (ng/mL)	150.1 ± 76.9	1196.9 ± 588.6	0.316

[a]include laparoscopic and robotic left lateral sectionectomy
[b]end-stage renal disease
[c]mean ± standard error of mean

Table 6 Comparison of surgical variables and outcome between laparoscopic stapleless left lateral sectionectomy (LH) and open left lateral sectionectomy (OH) for hepatocellular carcinoma less than 5 cm

Categorical variables	LH group [a] (n = 16)	OH group (n = 49)	p value
Inflow control (Yes (%))	5 (31.3)	27 (57.4)	0.088
Blood transfusion (Yes(%))	2 (12.5)	1 (2.0)	0.147
Complications (Yes (%))	5 (31.3)	13 (26.5)	0.753
Major complications [b] (Yes (%))	0 (0)	2 (4.1)	1.000
Thirty-day mortality (Yes (%))	0 (0)	0 (0)	N.A.
In-hospital mortality (Yes (%))	0 (0)	0 (0)	N.A.
Early recurrence [c](Yes (%))	3 (18.8)	16 (32.7)	0.357
Continuous variables [d]	LH group [a] (n = 16)	OH group (n = 49)	p value
Operative duration (minutes)	267.1 ± 23.96	219.1 ± 10.04	0.079
Blood loss (ml)	216.3 ± 50.33	172.5 ± 26.47	0.449
Duration of inflow control [e] (minutes)	85.6 ± 8.04	32.8 ± 3.51	< 0.001
Duration of parenchymal transection (minutes)	80.5 ± 9.30	50.5 ± 4.20	0.001
Post-OP hospital stay (days) (range)	8.4 ± 0.63 (5–15)	9.1 ± 0.54 (6–29)	0.474

[a]include laparoscopic and robotic left lateral sectionectomy
[b]major surgical complications include grade III-IV surgical complications
[c]recurrence within two years after the index operation
[d]mean ± standard error of mean
[e]mean duration among those who had inflow control

complication rate, mortality, and early recurrence rate were not different between the cirrhotic and non-cirrhotic groups. In addition to excellent surgical result, the surgical radicality was not compromised by the laparoscopic approach, whereby all patients in the laparoscopic group had an R0 resection and more than 60% of patients had their safety margin larger than 1 cm in width. This result was encouraging since the most prevailing doubt regarding laparoscopic cancer surgery is tumor radicality! The current study demonstrated that laparoscopic left lateral sectionectomy can provide complete HCC eradication, just as in the conventional open approach, even in the cirrhotic liver. Furthermore, regardless of the tumor size, the long-term oncological survival after LLS was equivalent to that after open surgery. Our study, as a result, is one of the first report in the English literature to demonstrate the surgical as well as oncological outcome of LLS for HCC. Given the inherent merits of smaller wounds, less pain, better cosmetics, and earlier postoperative ambulation and recovery, laparoscopic left lateral sectionectomy should be the standard treatment for HCC even when performed by less experienced surgeons. The recommendation concluded by the Louisville statement thus stands reappraised and validated [7].

The technique employed in the current study did not encourage the use of vascular staplers for parenchymal transection during LLS. Since the left lateral liver sector is usually thin and contributes only about 15–30% of total liver volume, the resection of this sector rarely results in postoperative hepatic failure. The relatively constant vascular anatomy and straight transection plane also render this operation less challenging to hepatobiliary surgeons [9]. Many liver surgeons, whether experienced or beginners, would thus apply vascular staplers for parenchymal transection during LLS in order to facilitate the operation. However, we hold the view that since the anatomy of the left lateral sector is constant and straight, it is a good opportunity for liver surgeons to familiarize themselves with the techniques required to perform laparoscopic liver

Table 7 Comparison of pathologic characteristics between laparoscopic stapleless left lateral sectionectomy (LH) and open left lateral sectionectomy (OH) for hepatocellular carcinoma less than 5 cm

Variables	LH group [a] (n = 16)	OH group (n = 49)	p value
Tumor size (cm)[b]	2.6 ± 0.27	2.9 ± 0.15	0.350
Encapsulation (Yes (%))	14 (87.5)	44 (89.8)	1.000
Capsular invasion (Yes (%))	10 (62.5)	30 (62.5)	1.000
Tumor rupture (Yes (%))	0 (0)	2 (4.1)	1.000
Vascular invasion (Yes (%))	4 (25.0)	13 (26.5)	1.000
Daughter nodules (Yes (%))	2 (12.5)	6 (12.2)	1.000
Resection margin (Negative (%))	16 (100)	48 (98.0)	1.000
Safety margin (≥1 cm (%))	10 (62.5)	27 (55.1)	0.773
Edmonson and Steiner grade (III and IV (%))	4 (26.7)	17 (36.2)	0.551
Cirrhosis (Yes (%))	8 (50.0)	32 (65.3)	0.376
T stage			
T1 (%)	11 (68.8)	28 (59.6)	0.816
T2 (%)	4 (25.0)	14 (29.8)	
T3a/T3b (%)	0/1 (0/6.3)	0/3 (0/6.4)	
T4 (%)	0 (0)	2 (4.3)	

[a]include laparoscopic and robotic left lateral sectionectomy
[b]mean ± standard error of mean

Table 8 Comparison of surgical variables and outcome between cirrhotic and non-cirrhotic livers when performing laparoscopic stapleless left lateral sectionectomy for hepatocellular carcinoma

Categorical variables	Cirrhotic (n = 8)	Non-cirrhotic (n = 10)	p value
Inflow control (Yes (%))	3 (37.5)	2 (20.0)	0.608
Blood transfusion (Yes(%))	2 (25.0)	1 (10.0)	0.559
Complications (Yes (%))	4 (50.0)	2 (20.0)	0.321
Major complications [a] (Yes (%))	0 (0)	0 (0)	N.A.
Thirty-day mortality (Yes (%))	0 (0)	0 (0)	N.A.
In-hospital mortality (Yes (%))	0 (0)	0 (0)	N.A.
Early recurrence [b](Yes (%))	1 (12.5)	2 (20.0)	1.000

Continuous variables [c]	Cirrhotic (n = 8)	Non-cirrhotic (n = 10)	p value
Operative duration (minutes)	270.9 ± 24.47	299.9 ± 49.28	0.607
Blood loss (ml)	321.3 ± 80.99	134.0 ± 32.70	0.060
Duration of inflow control[d] (minutes)	75.7 ± 9.24	100.5 ± 4.50	0.139
Duration of parenchymal transection (minutes)	82.8 ± 9.93	105.0 ± 25.06	0.521
Post-OP hospital stay (days) (range)	9.6 ± 0.96 (6–15)	7.5 ± 0.52 (5–10)	0.057

[a]major surgical complications include grade III-IV surgical complications
[b]recurrence within two years after the index operation
[c]mean ± standard error of mean
[d]mean duration among those who had inflow control

resection. We believe this stapleless approach is a safe and efficient opportunity for liver surgeons to gather the experience necessary to overcome the learning curve required for LH. This concept is similar to that established by Komatsu et al. [25]. Last but not the least, we found that laparoscopic Cavitron ultrasonic surgical aspirator (CUSA) was rarely indicated in LLS since the other energy devices such as Harmonic scalpels or Thunderbeat dissectors are capable enough to complete the parenchymal transection. This result is also comparable to that published by Liu et al. in 2017 [26]. Although our stapleless technique appears promising, some drawbacks still require considerations. First, to skeletonize the portal pedicles and hepatic veins, more time is necessary for such meticulous parenchymal transection in order to complete the entire operation. Moreover, to achieve such extensive dissection, the energy device would produce some smoke, which may blur the video laparoscope and hamper the operation. However, we believe these are only minor flaws and would not alter our commitment towards the stapleless LLS. As a result, through this stapleless stepwise approach, we provide liver surgeons with an opportunity to practice their techniques in preparation for more complicated major liver resections.

In the current study, the postoperative hospital stay was not significantly different between the two groups. We believe this may be attributed to several reasons. First, since we just started our laparoscopic program, our immature technique may result in prolonged postoperative stay. The lack of knowledge regarding post-laparoscopic recovery and care may also have resulted in delayed hospital discharge. Second, since our national health care insurance reimburses the cost of postoperative hospital stay, patients usually prefer not to be discharged until they have completely recovered. Lastly, the small number of patients in the current study renders the statistics less significant. We believe the trend towards shorter hospital stay for LLS will become more pronounced when more patients have accumulated.

The current study compared the outcome after laparoscopic and conventional open left lateral sectionectomy for HCC. It is often difficult to initiate a new surgical technique, especially when there has been an long-established equivalent counterpart. For minimally invasive surgery (MIS) per se, during the residency years of the index young surgeon, MIS in Taiwan were mostly limited to simple procedures such as LC, LA, and laparoscopic gastrorrhaphy. Laparoscopic major gastrointestinal or hepatobiliary surgeries, on the other hand, were relatively rare and performed mainly by several experienced surgeons. Thanks for the support from the institutions and related surgical associations in Taiwan, the index surgeon and other motivated surgeons, after finishing their residency training, gained access to more complicated laparoscopic procedures including laparoscopic hepatectomy. Almost a decade after, MIS in Taiwan is a booming technique that almost every medical center now is capable of performing laparoscopic gastrointestinal surgeries. Residents nowadays are able to observe and participate in more complicated laparoscopic procedures during their training period. Given the evidence obtained from previous study and the current research [27], senior residents or less experienced surgeons will have the opportunity to perform LLS as the first step toward laparoscopic hepatectomy.

Despite encouraging results, the current study still has some limitations. First, since it is a retrospective study based on clinical data retrieved from a database, incomplete data collection is inevitable when reviewing records many years ago. Second, the lack of randomization between LH and OH groups also introduced selection bias into our final statistical analysis. A prospective randomized control trial is thus warranted to validate our findings. Third, more than one surgeon conducted the conventional open hepatectomy, the results after OH may be less homogenous. Fourth, in some cases, the follow-up duration was not long enough. A longer follow-up period is thus required to give a more convincing result. Lastly, as mentioned above, we need more laparoscopic experience to demonstrate the significance of LH for HCC.

Conclusions

The current study demonstrated that our stapleless laparoscopic liver resection is a safe and feasible procedure for less experienced liver surgeons to resect HCC located at the left lateral liver sector, even for HCC in cirrhotic livers. It delivers comparable surgical results with similar operation time and blood loss, less need for inflow control, low complication rate, and zero mortality rate. The oncological disease-free survival and overall survival rates are also equivalent to the conventional open approach. As suggested by the Louisville statement, LLS should be the standard treatment of choice for HCC, especially when the tumor is less than 5 cm in diameter. In addition, our stapleless LLS can provide a platform for liver surgeons to apply laparoscopic technique before conducting more complicated liver resections. Further randomized prospective studies are warranted to determine the actual role of laparoscopic surgery in the treatment of HCC.

Acknowledgments
We are grateful to all our colleagues in the Department of Cancer Center, Department of Pathology, and Graduate Institute of Clinical Medical Sciences, Chang Gung University for their technical assistance. We are also grateful to Jo-Chu Chiu and Chun-Hsing Wu for their assistance in data retrieval and processing.

Funding
The collection of the clinical data, performance of the statistical analysis, interpretation of the results, and English proofread are funded by Chang Gung Memorial Hospital (CMRPG3F1991) and Ministry of Science and Technology, Taiwan, R.O.C. (MOST 106–2314-B-182A-018 / NMRPG3G0181).

Authors' contributions
CWL designed the study, conducted the laparoscopic surgery, and drafted the manuscript. HIT, HTC, and WTC collected the clinical data and revised the manuscript. HYH and YPL analyzed the clinicopathological data and performed the statistics. CCC assisted the laparoscopic surgery and revised the manuscript. MCY designed the study, performed the open hepatectomy, and drafted the manuscript. THW, WCL, and MFC conducted open hepatectomy, coordinated the study, and revised the manuscript. All authors read and approved the final manuscript.

Consent for publication
Not applicable.

Competing interests
Chao-Wei Lee, Hsin-I Tsai, Hao-Tsai Cheng, Wei-Ting Chen, Heng-Yuan Hsu, Chien-Chih Chiu, Yi-Ping Liu, Tsung-Han Wu, Ming-Chin Yu, Wei-Chen Lee, and Miin-Fu Chen have no conflicts of interest or financial ties to disclose.

Author details
[1]Department of Surgery, Linkou Chang Gung Memorial Hospital, No.5, Fuxing St, Guishan Dist, Taoyuan City 33305, Taiwan, Republic of China. [2]College of Medicine, Chang Gung University, Guishan, Taoyuan, Taiwan, Republic of China. [3]Graduate Institute of Clinical Medical Sciences, Chang Gung University, Guishan, Taoyuan, Taiwan, Republic of China. [4]Department of Anesthesiology, Linkou Chang Gung Memorial Hospital, No.5, Fuxing St, Guishan Dist, Taoyuan City 33305, Taiwan, Republic of China. [5]Department of Gastroenterology and Hepatology, Linkou Chang Gung Memorial Hospital, No.5, Fuxing St, Guishan Dist, Taoyuan City 33305, Taiwan, Republic of China. [6]Department of Nursing, Linkou Chang Gung Memorial Hospital, No.5, Fuxing St, Guishan Dist, Taoyuan City 33305, Taiwan, Republic of China. [7]Department of Surgery, Xiamen Chang Gung Hospital, Xiamen, China.

References
1. Salminen P, Hurme S, Ovaska J. Fifteen-year outcome of laparoscopic and open Nissen fundoplication: a randomized clinical trial. Ann Thorac Surg. 2012;93(1):228–33 PubMed PMID: 22098922. Epub 2011/11/22. eng.
2. Law WL, Poon JT, Fan JK, Lo SH. Comparison of outcome of open and laparoscopic resection for stage II and stage III rectal cancer. Ann Surg Oncol. 2009;16(6):1488–93 PubMed PMID: 19290491. Epub 2009/03/18. eng.
3. Lo CM, Liu CL, Fan ST, Lai EC, Wong J. Prospective randomized study of early versus delayed laparoscopic cholecystectomy for acute cholecystitis. Ann Surg. 1998;227(4):461–7 PubMed PMID: 9563529. Pubmed Central PMCID: PMC1191296. Epub 1998/05/01. eng.

4. Chen J, Li H, Liu F, Li B, Wei Y. Surgical outcomes of laparoscopic versus open liver resection for hepatocellular carcinoma for various resection extent. Medicine. 2017;96(12):e6460 PubMed PMID: 28328863. Pubmed Central PMCID: PMC5371500. Epub 2017/03/23. eng.

5. Nguyen KT, Gamblin TC, Geller DA. World review of laparoscopic liver resection-2,804 patients. Ann Surg. 2009;250(5):831–41 PubMed PMID: 19801936. Epub 2009/10/06. eng.

6. Lee CW, Tsai HI, Sung CM, Chen CW, Huang SW, Jeng WJ, et al. Risk factors for early mortality after hepatectomy for hepatocellular carcinoma. Medicine. 2016;95(39):e5028 PubMed PMID: 27684875. Epub 2016/09/30. eng.

7. Buell JF, Cherqui D, Geller DA, O'Rourke N, Iannitti D, Dagher I, et al. The international position on laparoscopic liver surgery: the Louisville statement, 2008. Ann Surg. 2009;250(5):825–30 PubMed PMID: 19916210. Epub 2009/11/17. eng.

8. Wakabayashi G, Cherqui D, Geller DA, Buell JF, Kaneko H, Han HS, et al. Recommendations for laparoscopic liver resection: a report from the second international consensus conference held in Morioka. Ann Surg. 2015;261(4): 619–29 PubMed PMID: 25742461. Epub 2015/03/06. eng.

9. Cheung TT, Poon RT, Dai WC, Chok KS, Chan SC, Lo CM. Pure laparoscopic versus open left lateral Sectionectomy for hepatocellular carcinoma: a single-center experience. World J Surg. 2016;40(1):198–205 PubMed PMID: 26316115. Epub 2015/09/01. eng.

10. Sobin LH, Gospodarowicz MK, Wittekind C. International Union Against Cancer (UICC): TNM Classification of Malignant Tumours. 7th ed. New Jersey: Wiley-Blackwell; 2009.

11. Lau H, Man K, Fan ST, Yu WC, Lo CM, Wong J. Evaluation of preoperative hepatic function in patients with hepatocellular carcinoma undergoing hepatectomy. Br J Surg. 1997;84(9):1255–9 PubMed PMID: 9313707. Epub 1997/10/06. eng.

12. Dindo D, Demartines N, Clavien P-A. Classification of surgical complications. Ann Surg. 2004;240(2):205–13.

13. Sherman M. Recurrence of hepatocellular carcinoma. N Engl J Med. 2008; 359(19):2045–47.

14. Torre LA, Bray F, Siegel RL, Ferlay J, Lortet-Tieulent J, Jemal A. Global cancer statistics, 2012. CA Cancer J Clin. 2015;65(2):87–108 PubMed PMID: 25651787.

15. Department of Health ROC. Report of leading cancer-related death in 2014. p. 2015.

16. Lin HM, Lei LM, Zhu J, Li GL, Min J. Risk factor analysis of perioperative mortality after ruptured bleeding in hepatocellular carcinoma. World J Gastroenterol. 2014;20(40):14921–6 PubMed PMID: 25356052. Pubmed Central PMCID: PMC4209555. Epub 2014/10/31. eng.

17. Yang T, Zhang J, Lu JH, Yang GS, Wu MC, Yu WF. Risk factors influencing postoperative outcomes of major hepatic resection of hepatocellular carcinoma for patients with underlying liver diseases. World J Surg. 2011; 35(9):2073–82 PubMed PMID: 21656309.

18. Wei AC, Tung-Ping Poon R, Fan ST, Wong J. Risk factors for perioperative morbidity and mortality after extended hepatectomy for hepatocellular carcinoma. Br J Surg. 2003;90(1):33–41 PubMed PMID: 12520572.

19. Fan ST, Lo CM, Liu CL, Lam CM, Yuen WK, Yeung C, et al. Hepatectomy for hepatocellular carcinoma: toward zero hospital deaths. Ann Surg. 1999; 229(3):322–30 PubMed PMID: 10077043. Pubmed Central PMCID: PMC1191696. English.

20. Hsu HY, Yu MC, Lee CW, Tsai HI, Sung CM, Chen CW, et al. RAM score is an effective predictor for early mortality and recurrence after hepatectomy for hepatocellular carcinoma. BMC Cancer. 2017;17(1):742 PubMed PMID: 29121890. Epub 2017/11/11. eng.

21. Guro H, Cho JY, Han HS, Yoon YS, Choi Y, Periyasamy M. Current status of laparoscopic liver resection for hepatocellular carcinoma. Clin Mol Hepatol. 2016;22(2):212–8 PubMed PMID: 27304550. Pubmed Central PMCID: PMC4946407. Epub 2016/06/16. eng.

22. Wong-Lun-Hing EM, van Dam RM, van Breukelen GJ, Tanis PJ, Ratti F, van Hillegersberg R, et al. Randomized clinical trial of open versus laparoscopic left lateral hepatic sectionectomy within an enhanced recovery after surgery programme (ORANGE II study). Br J Surg. 2017;104(5):525–35 PubMed PMID: 28138958. Epub 2017/02/01. eng.

23. Im C, Cho JY, Han HS, Yoon YS, Choi Y, Jang JY, et al. Laparoscopic left lateral sectionectomy in patients with histologically confirmed cirrhosis. Surg Oncol. 2016;25(3):132–8 PubMed PMID: 27566013. Epub 2016/08/28. eng.

24. Goh BK, Chan CY, Lee SY, Lee VT, Cheow PC, Chow PK, et al. Laparoscopic Liver Resection for Tumors in the Left Lateral Liver Section. JSLS. 2016;20(1)

PubMed PMID: 26877627. Pubmed Central PMCID: PMC4744999. Epub 2016/02/16. eng.

25. Komatsu S, Scatton O, Goumard C, Sepulveda A, Brustia R, Perdigao F, et al. Development Process and Technical Aspects of Laparoscopic Hepatectomy: Learning Curve Based on 15 Years of Experience. J Am Coll Surg. 2017; 224(5):841–50.

26. Liu F, Wei Y, Li H, Wang W, Wen T, Wu H, et al. LigaSure versus CUSA for parenchymal transection during laparoscopic hepatectomy in hepatocellular carcinoma patients with cirrhosis: a propensity score-matched analysis. Surg Endosc. 2017. PubMed PMID: 29124405. Epub 2017/11/11. eng.

27. Hasegawa Y, Nitta H, Sasaki A, Takahara T, Ito N, Fujita T, et al. Laparoscopic left lateral sectionectomy as a training procedure for surgeons learning laparoscopic hepatectomy. J Hepatobiliary Pancreat Sci. 2013;20(5):525–30.

14

Impact of antiviral therapy on hepatocellular carcinoma and mortality in patients with chronic hepatitis C

Chang Seok Bang[1] and Il Han Song[2*]

Abstract

Background: The long-term clinical outcomes of antiviral therapy for patients with chronic hepatitis C are uncertain in terms of hepatitis C virus (HCV)-related morbidity and mortality according to the response to antiviral therapy. This study aimed to assess the impact of antiviral treatment on the development of HCC and mortality in patients with chronic HCV infection.

Methods: A systematic review was conducted for studies that evaluated the antiviral efficacy for patients with chronic hepatitis C or assessed the development of HCC or mortality between SVR (sustained virologic response) and non-SVR patients. The methodological quality of the enrolled publications was evaluated using Risk of Bias table or Newcastle-Ottawa scale. Random-effect model meta-analyses and meta-regression were performed. Publication bias was assessed.

Results: In total, 59 studies (4 RCTs, 15 prospective and 40 retrospective cohort studies) were included. Antiviral treatment was associated with reduced development of HCC (vs. no treatment; OR 0.392, 95% CI 0.275–0.557), and this effect was intensified when SVR was achieved (vs. no SVR, OR: 0.203, 95% CI 0.164–0.251). Antiviral treatment was associated with lower all-cause mortality (vs. no treatment; OR 0.380, 95% CI 0.295–0.489) and liver-specific mortality (OR 0.363, 95% CI 0.260–0.508). This rate was also intensified when SVR was achieved [all-cause mortality (vs. no SVR, OR 0.255, 95% CI 0.199–0.326), liver-specific mortality (OR 0.126, 95% CI 0.094–0.169)]. Sensitivity analyses revealed robust results, and a small study effect was minimal.

Conclusions: In patients with chronic hepatitis C, antiviral therapy can reduce the development of HCC and mortality, especially when SVR is achieved.

Keywords: Antiviral therapy, Chronic hepatitis C, Hepatocellular carcinoma, Mortality, Sustained virologic response

Background

Antiviral treatment for chronic hepatitis C (CHC) aims to prevent hepatitis C virus (HCV)-related morbidity and mortality, including complications of liver fibrosis or cirrhosis and the development of hepatocellular carcinoma (HCC). Treatment reduces the degree of necroinflammation of the liver and induces regression of hepatic fibrosis [1]. Although direct-acting antivirals have recently emerged as a promising therapy, conventional interferon (IFN) or pegylated IFN (PegIFN) with or without ribavirin (RBV) has been used as the standard treatment for curing HCV.

A sustained virologic response (SVR) is the surrogate indicator for eradicating HCV and is considered to be "cure" [2]. SVR24 or SVR12, which is the state of undetectable HCV RNA in a sensitive assay with a lower limit of detection <50 IU/mL at week 24 or 12 after the end of treatment are accepted as an endpoint of treatment [3].

* Correspondence: ihsong21@dankook.ac.kr
[2]Division of Hepatology, Department of Internal Medicine, Dankook University College of Medicine, Cheonan, Korea, Republic of Korea
Full list of author information is available at the end of the article

The evolution of CHC is slow, and there is no specific symptom before progression to liver fibrosis. Due to delayed diagnosis of HCV-related chronic liver disease such as chronic hepatitis or liver fibrosis, it is difficult to start an anitviral treatment in the early stage of the disease. Previous study has demonstrated an achievement of SVR was associated with less risk for mortality (risk ratio 0.16) and development of HCC (risk ratio 0.37) [4]. However, the majority of studies assessed short-term prognosis and the long-term clinical outcomes of antiviral therapy for patients with chronic hepatitis C are uncertain in terms of HCV-related morbidity and mortality, including disease progression to advanced hepatic fibrosis or cirrhosis, hepatic decompensation, HCC, and liver-specific death, especially according to the response to antiviral therapy. Moreover, viral replication of HCV is not known to be directly related to HCC development [4].

The aim of this study was to assess the impact of antiviral treatment on the development of HCC and mortality in patients with CHC.

Methods

This systematic review and meta-analysis fully adhered to the principle of PRISMA (Preferred Reporting Items for Systematic reviews and Meta-Analyses) checklist.

Literature searching strategy

PubMed, Embase, and the Cochrane Library were searched using common keywords associated with chronic hepatitis C, HCC, or SVR (from inception to April 2016) by 2 independent evaluators (C.S.B. and Y.J.Y.). Medical Subject Headings (MeSH) or Emtree keywords were selected for searching of electronic databases. The keywords included 'hepatitis C', 'HCV', 'hepatocellular carcinoma', 'HCC', 'sustained virologic response', 'SVR' and 'mortality'. These keywords were combined for a searching strategy using Boolean operators. The abstracts of all identified studies were reviewed to exclude irrelevant articles. Full-text reviews were performed to determine whether the inclusion criteria were satisfied by the remaining studies and the bibliographies of relevant articles were reviewed to identify additional studies. Disagreements between the evaluators were resolved by discussion or consultation with a third evaluator (I.H.S.). The detailed searching strategy is described in Table 1.

Selection criteria

We included randomized or non-randomized studies that met the following criteria: 1. Study designed to evaluate the efficacy of antiviral treatment on the development of HCC or mortality in CHC patients and a control group, or in CHC patients with SVR and the no SVR group; 2. Publications on human subjects; 3. Full-text publication; and 4. English language. Studies that

Table 1 Clinical data of included studies

1. PubMed

1. Hepatitis C[Mesh] OR HCV
2. HCC OR "hepatocellular carcinoma"
3. SVR OR "sustained virologic response"
4. Mortality
(#1 AND #2) OR (#1 AND #3) OR (#1 AND #4) - > removed duplicated articles

2. Embase

1. (hepatitis C or hcv).mp
2. (hcc or hepatocellular carcinoma).mp
3. (svr or sustained virologic reponse).mp
4. mortality
After accumulation of (1 and 2), (1 and 3), and (1 and 4), and then removed duplicated articles

3. Cochrane library

1. Hepatitis C OR HCV
2. HCC OR "hepatocellular carcinoma"
3. SVR OR "sustained virologic response"
4. Mortality
(#1 AND #2) OR (#1 AND #3) OR (#1 AND #4) - > removed duplicated articles

met the all of the inclusion criteria were sought and selected. The exclusion criteria were as follows: 1. Incomplete data; 2. Review article; 3. Animal study; 4. Letter or case article; or 5. Abstract only publication. Studies meeting at least 1 of the exclusion criteria were excluded from this analysis.

Methodological quality

The methodological quality of the enrolled publications was assessed using the Risk of Bias table for randomized studies and the Newcastle-Ottawa Scale for non-randomized studies. The Risk of Bias was assessed as described in the Cochrane handbook by recording the method used to generate the randomization sequence, allocation concealment, determination of whether blinding was implemented for participants or staff, and evidence of selective reporting of the outcomes [5]. Review Manager version 5.3.3 (Revman for Windows 7, the Nordic Cochrane Centre, Copenhagen, Denmark) was used to generate the Risk of Bias table. The Newcastle-Ottawa scale is categorized into three parameters: the selection of the study population, the comparability of the groups, and the ascertainment of the exposure or outcome. Each parameter consists of subcategorized questions: selection ($n = 4$), comparability ($n = 1$), and exposure or outcome ($n = 3$) [6, 7]. Stars that are awarded for each item serve as a quick visual assessment of the methodological quality of the studies. A study can be graded a maximum of 9 stars, which indicates the highest quality. Two of the evaluators (C.S.B. and Y.J.Y.) independently assessed the methodological quality of all studies, and any disagreements between the evaluators were resolved by discussion or consultation with a third evaluator (I.H.S.).

Primary and modifier-based analyses

The following questions were primary topic of this meta-analyses: In patients with CHC, 1. Does the antiviral treatment reduce the development of HCC? 2. Does the antiviral treatment reduce all-cause or 3. liver-specific mortality? 4. Does the achievement of SVR reduce the development of HCC? 5. Does the achievement of SVR reduce all-cause or 6. liver-specific mortality?

The analysis was performed as 6 distinct meta-analyses to answer the 6 questions described above. Two evaluators (C.S.B. and Y.J.Y.) independently used the same data fill-up form to collect the primary summary outcome and modifiers in each study. The outcome was the relative rate of the development of HCC or mortality between antiviral treatment and the control groups, or the SVR and no SVR groups. These ratios were extracted and evaluated by odds ratios (ORs). Sensitivity analyses, including cumulative and one study removed analyses were performed to confirm the robustness of the main analysis results. These analyses were calculated in the order of publication year or effect size to find whether the time trend exists or which study is more or less influential in the pooled estimate. We also performed a meta-ANOVA and meta-regression to identify the reason of heterogeneity based on the multiple modifiers identified during systematic review. These reasons include study format (randomized/prospective cohort/retrospective cohort study), nationality, histology (degree of liver fibrosis), follow-up duration, Newcastle-Ottawa scale, age, and the regimen of the treatment (IFN, IFN with RBV, PegIFN with or without RBV). The follow-up duration of each study was categorized as long-term (≥5 years) or short-term (<5 years).

Statistics

Comprehensive Meta-Analysis software (version 3, Biostat; Borenstein M, Hedges L, Higgins J and Rothstein H. Englewood, NJ, USA) was used for this meta-analysis. We calculated the ORs with 95% confidence intervals (CIs) using 2×2 tables from the original articles to evaluate the efficacy of antiviral treatment between the treatment and control groups, or the SVR and no SVR groups whenever possible. Heterogeneity was determined using the I^2 test developed by Higgins, which measures the percentage of total variation across studies [8]. I^2 was calculated as follows: I^2 (%) = 100 × (Q-df)/Q, where Q is Cochrane's heterogeneity statistic and df signifies the degree of freedom. Negative values for I^2 were set to zero, and an I^2 value over 50% was considered to be of substantial heterogeneity (range: 0–100%) [9]. Pooled-effect sizes with 95% CIs were calculated using a random effects model and the method of DerSimonian and Laird due to methodological heterogeneity [10]. These results were confirmed by the I^2 test. Significance

was set at $p = 0.05$. Publication bias was evaluated using Begg's funnel plot, Egger's test of the intercept, Begg and Mazumdar's rank correlation test, and Duval and Tweedie's trim and fill method [11–15].

Results

Identification of relevant studies

Figure 1 presents a flow diagram of how relevant studies were identified. In total, 36,421 articles were identified by a search of 3 databases. In all, 7451 duplicate studies and an additional 28,481 studies were excluded during the initial screening through a review of the titles and abstracts. The full texts of the remaining 489 studies were then thoroughly reviewed. Among these studies, 431 articles were excluded from the final analysis. The reasons for study exclusion during the final review were as follows: review article ($n = 12$), incomplete data ($n = 7$), not meeting the inclusion criteria ($n = 409$), or abstract only study ($n = 3$). The remaining 58 studies [4 randomized controlled studies (RCTs), 15 prospective cohort, and 40 retrospective cohort studies] were included in the final analysis.

Characteristics of included studies

In each study topic, about 13–35 studies were enrolled. In terms of the study format, RCTs, prospective and retrospective cohort studies were mixed. The number of Western population-based studies and the number of Asian population-based studies were evenly distributed. The age of enrolled patients ranged from 37 to 64 years (median). The follow-up duration ranged from 32 months (mean) to 11.5 years (median). Most of the studies used IFN-based regimens with or without RBV in topic 1, 2 and 3. However, a PegIFN-based regimen and IFN-based regimens were evenly distributed in topic 4, 5, and 6. Underlying histology of liver was variable, but some studies exclusively assessing liver cirrhosis patients were included. The detailed characteristics of the included studies are described in Tables 2, 3, 4, 5, and 6.

Methodological quality

The methodological quality of cohort study is described in the Table 3, 4, 5 and 6. This feature was evaluated as modifiers in each analysis. The methodological quality of RCT is described in Additional file 1: Appendix 1. Given the similar methodological quality among RCTs, sensitivity analysis or subgroup analyses based on the methodological quality in RCTs were not performed.

Efficacy of antiviral treatment on the development of HCC in chronic hepatitis C patients

The overall efficacy of antiviral treatment on the development of HCC exhibited an OR of 0.392 (95% CI: 0.275–0.557, p <0.001) in a random effect model analysis (Fig. 2).

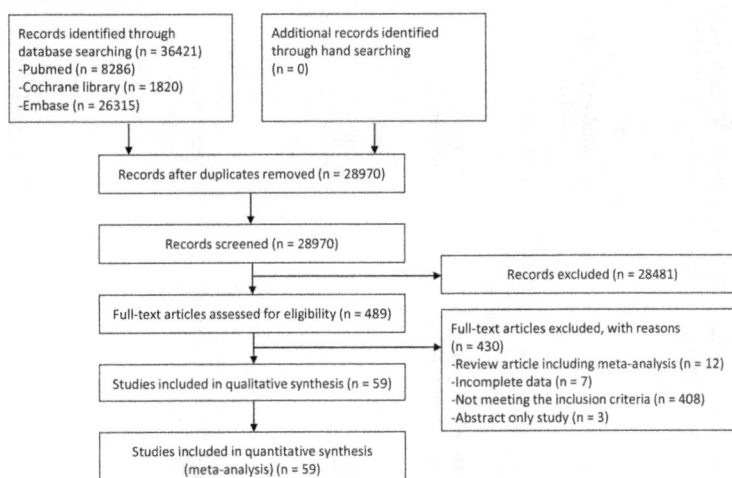

Fig. 1 Flow diagram for identification of relevant studies

The funnel plot showed asymmetry on the right lower quadrant area (Additional file 1: Appendix Figure S2). However, the Egger's test revealed an intercept of −2.131 (95% CI: −4.81–0.54, t-value: 1.64, df: 23, $p = 0.11$ (2-tailed)). The rank correlation test also showed a Kendall's tau of −0.19 with a continuity correction ($p = 0.17$). The trim and fill method indicated that no study was trimmed. Overall, there was no evidence of publication bias.

A cumulative meta-analysis of enrolled studies based on publication year showed no specific time trend (Additional file 1: Appendix 3). A cumulative meta-analysis based on effect size showed no small study bias (Additional file 1: Appendix 4). One study removed meta-analysis revealed a stable feature (Additional file 1: Appendix 5). Overall, the sensitivity meta-analyses revealed robust results.

Methodological quality of Newcastle-Ottawa scale potentially explained heterogeneity in meta-ANOVA tests ($p = 0.027$) (Additional file 1: Appendix 6). A meta-regression revealed a Newcastle-Ottawa scale score of 8 for the reason of heterogeneity ($p = 0.027$) (Additional file 2: Table S1). After excluding 10 studies (Newcastle-Ottawa scale 8), no covariates explained heterogeneity in meta-regression tests. Therefore, methodological quality was the reason of heterogeneity in this analysis.

Efficacy of antiviral treatment on All-cause mortality in patients with chronic hepatitis C

The overall efficacy of antiviral treatment on all-cause mortality revealed an OR of 0.380 (95% CI: 0.295–0.489, $p < 0.001$) in a random effect model analysis (Fig. 3). The funnel plot showed asymmetry on the right lower quadrant area (Additional file 1: Appendix 7). However, the Egger's test revealed an intercept of 0.266 (95% CI: −2.010–2.542, t-value: 0.25, df: 15, $p = 0.81$ (2-tailed)). The rank correlation test also showed a Kendall's tau of 0.04 with a continuity correction ($p = 0.84$). The trim and fill method indicated that 1 study was trimmed. After excluding the study by Testino et al. [16] located on the left lower quadrant in funnel plot, the OR was 0.385 (95% CI: 0.298–0.496, $p < 0.001$). Overall, the impact of bias was minimal.

A cumulative meta-analysis of enrolled studies based on publication year showed no specific time trend (Additional file 1: Appendix 8). A cumulative meta-analysis based on effect size showed no small study bias (Additional file 1: Appendix 9). One study removed meta-analysis revealed a stable feature (Additional file 1: Appendix 10). Overall, the sensitivity meta-analyses revealed robust results.

Meta-ANOVA or meta-regression showed no specific modifier for the reason of heterogeneity (Additional file 1: Appendix 11) (Additional file 2: Table S2). Overall, no covariates were found to be explaining heterogeneity in this meta-analysis.

Efficacy of antiviral treatment on liver-specific mortality in chronic hepatitis C patients

The overall efficacy of antiviral treatment on liver-specific mortality exhibited an OR of 0.363 (95% CI: 0.260–0.508, $p < 0.001$) in a random effect model analysis (Additional file 1: Appendix 12). The funnel plot showed symmetry (Additional file 1: Appendix 13). However, the Egger's test revealed that intercept was 3.06 (95% CI: 0.295–5.831, t-value: 2.43, df: 11, $p = 0.03$ (2-tailed)). The rank correlation test showed a Kendall's tau of 0.28 with a continuity correction ($p = 0.20$). The trim and fill method indicated that no study was trimmed. After excluding an outlier (study by Kasahara A et al. [17]) located on the left upper quadrant area in funnel plot, the OR was 0.398 (95% CI: 0.314–0.504, $p < 0.001$). Overall, the impact of bias was minimal.

Table 2 Clinical data summary of all included studies

Topic	Number of enrolled studies and population	Study format	Nationality	Age	Follow-up duration	Treatment regimen	Histology
Topic 1	25 studies (9691 treated vs. 6010 control)	3 RCTs, 8 prospective cohort studies, 14 retrospective cohort studies	15 Western population-based studies, 10 Asian population-based studies	37 to 61 years (median)	32 months to 10 years (mean)	IFN-based regimens with or without RBV, except 4 studies with a PegIFN-based regimen	10 studies exclusively assessing LC patients
Topic 2	17 studies (9868 treated vs. 4700 controls)	1 RCT, 5 prospective cohort studies, 11 retrospective cohort studies	8 Western population-based studies, 9 Asian population-based studies	37 to 61 years (median)	55 months to 11.5 years (median)	IFN-based regimen with or without RBV, except 3 studies with a PegIFN-based regimen	3 studies exclusively assessing LC patients
Topic 3	13 studies (8671 treated vs. 2831 controls)	5 prospective cohort studies, 8 retrospective cohort studies	5 Western population-based studies, 8 Asian population-based studies	37 to 61 years (median)	55 months to 11.5 years (median)	IFN-based regimen with or without RBV, except 2 studies with a PegIFN-based regimen	4 studies exclusively assessing LC patients
Topic 4	35 studies (14756 patients with SVR vs. 12741 patients with no SVR)	1 RCT, 8 prospective cohort studies, 26 retrospective cohort studies	17 Western population-based studies, 17 Asian population-based studies, 1 Saudi Arabia and Egypt population-based study	37 to 64 years (median)	2.1 (median) to 10 years (mean)	20 studies with PegIFN-based regimen, 15 studies with IFN-based regimen	9 studies exclusively assessing LC patients
Topic 5	22 studies (12440 patients with SVR vs. 18980 patients with no SVR)	4 prospective cohort studies, 18 retrospective cohort studies	12 Western population-based studies, 9 Asian population-based studies, 1 Saudi Arabia and Egypt population-based study	41.8 to 64 years (mean)	2.1 to 11.5 years (median)	11 studies with PegIFN-based regimen, 11 studies with IFN-based regimen	3 studies exclusively assessing LC patients
Topic 6	23 studies (5148 patients with SVR vs. 10356 patients with no SVR)	7 prospective cohort studies, 16 retrospective cohort studies	14 Western population-based studies, 9 Asian population-based studies	41.8 to 64 (mean)	2.1 to 11.5 years (median)	12 studies with PegIFN-based regimen, 11 studies with IFN-based regimen	6 studies exclusively assessing LC patients

RCT randomized controlled study, *IFN* interferon, *PegIFN* pegylated interferon, *RBV* ribavirin, *LC* liver cirrhosis, *SVR* sustained virologic response

Table 3 Clinical data of included studies for the efficacy of antiviral treatment on the development of HCC in patients with CHC

Study	Nationality	Age	Duration of follow up	Study format	Genotype	NOS	Treatment	HCC/Total treatment	HCC/Control	Histology
Mazella G et al. (1996) [23]	Italy	Tx: 53, control: 54 (mean)	mean 32 months	P	unknown	7	IFN-α or lymphoblastoid	5/193	9/92	Child A LC
Bruno S et al.(1997) [24]	Italy	Tx: 56, control: 59 (mean)	median 68 months	P	62% type 1b	7	IFN-α	6/83	16/80	LC (mainly Child A)
Fattovich G et al. (1997) [25]	Italy	Tx: 53, control: 57 (mean)	mean 60 months	R	unknown	8	IFN-α	7/193	16/136	LC
Serfaty L et al. (1998) [26]	France	Tx: 55, control: 56 (mean)	median 40 months	P	48% 1b	7	IFN-α	2/59	9/44	Knodell 10 (mean)
Benvegnù L et al.(1998) [27]	Italy	Tx: 56.7, control: 59.5 (mean)	mean 71.5 months	P	unknown	8	IFN	4/75	20/77	Child A LC
International Interferon-α Hepatocellular Carcinoma Study Group (1998) [28]	Italy and Argentina	54 (median)	36 months	R	unknown	7	IFN-α or lymphoblastoid	21/232	48/259	unknown
Imai Y et al.(1998) [29]	Japan	unknown	Tx: 47.6, control: 46.8 (median)	R	unknown	7	IFN-α	28/419	19/144	F3,4: 37% in Tx, 53% in control
Yoshida H et al. (1999) [30]	Japan	Tx: 49.5, control: 53.6 (mean)	median 4.3 years	R	70.3% type 1	7	IFN-α or IFN-β or combination	89/2400	59/490	F3,4: 33.1% in Tx, 33.8% in control
Okanoue T et al. (1999) [31]	Japan	42.6–57.6 (mean)	mean 39.5–67.1 months	R	unknown	7	IFN-α or lymphoblastoid	52/1148	22/55	F3,4: 34% in Tx, F4: 100% in control
Valla DC et al. (1999) [32]	France	Tx: 57, control: 56 (mean)	mean 160 weeks	RCT	unknown	7	IFN-α	5/47	9/52	compensated LC
Ikeda K et al. (2001) [33]	Japan	57 (median)	median 7.6 years	R	unknown	7	IFN-α or IFN-β	32/113	271/581	LC
Gramenzi A et al. (2001) [34]	Italy	Tx: 57.9, control: 58.1 (mean)	median 55–58 months	P	unknown	7	IFN-α	6/72	19/72	LC (mainly Child A)
Nishiguchi S et al. (2001) [35]	Japan	Tx: 54.7, control: 57.3 (mean)	mean 8.2 years	RCT	75.6% type 2	7	IFN-α	12/45	33/45	unknown
Testino G et al. (2002) [16]	Italy	Tx: 55.3, control: 56.8 (mean)	mean 95.4 months	R	55% type 1b, 45% type 2	8	IFN-α	12/51	24/71	Child A LC
Coverdale SA et al. (2004) [36]	Australia	Tx: 37, control: 38 (median)	median 9 years	P	39.6% type 1	7	IFN-α	26/384	7/71	Scheuer fibrosis score 2
Azzaroli F et al. (2004) [37]	Italy	55.1 (mean)	5 years	RCT	64.4% type 1b	7	IFN-α with RBV	2/71	9/30	LC
Shiratori Y et al. (2005) [38]	Japan	Tx: 57, control: 61 (median)	median 6.8 years	P	71.9% type 1b	8	IFN-α or lymphoblastoid	84/271	35/74	unknown
Yu ML et al. (2006) [39]	Taiwan	Tx: 46.9, control: 43.6 (mean)	mean 5.18–5.15 years	R	46.2% type 1	8	IFN-α with or without RBV	51/1057	54/562	LC 15.6% in Tx, 12.1% in control
Sinn DH et al. (2008) [40]	Korea	48.4–58.2 (mean)	median 55.2 months	R	48.6% type 2	7	IFN/PegIFN with or without RBV	14/490	122/647	F3,4: 49% in Tx, F4: 33% in control
Di Martino V et al. (2011) [41]	France	unknown	median 59 months	R	57.9% type 1	7	IFN with or without RBV, or PegIFN with RBV	9/184	5/184	55.5% F2 or greater

Table 3 Clinical data of included studies for the efficacy of antiviral treatment on the development of HCC in patients with CHC (*Continued*)

Tateyama M et al. (2011) [42]	Japan	57 (median)	mean 8.2 years	R	72.1% type 1b	8	IFN/PegIFN with or without RBV	110/373	63/334	F3,4: 34.1%
Maruoka D et al. (2012) [43]	Japan	50.4–54 (mean)	mean 9.9 years	R	73.6% type 1	8	IFN-α/IFN-β with or without RBV	85/577	35/144	F3,4: 24.3% in Tx, F4: 43.1% in control
Cozen ML et al. (2013) [44]	US	50.98 (mean)	mean 10 years	R	68.7% type 1	8	IFN-α with or without RBV	11/159	9/199	F3,4: 19% (30.2% in Tx, 10.1% in control)
Aleman S et al. (2013) [45]	Sweden	51 (mean)	mean 5.3 years	R	50% type 1	8	PegIFN with RBV	32/303	14/48	LC
Cozen ML et al. (2016) [46]	US	51.4 (mean)	mean 8.5 years	P	71.6% type 1 or 4	8	IFN-α with RBV	43/692	84/1519	LC 15.8% in Tx, 5.3% in control

HCC hepatocellular carcinoma, *CHC* chronic hepatitis C, *NOS* Newcastle-Ottawa scale, *Tx* treatment group, *R* retrospective cohort study, *P* prospective cohort study, *RCT* randomized controlled study, *IFN* interferon, *PegIFN* pegylated interferon, *RBV* ribavirin, *LC* liver cirrhosis

Table 4 Clinical data of included studies for the efficacy of antiviral treatment on all-cause and liver-specific mortality in patients with CHC

Study	Nationality	Age	Duration of follow up	Study format	Genotype	NOS	Treatment	Death/Total treatment	Death/Control	Histology
Benvegnù L et al. (1998) [27]	Italy	Tx: 56.7, control: 59.5 (mean)	mean 71.5 months	P	unknown	8	IFN	[a]3/75	[a]15/77	Child A LC
Ikeda K et al. (2001) [33]	Japan	57 (median)	median 7.6 years	R	unknown	7	IFN-α or IFN-β	20/113 [a]12/113	266/581 [a]124/581	LC
Gramenzi A et al. (2001) [34]	Italy	Tx: 57.9, control: 58.1 (mean)	median 55–58 months	P	unknown	7	IFN-α	[a]7/72	9/72 [a]8/72	LC (mainly Child A)
Nishiguchi S et al. (2001) [35]	Japan	Tx: 54.7, control: 57.3 (mean)	mean 8.2 years	RCT	75.6% type 2	8	IFN-α	5/45	26/45	unknown
Testino G et al. (2002) [16]	Italy	Tx: 55.3, control: 56.8 (mean)	mean 95.4 months	R	55% type 1b, 45% type 2	8	IFN-α	1/51	9/71	Child A LC
Yosida H et al. (2002) [47]	Japan	Tx: 49.5, control: 54.6 (mean)	mean 5.4 years	R	unknown	8	IFN-α or IFN-β	56/2430 [a]35/2430	30/459 [a]23/459	F3,4: 32.2% in Tx, 31.6% in control, 26.3% in SVR, 35.2% in no SVR
Imazeki F et al. (2003) [48]	Japan	Tx: 49.2, control: 53.1 (mean)	mean 8.2 years	R	73.9% type 1	8	IFN-α or IFN-β	33/355 [a]19/355	15/104 [a]12/104	F3,4: 26.7% in Tx, 29.8% in control
Coverdale SA et al. (2004) [36]	Australia	Tx: 37, control: 38 (median)	median 9 years	P	39.6% type 1	7	IFN-α	[a]36/384	[a]12/71	Scheuer fibrosis score 2
Kasahara A et al. (2004) [17]	Japan	Tx: 53, control: 54 (median)	mean 6 years	R	unknown	8	IFN	101/2698 [a]69/2698	52/256 [a]42/256	F3,4: 38.7% in Tx, 48% in control, 28.6% in SVR, 43% in no SVR
Shiratori Y et al. (2005) [38]	Japan	Tx: 57, control: 61 (median)	median 6.8 years	P	71.9% type 1b	8	IFN-α or lymphoblastoid	45/271 [a]32/271	24/74 [a]19/74	unknown
Yu ML et al. (2006) [39]	Taiwan	Tx: 46.9, control: 43.6 (mean)	mean 5.18–5.15 years	R	46.2% type 1	8	IFN-α with or without RBV	16/1057 [a]14/1057	12/562 [a]10/562	LC 15.6% in Tx, 12.1% in control
Di Martino V et al. (2011) [41]	France	unknown	median 59 months	R	57.9% type 1	7	IFN with or without RBV, or PegIFN with RBV	9/184 [a]5/184	20/194 [a]4/184	55.5% F2 or greater
Yamasaki K et al. (2012) [49]	Japan	60.9 (mean)	median 11.5 years	P	59.9% type 1b	7	IFN-α or β or lymphoblastoid with or without RBV	25/152 [a]6/152	90/199 [a]32/199	unknown
Maruoka D et al. (2012) [43]	Japan	50.4–54 (mean)	mean 9.9 years	R	73.6% type 1	8	IFN-α/IFN-β with or without RBV	84/577 [a]52/577	37/144 [a]30/144	F3,4: 24.3% in Tx, F4: 43.1% in control
Cozen ML et al. (2013) [44]	US	50.98 (mean)	mean 10 years	R	68.7% type 1	8	IFN-α with or without RBV	31/159	47/199	F3,4: 19% (30.2% in Tx, 10.1% in control)
Aleman S et al. (2013) [45]	Sweden	51 (mean)	mean 5.3 years	R	50% type 1	8	PegIFN with RBV	59/303 [a]39/303	18/48 [a]16/48	LC
Kutala BK et al. (2015) [50]	France	50 (median)	median 5.5 years	R	55.7% type 1	8	IFN/PegIFN with or without RBV	30/325	19/102	F3,4: 100%
Cozen ML et al. (2016) [46]	US	51.4 (mean)	mean 8.5 years	P	71.6% type 1 or 4	8	IFN-α with RBV	112/692	488/1519	LC 15.8% in Tx, 5.3% in control

[a]: Liver-specific death, CHC chronic hepatitis C, NOS Newcastle-Ottawa scale, Tx treatment group, R retrospective cohort study, P prospective cohort study, RCT randomized controlled study, IFN interferon, PegIFN pegylated interferon, RBV ribavirin, LC liver cirrhosis, SVR sustained virologic response

Table 5 Clinical data of included studies for the efficacy of SVR on the development of HCC in patients with CHC

Study	Nationality	Age	Duration of follow up	Study format	Genotype	NOS	Treatment	HCC/Total SVR	HCC/No SVR	Histology
Nishiguchi S et al. (1995) [51]	Japan	Tx: 54.7, control: 57.3 (mean)	2–7 years	RCT	75.6% type 2		IFN-α	0/7	2/38	HAI 11.7 in Tx, 11.8 in control (mean)
Tanaka K et al. (1998) [52]	Japan	SVR: 47.7, no SVR: 51 (mean)	about 40 months	P	unknown	7	lymphoblastoid IFN	0/8	10/47	LC
Yoshida H et al. (1999) [30]	Japan	Tx: 49.5, control: 53.6 (mean)	median 4.3 years	R	70.3% type 1	7	IFN-α or IFN-β or combination	10/789	79/1611	F3,4: 33.1% in Tx, 33.8% in control
Testino G et al. (2002) [16]	Italy	Tx: 55.3, control: 56.8 (mean)	mean 95.4 months	R	55% type 1b, 45% type 2	8	IFN-α	3/11	12/40	Child A LC
Okanoue T et al. (2002) [53]	Japan	Tx: 50.4, control: 58.1 (mean)	Mean 5.6 years	R	unknown	7	IFN-α or lymphoblastoid	4/426	110/994	F3,4: 20.9% in SVR, 34.4% in control
Coverdale SA et al. (2004) [36]	Australia	Tx: 37, control: 38 (median)	median 9 years	P	39.6% type 1	7	IFN-α	1/50	25/334	Scheuer fibrosis score 2
Shiratori Y et al. (2005) [38]	Japan	Tx: 57, control: 61 (median)	median 6.8 years	P	71.9% type 1b	8	IFN-α or lymphoblastoid	11/64	73/207	unknown
Yu ML et al. (2006) [39]	Taiwan	Tx: 46.9, control: 43.6 (mean)	mean 5.18–5.15 years	R	46.2% type 1	8	IFN-α with or without RBV	12/715	39/342	LC 15.6% in Tx, 12.1% in control
Pradat P et al. (2007) [54]	Europe	45–47 (mean)	5–7 years	P	49.2% type 1	6	IFN/PegIFN with or without RBV	0/91	17/266	unknown
Braks RE et al. (2007) [55]	France	54.1 (mean)	mean 7.7 years	R	61.1% type 1	8	IFN-α with or without RBV, or PegIFN with RBV	1/37	24/76	Child A LC
Bruno S et al. (2007) [56]	Italy	54.7 (mean)	Mean 96.1 months	R	71.8% type 1	8	IFN-α	7/124	122/759	Child A LC
Hasegawa E et al. (2007) [57]	Japan	56 (median)	median 4.6 years	R	65% 2a	7	IFN-α,β/lymphoblastoid with or without RBV	3/48	16/57	LC
Veldt BJ et al. (2007) [58]	Europe and Canada	48 (median)	median 2.1 years	R	59% type 1	8	IFN/PegIFN with or without RBV	3/142	32/337	Ishak 4–6
Floreani A et al. (2008) [59]	Italy	44.5–55.7 (mean)	mean 23.4–25.2 months	R	41.3% type 1	7	PegIFN with RBV	0/40	5/38	unknown
Sinn DH et al. (2008) [40]	Korea	48.4–58.2 (mean)	median 55.2 months	R	48.6% type 2	7	IFN/PegIFN with or without RBV	4/296	10/194	F3,4: 49% in Tx, F4: 33% in control
Kurokawa M et al. (2009) [60]	Japan	55.8 (mean)	median 36.5 months	R	72.9% type 1	7	IFN-α with RBV	4/139	21/264	F3,4: 31.3%
Asahina Y et al. (2010) [61]	Japan	55.4 (mean)	mean 7.5 years	R	69.6% type 1b	8	IFN-α,β with or without RBV, or PegIFN with RBV	22/686	149/1356	F3,4: 25.2%
Kawamura Y et al. (2010) [62]	Japan	50 (median)	median 6.7 years	R	unknown	8	IFN-α,β with or without RBV	12/1081	61/977	F1,2: 93.1%
Cardoso AC et al. (2010) [63]	France	55 (mean)	median 3.5 years	R	60% type 1	7	IFN/PegIFN with or without RBV	6/103	40/204	F3,4: 100%
	US	48.6–49.6 (mean)		P	87.2% type 1	8	PegIFN with or without RBV	2/140	33/386	F3,4: 100%

Table 5 Clinical data of included studies for the efficacy of SVR on the development of HCC in patients with CHC *(Continued)*

Study	Country	Age	Follow-up	Design	Genotype	NOS	Treatment	HCC/SVR	HCC/no SVR	Fibrosis/cirrhosis
Morgan TR et al. (2010) [64]			median 79–96 months							
Di Martino V et al. (2011) [41]	France	unknown	median 59 months	R	57.9% type 1	7	IFN with or without RBV, or PegIFN with RBV	1/59	8/125	55.5% F2 or greater
Velosa J et al. (2011) [65]	Portugal	51.7 (mean)	mean 6.4 years	R	61% type 1	7	IFN/PegIFN with or without RBV	1/39	20/91	compensated LC
Iacobellis A et al. (2011) [66]	Italy	59–62 (mean)	mean 51 months	P	57.3% type 1	7	PegIFN with RBV	5/24	11/51	decompensated LC
Hung CH et al. (2011) [67]	Taiwan	53 (median)	median 4.3 years	R	49% type 1	7	IFN/PegIFN with or without RBV	33/1027	54/443	unknown
Takahashi H et al. (2011) [68]	Japan	55.4 (mean)	Mean 52 months	R	74.9% type 1b	7	IFN-α,β/PegIFN with RBV	1/89	12/114	F3,4: 23.2%
Backus LI et al. (2011) [69]	US	51–53 (mean)	median 3.8 years	R	72.1% type 1	6	PegIFN with RBV	223/7434	283/1440	13% LC
Tateyama M et al. (2011) [42]	Japan	57 (median)	mean 8.2 years	R	72.1% type 1b	8	IFN/PegIFN with or without RBV	3/139	44/234	F3,4: 34.1%
Osaki Y et al. (2012) [70]	Japan	59 (median)	median 4.1 years	R	59.9% type 1	7	IFN/PegIFN with RBV	1/185	22/197	unknown
van der Meer AJ et al. (2012) [71]	Europe and Canada	48 (mean)	median 8.4 years	R	68% type 1	8	IFN/PegIFN with or without RBV	7/125	76/405	Ishak 4–6
Maruoka D et al. (2012) [43]	Japan	50.4–54 (mean)	mean 9.9 years	R	73.6% type 1	8	IFN-α/IFN-β with or without RBV	5/221	80/356	F3,4: 24.3% in Tx, F4: 43.1% in control
Cozen ML et al. (2013) [44]	US	50.98 (mean)	mean 10 years	R	68.7% type 1	8	IFN-α with or without RBV	2/69	9/90	F3,4: 19% (30.2% in Tx, 10.1% in control)
Alfaleh FZ et al. (2013) [72]	Saudi Arabia, Egypt	48 (mean)	mean 63.8 months	P	30.6% type 4	8	PegIFN with or without RBV	0/62	4/95	F3,4: 24.6% (27.1% in SVR, 31.1% in no SVR)
Aleman S et al. (2013) [45]	Sweden	51 (mean)	mean 5.3 years	R	50% type 1	8	PegIFN with RBV	6/110	26/193	LC
Di Marco V et al. (2016) [73]	Italy	58 (mean)	median 7.6 years	P	83.4% type 1	8	PegIFN with RBV	7/108	92/336	compensated LC
Ikezaki H et al. (2016) [74]	Japan	60–64 (median)	median 2.8 years	R	52.7% in type 1	7	IFN-β with RBV	2/68	7/44	F3,4: 30.9% in SVR, 72.7% in no SVR

SVR sustained virologic response, *HCC* hepatocellular carcinoma, *CHC* chronic hepatitis C, *NOS* Newcastle-Ottawa scale, *Tx* treatment group, *R* retrospective cohort study, *P* prospective cohort study, *RCT* randomized controlled study, *IFN* interferon, *PegIFN* pegylated interferon, *RBV* ribavirin, *LC* liver cirrhosis

Table 6 Clinical data of included studies for the efficacy of SVR on all-cause and liver-specific mortality in patients with CHC

Study	Nationality	Age	Duration of follow up	Study format	Genotype	NOS	Treatment	Death/ Total SVR	Death/No SVR	Histology
Yosida H et al. (2002) [47]	Japan	Tx: 49.5, control: 54.6 (mean)	mean 5.4 years	R	unknown	8	IFN-α or IFN-β	[a]7/817	[a]49/1613	F3,4: 32.2% in Tx, 31.6% in control, 26.3% in SVR, 35.2% in no SVR
Okanoue T et al. (2002) [53]	Japan	Tx: 50.4, control: 58.1 (mean)	Mean 5.6 years	R	unknown	7	IFN-α or lymphoblastoid	2/426 [a]0/ 426	47/994 [a]34/994	F3,4: 20.9% in SVR, 34.4% in control
Imazeki F et al. (2003) [48]	Japan	Tx: 49.2, control: 53.1 (mean)	mean 8.2 years	R	73.9% type 1	8	IFN-α or IFN-β	4/116 [a]1/ 116	29/239 [a]18/239	F3,4: 26.7% in Tx, 29.8% in control
Coverdale SA et al. (2004) [36]	Australia	Tx: 37, control: 38 (median)	median 9 years	P	39.6% type 1	7	IFN-α	[a]1/50	[a]35/334	Scheuer fibrosis score 2
Kasahara A et al. (2004) [17]	Japan	Tx: 53, control: 54 (median)	mean 6 years	R	unknown	8	IFN	7/738 [a]1/ 738	94/1930 [a]68/1930	F3,4: 38.7% in Tx, 48% in control, 28.6% in SVR, 43% in no SVR
Shiratori Y et al. (2005) [38]	Japan	Tx: 57, control: 61 (median)	median 6.8 years	P	71.9% type 1b	8	IFN-α or lymphoblastoid	1/64 [a]0/ 64	44/207 [a]32/207	unknown
Yu ML et al. (2006) [39]	Taiwan	Tx: 46.9, control: 43.6 (mean)	mean 5.18– 5.15 years	R	46.2% type 1	8	IFN-α with or without RBV	4/715 [a]3/ 715	12/342 [a]11/342	LC 15.6% in Tx, 12.1% in control
Arase Y et al. (2007) [75]	Japan	SVR: 63, no SVR: 64 (mean)	mean 7.4 years	R	60.4% type 1b	8	IFN-α/β with or without RBV	9/140 [a]2/ 140	44/360 [a]32/360	F3,4: 14.5 in SVR, 27.5 in no SVR
Bruno S et al. (2007) [56]	Italy	54.7 (mean)	Mean 96.1 months	R	71.8% type 1	8	IFN-α	6/124 [a]2/ 120	114/759 [a]83/728	Child A LC
Veldt BJ et al. (2007) [58]	Europe and Canada	48 (median)	median 2.1 years	R	59% type 1	8	IFN/PegIFN with or without RBV	2/142 [a]1/ 142	24/337 [a]19/337	Ishak 4–6
Cardoso AC et al. (2010) [63]	France	55 (mean)	median 3.5 years	R	60% type 1	7	IFN/PegIFN with or without RBV	[a]3/103	[a]18/204	F3,4: 100%
Morgan TR et al. (2010) [64]	US	48.6–49.6 (mean)	median 79–96 months	P	87.2% type 1	8	PegIFN with or without RBV	[a]1/140	[a]23/386	F3,4: 100%
Innes HA et al. (2011) [76]	UK	41.8 (mean)	mean 5.3 years	R	35.6% type 1	8	IFN/PegIFN with or without RBV	13/560 [a]5/560	75/655 [a]50/655	85.8% no LC
Di Martino V et al. (2011) [41]	France	unknown	median 59 months	R	57.9% type 1	7	IFN with or without RBV, or PegIFN with RBV	0/59 [a]0/ 59	9/125 [a]5/ 125	55.5% F2 or greater
Velosa J et al. (2011) [65]	Portugal	51.7 (mean)	mean 6.4 years	R	61% type 1	7	IFN/PegIFN with or without RBV	[a]0/39	[a]15/91	compensated LC
Iacobellis A et al. (2011) [66]	Italy	59–62 (mean)	median 51 months	P	57.3% type 1	7	PegIFN with RBV	[a]2/24	[a]23/51	decompensated LC
Backus LI et al. (2011) [69]	US	51–53 (mean)	median 3.8 years	R	72.1% type 1	6	PegIFN with RBV	525/7434	1440/9430	13% LC
Yamasaki K et al. (2012) [49]	Japan	60.9 (mean)	median 11.5 years	P	59.9% type 1b	7	IFN-α or β or lymphoblastoid with or without RBV	9/72 [a]1/ 72	16/80 [a]5/ 80	unknown
van der Meer AJ et al. (2012) [71]	Europe and Canada	48 (mean)	median 8.4 years	R	68% type 1	8	IFN/PegIFN with or without RBV	13/125 [a]3/125	100/405 [a]103/405	Ishak 4–6
	Japan	50.4–54 (mean)		R		8				F3,4: 24.3% in Tx, F4: 43.1% in control

Table 6 Clinical data of included studies for the efficacy of SVR on all-cause and liver-specific mortality in patients with CHC (Continued)

Study	Country	Age	Design	Follow-up	Genotype	NOS	Treatment			Cirrhosis
Maruoka D et al. (2012) [43]				mean 9.9 years	73.6% type 1	8	IFN-α/IFN-β with or without RBV	10/221 [a]2/221	74/356 [a]50/356	
Cozen ML et al. (2013) [44]	US	50.98 (mean)	R	mean 10 years	68.7% type 1	8	IFN-α with or without RBV	6/69	25/90	F3,4: 19% (30.2% in Tx, 10.1% in control)
Alfaleh FZ et al. (2013) [72]	Saudi Arabia, Egypt	48 (mean)	P	mean 63.8 months	30.6% type 4	8	PegIFN with or without RBV	0/62 [a]0/62	4/95 [a]8/95	F3,4: 24.6% (27.1% in SVR, 31.1% in no SVR)
Aleman S et al. (2013) [45]	Sweden	51 (mean)	R	mean 5.3 years	50% type 1	8	PegIFN with RBV	11/110 [a]4/110	48/193 [a]35/193	LC
Singal AG et al. (2013) [77]	US	48 (median)	R	median 36–72 months	68.6% type 1	7	PegIFN with RBV	2/83	41/159	17.3% LC
Dieperink E et al. (2014) [78]	US	51.4 (mean)	R	median 7.5 years	70% type 1	8	IFN/PegIFN with or without RBV	19/222 [a]6/222	81/314 [a]56/314	F3,4: 54.5% (41.3% in SVR, 64.7% in no SVR)
Kutala BK et al. (2015) [50]	France	50 (median)	R	median 5.5 years	55.7% type 1	8	IFN/PegIFN with or without RBV	3/104	27/221	F3,4: 100%
Di Marco V et al. (2016) [73]	Italy	58 (mean)	P	median 7.6 years	83.4% type 1	8	PegIFN with RBV	[a]8/108	[a]98/336	compensated LC

[a]: Liver-specific death, *SVR* sustained virologic response, *CHC* chronic hepatitis C, *NOS* Newcastle-Ottawa scale, *Tx* treatment group, *R* retrospective cohort study, *P* prospective cohort study, *RCT* randomized controlled study, *IFN* interferon, *PegIFN* pegylated interferon, *RBV* ribavirin, *LC* liver cirrhosis

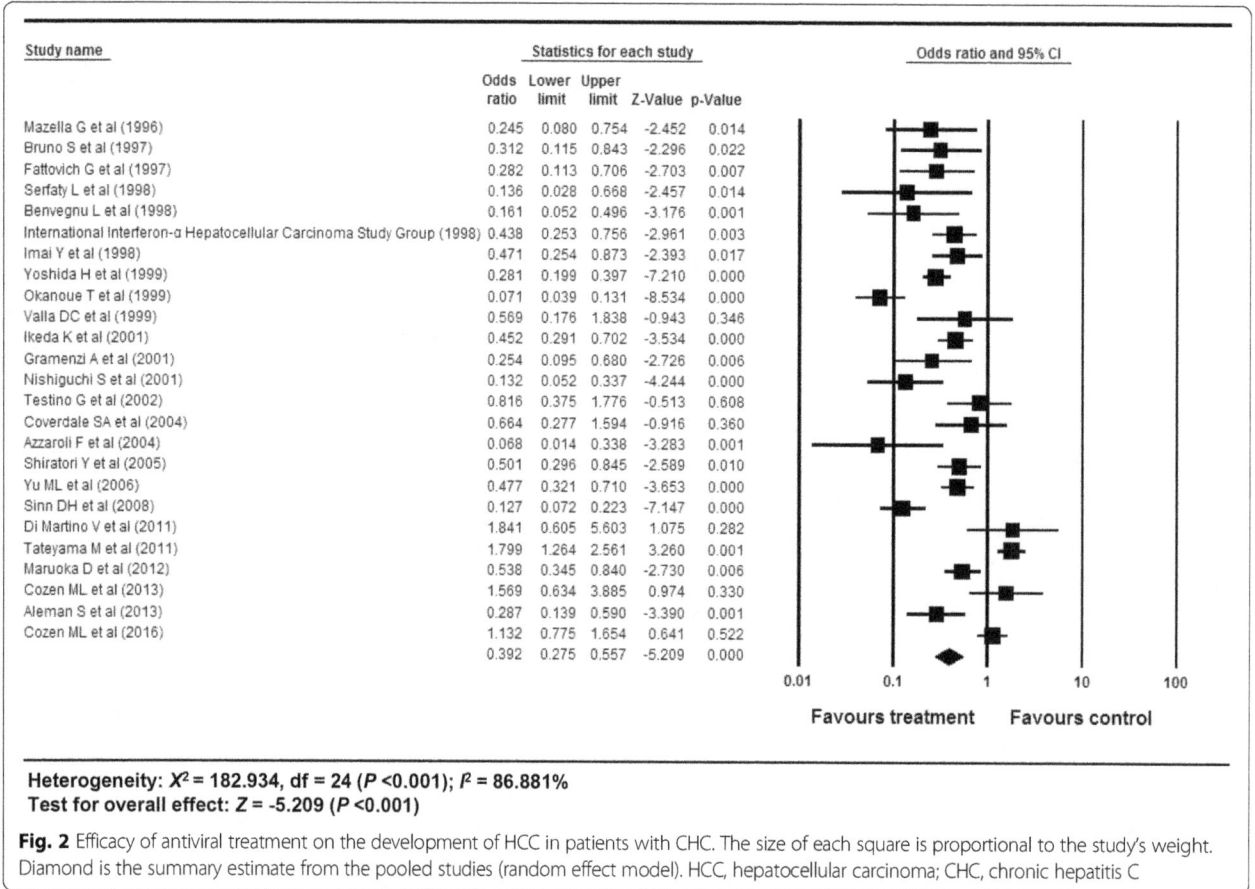

Study name	Odds ratio	Lower limit	Upper limit	Z-Value	p-Value
Mazella G et al (1996)	0.245	0.080	0.754	-2.452	0.014
Bruno S et al (1997)	0.312	0.115	0.843	-2.296	0.022
Fattovich G et al (1997)	0.282	0.113	0.706	-2.703	0.007
Serfaty L et al (1998)	0.136	0.028	0.668	-2.457	0.014
Benvegnu L et al (1998)	0.161	0.052	0.496	-3.176	0.001
International Interferon-α Hepatocellular Carcinoma Study Group (1998)	0.438	0.253	0.756	-2.961	0.003
Imai Y et al (1998)	0.471	0.254	0.873	-2.393	0.017
Yoshida H et al (1999)	0.281	0.199	0.397	-7.210	0.000
Okanoue T et al (1999)	0.071	0.039	0.131	-8.534	0.000
Valla DC et al (1999)	0.569	0.176	1.838	-0.943	0.346
Ikeda K et al (2001)	0.452	0.291	0.702	-3.534	0.000
Gramenzi A et al (2001)	0.254	0.095	0.680	-2.726	0.006
Nishiguchi S et al (2001)	0.132	0.052	0.337	-4.244	0.000
Testino G et al (2002)	0.816	0.375	1.776	-0.513	0.608
Coverdale SA et al (2004)	0.664	0.277	1.594	-0.916	0.360
Azzaroli F et al (2004)	0.068	0.014	0.338	-3.283	0.001
Shiratori Y et al (2005)	0.501	0.296	0.845	-2.589	0.010
Yu ML et al (2006)	0.477	0.321	0.710	-3.653	0.000
Sinn DH et al (2008)	0.127	0.072	0.223	-7.147	0.000
Di Martino V et al (2011)	1.841	0.605	5.603	1.075	0.282
Tateyama M et al (2011)	1.799	1.264	2.561	3.260	0.001
Maruoka D et al (2012)	0.538	0.345	0.840	-2.730	0.006
Cozen ML et al (2013)	1.569	0.634	3.885	0.974	0.330
Aleman S et al (2013)	0.287	0.139	0.590	-3.390	0.001
Cozen ML et al (2016)	1.132	0.775	1.654	0.641	0.522
	0.392	0.275	0.557	-5.209	0.000

Heterogeneity: X^2 = 182.934, df = 24 (P <0.001); I^2 = 86.881%
Test for overall effect: Z = -5.209 (P <0.001)

Fig. 2 Efficacy of antiviral treatment on the development of HCC in patients with CHC. The size of each square is proportional to the study's weight. Diamond is the summary estimate from the pooled studies (random effect model). HCC, hepatocellular carcinoma; CHC, chronic hepatitis C

A cumulative meta-analysis of enrolled studies based on publication year showed no specific time trend (Additional file 1: Appendix 14). A cumulative meta-analysis based on effect size showed no small study bias (Additional file 1: Appendix 15). One study removed meta-analysis revealed a stable feature (Additional file 1: Appendix 16). Overall, the sensitivity meta-analyses showed robust results.

A meta-ANOVA indicated that follow-up duration (p = 0.036) and methodological quality (p = 0.029) were suspicious for the reason of heterogeneity (Additional file 1: Appendix 17). A meta-regression indicated that follow-up duration (p = 0.036) and Newcastle-Ottawa scale score of 8 (p = 0.029) explained the heterogeneity (Additional file 2: Table S3). After excluding 2 studies (short-term follow-up duration), no covariates explained heterogeneity in meta-regression tests. After excluding 7 studies (Newcastle-Ottawa scale 8), no covariates explained heterogeneity in meta-regression tests. Therefore, follow-up duration and methodological quality were the reasons of heterogeneity in this analysis.

Efficacy of SVR on the development of HCC in patients with chronic hepatitis C
The overall efficacy of SVR on the development of HCC exhibited an OR of 0.203 (95% CI: 0.164–0.251, p <0.001)

in a random effect model analysis (Fig. 4). The funnel plot showed symmetry (Additional file 1: Appendix 18). The Egger's test showed that intercept was 0.56 (95% CI: −0.099–1.217, t-value: 1.73, df: 33, p = 0.09 (2-tailed)). The rank correlation test showed a Kendall's tau of −0.17 with a continuity correction (p = 0.16). The trim and fill method indicated that no study was trimmed. Overall, there was no evidence of publication bias.

A cumulative meta-analysis of enrolled studies based on publication year showed no specific time trend (Additional file 1: Appendix 19). A cumulative meta-analysis based on effect size showed no small study bias (Additional file 1: Appendix 20). One study removed meta-analysis showed a stable feature (Additional file 1: Appendix 21). Overall, the sensitivity meta-analyses revealed robust results.

Meta-ANOVA or meta-regression identified no specific modifier for the reason of heterogeneity (Additional file 1: Appendix 22) (Additional file 2: Table S4). Overall, no covariates explained heterogeneity.

Efficacy of SVR on all-cause mortality in patients with chronic hepatitis C
The overall efficacy of SVR on all-cause mortality revealed an OR of 0.255 (95% CI: 0.199–0.326, p < 0.001) in a random effect model analysis (Fig. 5). The funnel

Study name	Statistics for each study					Odds ratio and 95% CI
	Odds ratio	Lower limit	Upper limit	Z-Value	p-Value	
Ikeda K et al (2001)	0.255	0.153	0.424	-5.257	0.000	
Gramenzi A et al (2001)	0.754	0.265	2.147	-0.529	0.597	
Nishiguchi S et al (2001)	0.091	0.030	0.275	-4.257	0.000	
Testino G et al (2002)	0.138	0.017	1.124	-1.851	0.064	
Yoshida H et al (2002)	0.337	0.214	0.532	-4.679	0.000	
Imazeki F et al (2003)	0.608	0.316	1.169	-1.491	0.136	
Coverdale SA et al (2004)	0.509	0.250	1.034	-1.868	0.062	
Kasahara A et al (2004)	0.153	0.106	0.219	-10.134	0.000	
Shiratori Y et al (2005)	0.415	0.232	0.743	-2.961	0.003	
Yu ML et al (2006)	0.704	0.331	1.500	-0.909	0.363	
Di Martino V et al (2011)	0.447	0.198	1.010	-1.936	0.053	
Yamasaki K et al (2012)	0.238	0.143	0.398	-5.492	0.000	
Maruoka D et al (2012)	0.493	0.317	0.765	-3.156	0.002	
Cozen ML et al (2013)	0.783	0.470	1.305	-0.937	0.349	
Aleman S et al (2013)	0.403	0.210	0.772	-2.741	0.006	
Kutala BK et al (2015)	0.444	0.238	0.829	-2.548	0.011	
Cozen ML et al (2016)	0.408	0.324	0.513	-7.668	0.000	
	0.380	0.295	0.489	-7.532	0.000	

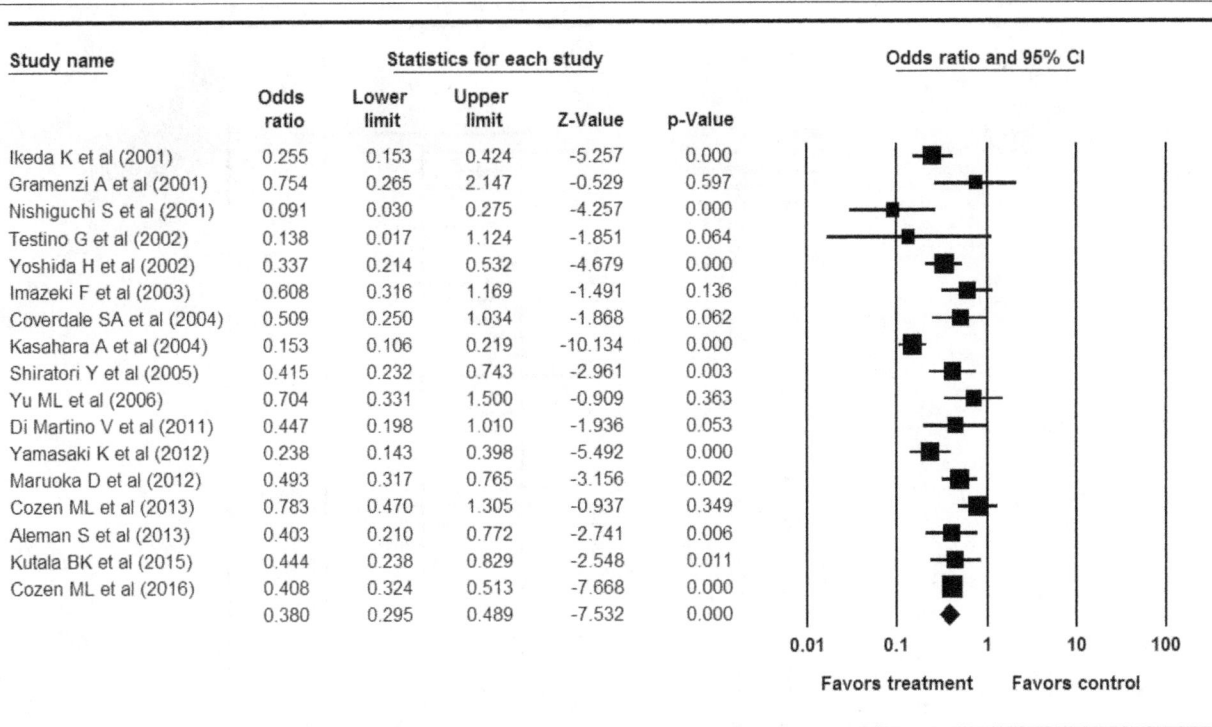

Heterogeneity: X^2 = 53.796, df = 16 (*P* <0.001); I^2 = 70.258%
Test for overall effect: Z = -7.532 (*P* <0.001)

Fig. 3 Efficacy of antiviral treatment on all-cause mortality in patients with CHC. The size of each square is proportional to the study's weight. Diamond is the summary estimate from the pooled studies (random effect model). CHC, chronic hepatitis C

plot showed asymmetry on the right lower quadrant area (Additional file 1: Appendix 23). The Egger's test showed that the intercept was −1.44 (95% CI: −1.921− −0.949, t-value: 6.16, df: 20, *p* <0.001 (2-tailed)). The rank correlation test showed a Kendall's tau of −0.23 with a continuity correction (*p* = 0.14). The trim and fill method indicated 11 studies were trimmed. Overall, there was evidence of publication bias.

A cumulative meta-analysis of enrolled studies based on publication year showed no specific time trend (Additional file 1: Appendix 24). A cumulative meta-analysis based on effect size showed no small study bias (Additional file 1: Appendix 25). One study removed meta-analysis revealed a stable feature (Additional file 1: Appendix 26). Overall, the sensitivity meta-analyses showed robust results.

Meta-ANOVA indicated that methodological quality potentially explained heterogeneity (*p* = 0.030) (Additional file 1: Appendix 27). Meta-regression revealed a Newcastle-Ottawa scale score of 8 for the reason of heterogeneity (Additional file 2: Table S5). After excluding 16 studies (Newcastle-Ottawa scale 8), no covariates explained heterogeneity in meta-regression tests. Therefore, methodological quality was the reasons of heterogeneity in this analysis.

Efficacy of SVR on liver-specific mortality in chronic hepatitis C patients

The overall efficacy of SVR on liver-specific mortality exhibited an OR of 0.126 (95% CI: 0.094–0.169, *p* < 0.001) in a random effect model analysis (Additional file 1: Appendix 28). The funnel plot showed asymmetry on the right lower quadrant area (Additional file 1: Appendix 29). The Egger's test indicated that intercept was −0.77 (95% CI: −1.473 − −0.057, t-value: 2.25, df: 21, *p* = 0.036 (2-tailed)). The rank correlation test revealed a Kendall's tau of −0.19 with a continuity correction (*p* = 0.20). The trim and fill method showed 6 studies were trimmed. Overall, there was evidence of publication bias.

A cumulative meta-analysis of enrolled studies based on publication year showed no specific time trend (Additional file 1: Appendix 30). A cumulative meta-analysis based on effect size showed no small study bias (Additional file 1: Appendix 31). One study removed meta-analysis revealed a stable feature (Additional file 1: Appendix 32). Overall, the sensitivity meta-analyses showed robust results.

Meta-ANOVA or meta-regression revealed no specific modifier for the reason of heterogeneity (Additional file 1: Appendix 33) (Additional file 2: Table S6). Overall, no covariates explained heterogeneity.

Study name	Statistics for each study					Odds ratio and 95% CI
	Odds ratio	Lower limit	Upper limit	Z-Value	p-Value	
Nishiguchi S et al (1995)	0.973	0.042	22.407	-0.017	0.987	
Tanaka K et al (1998)	0.210	0.011	3.947	-1.043	0.297	
Yoshida H et al (1999)	0.249	0.128	0.483	-4.108	0.000	
Testino G et al (2002)	0.875	0.197	3.880	-0.176	0.861	
Okanoue T et al (2002)	0.076	0.028	0.208	-5.024	0.000	
Coverdale SA et al (2004)	0.252	0.033	1.904	-1.336	0.182	
Shiratori Y et al (2005)	0.381	0.187	0.774	-2.667	0.008	
Yu ML et al (2006)	0.133	0.068	0.257	-5.992	0.000	
Pradat P et al (2007)	0.078	0.005	1.309	-1.773	0.076	
Braks RE et al (2007)	0.060	0.008	0.465	-2.693	0.007	
Bruno S et al (2007)	0.312	0.142	0.686	-2.898	0.004	
Hasegawa E et al (2007)	0.171	0.046	0.629	-2.657	0.008	
Veldt BJ et al (2007)	0.206	0.062	0.683	-2.582	0.010	
Floreani A et al (2008)	0.075	0.004	1.410	-1.730	0.084	
Sinn DH et al (2008)	0.252	0.078	0.815	-2.300	0.021	
Kurokawa M et al (2009)	0.343	0.115	1.019	-1.925	0.054	
Asahina Y et al (2010)	0.268	0.170	0.424	-5.634	0.000	
Kawamura Y et al (2010)	0.169	0.090	0.315	-5.581	0.000	
Cardoso AC et al (2010)	0.254	0.104	0.620	-3.008	0.003	
Morgan TR et al (2010)	0.155	0.037	0.655	-2.536	0.011	
Di Martino V et al (2011)	0.252	0.031	2.064	-1.284	0.199	
Velosa J et al (2011)	0.093	0.012	0.723	-2.270	0.023	
Iacobellis A et al (2011)	0.957	0.291	3.145	-0.073	0.942	
Hung CH et al (2011)	0.239	0.153	0.375	-6.250	0.000	
Takahashi H et al (2011)	0.097	0.012	0.758	-2.224	0.026	
Backus LI et al (2011)	0.126	0.105	0.152	-21.774	0.000	
Tateyama M et al (2011)	0.095	0.029	0.313	-3.872	0.000	
Osaki Y et al (2012)	0.043	0.006	0.324	-3.056	0.002	
van der Meer AJ et al (2012)	0.257	0.115	0.573	-3.321	0.001	
Maruoka D et al (2012)	0.080	0.032	0.201	-5.379	0.000	
Cozen ML et al (2013)	0.269	0.056	1.286	-1.645	0.100	
Alfaleh FZ et al (2013)	0.163	0.009	3.075	-1.211	0.226	
Aleman S et al (2013)	0.371	0.148	0.931	-2.113	0.035	
Di Marco V et al (2016)	0.184	0.082	0.410	-4.136	0.000	
Ikezaki H et al (2016)	0.160	0.032	0.811	-2.213	0.027	
	0.203	0.164	0.251	-14.759	0.000	

Favours SVR   Favours no SVR

Heterogeneity: $X^2 = 56.031$, df = 34 ($P = 0.010$); $I^2 = 39.319\%$
Test for overall effect: $Z = -14.759$ ($P < 0.001$)

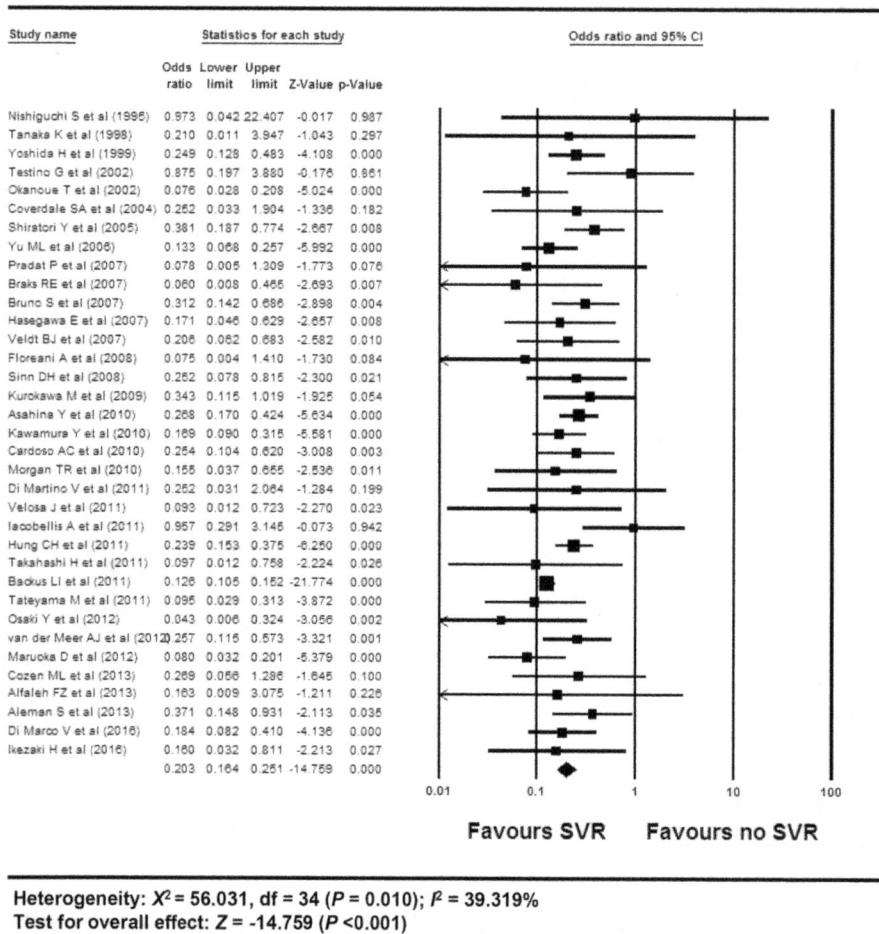

Fig. 4 Efficacy of SVR on the development of HCC in patients with CHC. The size of each square is proportional to the study's weight. Diamond is the summary estimate from the pooled studies (random effect model). SVR, sustained virologic response; HCC, hepatocellular carcinoma; CHC, chronic hepatitis C

The results of meta-regression analyses for each topic are summarized in Table 7.

Discussion

This meta-analyses confirmed the long-term efficacy of antiviral treatment in terms of prevention of HCC and reduction in all-cause and liver-specific mortality in patients with chronic HCV infection. This long-term efficacy was also intensified when SVR was achieved. Clinical outcomes regarding the efficacy of antiviral therapy in CHC patients have been continuously investigated by previous studies with a small number of patients or short-term follow-up duration. The reasons for performing this meta-analysis were a persistent risk of HCC even after attainment of SVR and a lack of sufficient data regarding long-term efficacy [18]. Persistent low-level of viremia and dysplastic hepatocyte regeneration are representative grounds for persistent risk of HCC after antiviral treatment [19, 20]. Interestingly, a recent meta-analysis revealed that IFN nonresponders exhibited a decreased risk of HCC recurrence after curative treatment of HCC, compared with no treatment patients, thus indicating that reduced necroinflammation and an inhibition of hepatic fibrosis progression prevent the development of HCC [21]. This results is consistent with that of our study and emphasized the importance of screening strategy of chronic hepatitis C.

Early antiviral treatment before progression to advanced fibrosis or cirrhosis is associated with an increasing probability of achieving SVR [22]. However, an indolent course of chronic hepatitis C makes it difficult for early diagnosis and treatment. Authors have revealed that favorable antiviral efficacy persists in all patients with chronic hepatitis C, regardless of histology. This result was also confirmed by a previous study indicating favorable antiviral efficacy even in patients with LC [18]. Considering the advanced fibrosis or cirrhosis is the sequelae of long-standing inflammation of liver, our study confirmed antiviral treatment is still valid in the late course of chronic hepatitis C. Although histology was

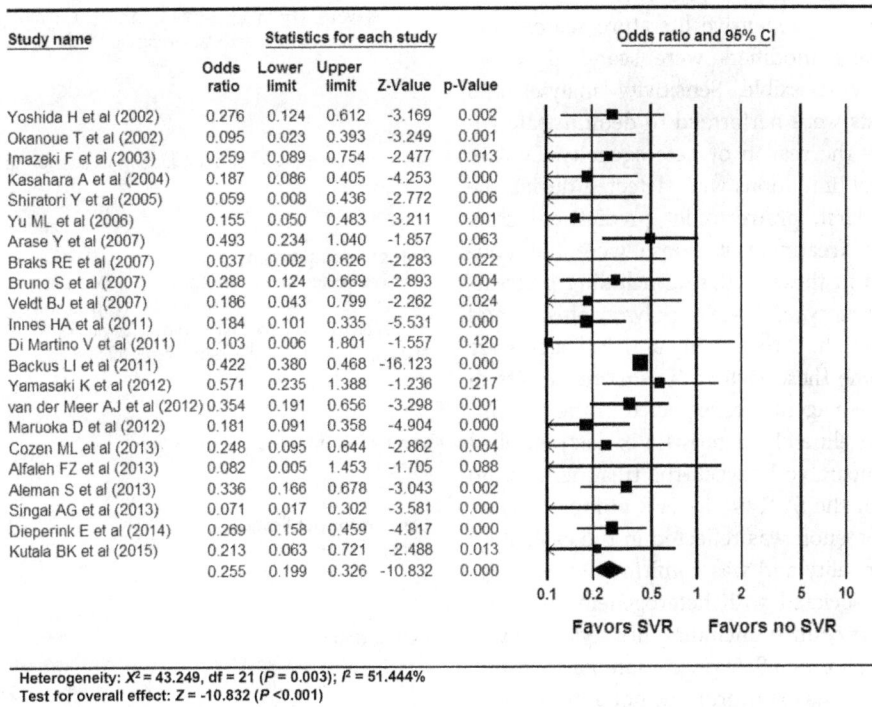

Fig. 5 Efficacy of SVR on all-cause mortality in patients with CHC. The size of each square is proportional to the study's weight. Diamond is the summary estimate from the pooled studies (random effect model). SVR, sustained virologic response; CHC, chronic hepatitis C

not a significant modifier in our meta-analysis, all of the included studies have substantially heterogeneous populations regarding the degree of fibrosis or cirrhosis of the liver. This finding was commonly detected in a previous meta-analysis [18]. However, considering the expanding treatment indication, including decompensated LC by the advent of direct-acting antiviral agents, histology is not expected to affect the long-term efficacy of antiviral treatment in the near future.

Despite the favorable efficacy of antiviral treatment, 2 modifiers associated with heterogeneity were identified in the meta-ANOVA and meta-regression analyses. Studies with Newcastle-Ottawa scale of 8 were modifier in the analysis of association between antiviral treatment and the development of HCC (Additional file 2: Table S1), in the analysis of association between antiviral treatment and the

liver-specific mortality (Additional file 2: Table S3), and in the analysis of association between SVR and all-cause mortality (Additional file 2: Table S5). Studies with a short-term follow-up duration were also modifier in the analysis of association between antiviral treatment and liver-specific mortality (Additional file 2: Table S3). Although these modifiers were confirmed as not significantly affecting the results of main analyses, this finding indicated the need for more number of high-quality and long-term follow-up studies on this topic.

Publication bias was detected in 2 topics (topic 5 and 6). Sensitivity analyses including cumulative and one study removed meta-analyses were rigorously performed to find the small study effect associated with publication bias, and these analyses showed no small study effect. Overall, the impact of publication bias was minimal.

Table 7 Results of meta-regression analyses

Modifier	Coefficient	Standard error	P value
NOS (topic 1)	NOS 8: 1.203	0.565	0.033
	NOS 7: 0.501	0.561	0.372
			Q: 7.24, df: 2, P = 0.027
Follow-up duration (topic 3)	1.140	0.542	0.036
NOS (topic 3)	NOS 8: −0.659	0.302	0.029
NOS (topic 5)	NOS 8: −0.540	0.209	0.010
	NOS 7: −0.544	0.322	0.091
			Q: 7.03, df: 2, P = 0.030

NOS Newcastle-Ottawa scale

This meta-analysis included the largest number of articles identified by a comprehensive literature search, and potential confounding modifiers were searched within each study whenever possible. Sensitivity analyses and meta-regression tests were performed to demonstrate robustness or identify the reason of heterogeneity. Despite the strengths, several limitations were detected during the systematic review. First, pretreatment predictive factors associated with the treatment response were not controlled or evaluated in these analyses, including pretreatment viral load, genotype, IL-28β polymorphism, and HBV or HIV coinfection. Direct-acting antiviral agents are expected to overcome these factors. Therefore, results of studies including these agents are expected in the near future. Second, the baseline characteristics of each enrolled study were not comparable between the treatment vs. no treatment groups, or the SVR vs. no SVR groups in some studies. This phenomenon was reflected in the evaluation of methodological quality and was confirmed to be a significant modifier associated with heterogeneity. Notably, difference by race or country including life style (obesity, consumption of alcohol or aflatoxin-contaminated foods, and chemical carcinogens exposure) was not appropriately investigated in our study. Considering the HCC is a heterogenous malignancy resulting from diverse causes of liver injury, different mechanisms or molecular pathways on the basis of country could be a cause of different treatment response. However, due to the heterogenous baseline characteristics including genotype and lacking of enough data about risk factors of HCC, the subgroup analyses by country could not present meaningful data. The limitations described above could be a cause of potential heterogeneity and bias. Therefore, studies controlling for various risk factors are needed to confirm these findings.

Conclusion

In conclusion, antiviral treatment for chronic hepatitis C showed improved outcome in the development of HCC and mortality, especially when SVR is achieved, although studies controlling for various risk factors of HCC and mortality are still lacking.

Abbreviations

CHC: Chronic hepatitis C; CI: Confidence interval; HCC: Hepatocellular carcinoma; HCV: Hepatitis C virus; IFN: Interferon; OR: Odds ratio; PegIFN: Pegylated interferon; RBV: Ribavirin; RCT: Randomized controlled studies; SVR: Sustained virologic response

Acknowledgements

Authors would like to appreciate Dr. Young Joo Yang's effort for helping manuscript searching and data filling up for this study.

Funding

There was no financial or grant support related to this article.

Author's contributions

CSB participated study concept, design, literature search, data abstraction, data analysis and manuscript writing. IHS participated study concept, design, data analysis and gave final approval for publication. All authors have read and approved the final version of this manuscript.

Competing interests

None

Consent for publication

Not applicable.

Author details

[1]Department of Internal Medicine, Hallym University College of Medicine, Chuncheon, Republic of Korea. [2]Division of Hepatology, Department of Internal Medicine, Dankook University College of Medicine, Cheonan, Korea, Republic of Korea.

References

1. AASLD/IDSA HCV Guidance Panel. Hepatitis C guidance: AASLD-IDSA recommendations for testing, managing, and treating adults infected with hepatitis C virus. Hepatology. 2015;62:932–54.
2. Swain MG, Lai M, Shiffman ML, Cooksley WG, Zeuzem S, Dieterich DT, Abergel A, Pessôa MG, Lin A, Tietz A, et al. A sustained virologic response is durable in patients with chronic hepatitis C treated with peginterferon Alfa-2a and ribavirin. Gastroenterology. 2010;139:1593–601.
3. Martinot-Peignoux M, Stern C, Maylin S, Ripault MP, Boyer N, Leclere L, Castelnau C, Giuily N, El Ray A, Cardoso AC, et al. Twelve weeks posttreatment follow-up is as relevant as 24 weeks to determine the sustained virologic response in patients with hepatitis c virus receiving pegylated interferon and ribavirin. Hepatology. 2010;51:1122–6.
4. Wen Y, Zheng YX, de Tan M. A comprehensive long-term prognosis of chronic hepatitis C patients with antiviral therapy: a meta-analysis of studies from 2008 to 2014. Hepat Mon. 2015;15:e27181.
5. Higgins JP, Green S. Cochrane handbook for systematic reviews of interventions. Version 5.1.0. The Cochrane Collaboration; 2011, 2013.
6. Stang A. Critical evaluation of the Newcastle-Ottawa scale for the assessment of the quality of nonrandomized studies in meta-analyses. Eur J Epidemiol. 2010;25:603–5.
7. Deeks JJ, Dinnes J, D'Amico R, Sowden AJ, Sakarovitch C, Song F, Petticrew M, Altman DG. Evaluating non-randomised intervention studies. Health Technol Assess. 2003;7:1–173. iii-x.
8. Higgins JP, Thompson SG. Quantifying heterogeneity in a meta-analysis. Stat Med. 2002;21:1539–58.
9. Higgins JP, Thompson SG, Deeks JJ, Altman DG. Measuring inconsistency in meta-analyses. BMJ. 2003;327:557–60.
10. DerSimonian R, Laird N. Meta-analysis in clinical trials. Control Clin Trials. 1986;7:177–88.

11. Duval S, Tweedie R. Trim and fill: a simple funnel-plot-based method of testing and adjusting for publication bias in meta-analysis. Biometrics. 2000;56:455–63.

12. Sutton AJ, Abrams KR, Jones DR, Sheldon TA, Song F. Methods for meta-analysis in medical research. Chichester (UK): Wiley; 2000.

13. Sterne JA, Egger M. Funnel plots for detecting bias in meta-analysis: guidelines on choice of axis. J Clin Epidemiol. 2001;54:1046–55.

14. Begg CB, Mazumdar M. Operating characteristics of a rank correlation test for publication bias. Biometrics. 1994;50:1088–101.

15. Egger M, Davey Smith G, Schneider M, Minder C. Bias in meta-analysis detected by a simple, graphical test. BMJ. 1997;315:629–34.

16. Testino G, Ansaldi F, Andorno E, Ravetti GL, Ferro C, De Iaco F, Icardi G, Valente U. Interferon therapy does not prevent hepatocellular carcinoma in HCV compensated cirrhosis. Hepatogastroenterology. 2002;49:1636–8.

17. Kasahara A, Tanaka H, Okanoue T, Imai Y, Tsubouchi H, Yoshioka K, Kawata S, Tanaka E, Hino K, Hayashi K, et al. Interferon treatment improves survival in chronic hepatitis C patients showing biochemical as well as virological responses by preventing liver-related death. J Viral Hepat. 2004;11:148–56.

18. Singal AK, Singh A, Jaganmohan S, Guturu P, Mummadi R, Kuo YF, Sood GK. Antiviral therapy reduces risk of hepatocellular carcinoma in patients with hepatitis C virus-related cirrhosis. Clin Gastroenterol Hepatol. 2010;8:192–9.

19. Hung CH, Lee CM, Lu SN, Wang JH, Hu TH, Tung HD, Chen CH, Chen WJ, Changchien CS. Long-term effect of interferon alpha-2b plus ribavirin therapy on incidence of hepatocellular carcinoma in patients with hepatitis C virus-related cirrhosis. J Viral Hepat. 2006;13:409–14.

20. Gerotto M, Dal Pero F, Bortoletto G, Ferrari A, Pistis R, Sebastiani G, Fagiuoli S, Realdon S, Alberti A. Hepatitis C minimal residual viremia (MRV) detected by TMA at the end of Peg-IFN plus ribavirin therapy predicts post-treatment relapse. J Hepatol. 2006;44:83–7.

21. Miyake Y, Iwasaki Y, Yamamoto K. Meta-analysis: reduced incidence of hepatocellular carcinoma in patients not responding to interferon therapy of chronic hepatitis C. Int J Cancer. 2010;127:989–96.

22. Everson GT, Hoefs JC, Seeff LB, Bonkovsky HL, Naishadham D, Shiffman ML, Kahn JA, Lok AS, Di Bisceglie AM, Lee WM, et al. Impact of disease severity on outcome of antiviral therapy for chronic hepatitis C: lessons from the HALT-C trial. Hepatology. 2006;44:1675–84.

23. Mazzella G, Accogli E, Sottili S, Festi D, Orsini M, Salzetta A, Novelli V, Cipolla A, Fabbri C, Pezzoli A, et al. Alpha interferon treatment may prevent hepatocellular carcinoma in HCV-related liver cirrhosis. J Hepatol. 1996;24:141–7.

24. Bruno S, Silini E, Crosignani A, Borzio F, Leandro G, Bono F, Asti M, Rossi S, Larghi A, Cerino A, et al. Hepatitis C virus genotypes and risk of hepatocellular carcinoma in cirrhosis: a prospective study. Hepatology. 1997; 25:754–8.

25. Fattovich G, Giustina G, Degos F, Diodati G, Tremolada F, Nevens F, Almasio P, Solinas A, Brouwer JT, Thomas H, et al. Effectiveness of interferon Alfa on incidence of hepatocellular carcinoma and decompensation in cirrhosis type C. European concerted action on viral hepatitis (EUROHEP). J Hepatol. 1997;27:201–5.

26. Serfaty L, Aumaitre H, Chazouilleres O, Bonnand AM, Rosmorduc O, Poupon RE, Poupon R. Determinants of outcome of compensated hepatitis C virus-related cirrhosis. Hepatology. 1998;27:1435–40.

27. Benvegnu L, Chemello L, Noventa F, Fattovich G, Pontisso P, Alberti A. Retrospective analysis of the effect of interferon therapy on the clinical outcome of patients with viral cirrhosis. Cancer. 1998;83:901–9.

28. International Interferon-alpha Hepatocellular Carcinoma Study Group. Effect of interferon-alpha on progression of cirrhosis to hepatocellular carcinoma: a retrospective cohort study. Lancet. 1998;351:1535–9.

29. Imai Y, Kawata S, Tamura S, Yabuuchi I, Noda S, Inada M, Maeda Y, Shirai Y, Fukuzaki T, Kaji I, et al. Relation of interferon therapy and hepatocellular carcinoma in patients with chronic hepatitis C. Osaka hepatocellular carcinoma prevention study group. Ann Internal Med. 1998;129:94–9.

30. Yoshida H, Shiratori Y, Moriyama M, Arakawa Y, Ide T, Sata M, Inoue O, Yano M, Tanaka M, Fujiyama S, et al. Interferon therapy reduces the risk for hepatocellular carcinoma: national surveillance program of cirrhotic and noncirrhotic patients with chronic hepatitis C in Japan. IHIT study group. Inhibition of hepatocarcinogenesis by interferon therapy. Ann Internal Med. 1999;131:174–81.

31. Okanoue T, Itoh Y, Minami M, Sakamoto S, Yasui K, Sakamoto M, Nishioji K, Murakami Y, Kashima K. Interferon therapy lowers the rate of progression to hepatocellular carcinoma in chronic hepatitis C but not significantly in an advanced stage: a retrospective study in 1148 patients. Viral hepatitis therapy study group. J Hepatol. 1999;30:653–9.

32. Valla DC, Chevallier M, Marcellin P, Payen JL, Trepo C, Fonck M, Bourliere M, Boucher E, Miguet JP, Parlier D, et al. Treatment of hepatitis C virus-related cirrhosis: a randomized, controlled trial of interferon alfa-2b versus no treatment. Hepatology. 1999;29:1870–5.

33. Ikeda K, Saitoh S, Kobayashi M, Suzuki Y, Suzuki F, Tsubota A, Arase Y, Murashima N, Chayama K, Kumada H. Long-term interferon therapy for 1 year or longer reduces the hepatocellular carcinogenesis rate in patients with liver cirrhosis caused by hepatitis C virus: a pilot study. J Gastroenterol Hepatol. 2001;16:406–15.

34. Gramenzi A, Andreone P, Fiorino S, Cammà C, Giunta M, Magalotti D, Cursaro C, Calabrese C, Arienti V, Rossi C, et al. Impact of interferon therapy on the natural history of hepatitis C virus related cirrhosis. Gut. 2001;48:843–8.

35. Nishiguchi S, Shiomi S, Nakatani S, Takeda T, Fukuda K, Tamori A, Habu D, Tanaka T. Prevention of hepatocellular carcinoma in patients with chronic active hepatitis C and cirrhosis. Lancet. 2001;357:196–7.

36. Coverdale SA, Khan MH, Byth K, Lin R, Weltman M, George J, Samarasinghe D, Liddle C, Kench JG, Crewe E, et al. Effects of interferon treatment response on liver complications of chronic hepatitis C: 9-years follow-up study. Am J Gastroenterol. 2004;99:636–44.

37. Azzaroli F, Accogli E, Nigro G, Trere D, Giovanelli S, Miracolo A, Lodato F, Montagnani M, Tamé M, Colecchia A, et al. Interferon plus ribavirin and interferon alone in preventing hepatocellular carcinoma: a prospective study on patients with HCV related cirrhosis. World J Gastroenterol. 2004;10: 3099–102.

38. Shiratori Y, Ito Y, Yokosuka O, Imazeki F, Nakata R, Tanaka N, Arakawa Y, Hashimoto E, Hirota K, Yoshida H, et al. Antiviral therapy for cirrhotic hepatitis C: association with reduced hepatocellular carcinoma development and improved survival. Ann Internal Med. 2005;142:105–14.

39. Yu ML, Lin SM, Chuang WL, Dai CY, Wang JH, Lu SN, Sheen IS, Chang WY, Lee CM, Liaw YF. A sustained virological response to interferon or interferon/ribavirin reduces hepatocellular carcinoma and improves survival in chronic hepatitis C: a nationwide, multicentre study in Taiwan. Antivir Ther. 2006;11:985–94.

40. Sinn DH, Paik SW, Kang P, Kil JS, Park SU, Lee SY, Song SM, Gwak GY, Choi MS, Lee JH, et al. Disease progression and the risk factor analysis for chronic hepatitis C. Liver Int. 2008;28:1363–9.

41. Di Martino V, Crouzet J, Hillon P, Thévenot T, Minello A, Monnet E. Long-term outcome of chronic hepatitis C in a population-based cohort and impact of antiviral therapy: a propensity-adjusted analysis. J Viral Hepat. 2011;18:493–505.

42. Tateyama M, Yatsuhashi H, Taura N, Motoyoshi Y, Nagaoka S, Yanagi K, Abiru S, Yano K, Komori A, Migita K, et al. Alpha-fetoprotein above normal levels as a risk factor for the development of hepatocellular carcinoma in patients infected with hepatitis C virus. J Gastroenterol. 2011;46:92–100.

43. Maruoka D, Imazeki F, Arai M, Kanda T, Fujiwara K, Yokosuka O. Long-term cohort study of chronic hepatitis C according to interferon efficacy. J Gastroenterol Hepatol. 2012;27:291–9.

44. Cozen ML, Ryan JC, Shen H, Lerrigo R, Yee RM, Sheen E, Wu R, Monto A. Nonresponse to interferon-alpha based treatment for chronic hepatitis C infection is associated with increased hazard of cirrhosis. PLoS One. 2013;8: e61568.

45. Aleman S, Rahbin N, Weiland O, Davidsdottir L, Hedenstierna M, Rose N, Verbaan H, Stål P, Carlsson T, Norrgren H, et al. A risk for hepatocellular carcinoma persists long-term after sustained virologic response in patients with hepatitis C-associated liver cirrhosis. Clin Infect Dis. 2013;57:230–6.

46. Cozen ML, Ryan JC, Shen H, Cheung R, Kaplan DE, Pocha C, Brau N, Aytaman A, Schmidt WN, Pedrosa M, et al. Improved survival among all interferon-alpha-treated patients in HCV-002, a veterans affairs hepatitis C cohort of 2211 patients, despite increased cirrhosis among nonresponders. Dig Dis Sci. 2016;61:1744–56.

47. Yoshida H, Arakawa Y, Sata M, Nishiguchi S, Yano M, Fujiyama S, Yamada G, Yokosuka O, Shiratori Y, Omata M. Interferon therapy prolonged life expectancy among chronic hepatitis C patients. Gastroenterology. 2002;123:483–91.

48. Imazeki F, Yokosuka O, Fukai K, Saisho H. Favorable prognosis of chronic hepatitis C after interferon therapy by long-term cohort study. Hepatology. 2003;38:493–502.

49. Yamasaki K, Tomohiro M, Nagao Y, Sata M, Shimoda T, Hirase K, Shirahama S. Effects and outcomes of interferon treatment in Japanese hepatitis C patients. BMC Gastroenterol. 2012;12:139.

50. Kutala BK, Guedj J, Asselah T, Boyer N, Mouri F, Martinot-Peignoux M, Valla D, Marcellin P, Duval X. Impact of treatment against hepatitis C virus on overall survival of naive patients with advanced liver disease. Antimicrob Agents Chemother. 2015;59:803–10.

51. Nishiguchi S, Kuroki T, Nakatani S, Morimoto H, Takeda T, Nakajima S, Shiomi S, Seki S, Kobayashi K, Otani S. Randomised trial of effects of interferon-alpha on incidence of hepatocellular carcinoma in chronic active hepatitis C with cirrhosis. Lancet. 1995;346:1051–5.

52. Tanaka K, Sata M, Uchimura Y, Suzuki H, Tanikawa K. Long-term evaluation of interferon therapy in hepatitis C virus-associated cirrhosis: does IFN prevent development of hepatocellular carcinoma? Oncol Rep. 1998;5:205–8.

53. Okanoue T, Itoh Y, Kirishima T, Daimon Y, Toyama T, Morita A, Nakajima T, Minami M. Transient biochemical response in interferon therapy decreases the development of hepatocellular carcinoma for 5 years and improves the long-term survival of chronic hepatitis C patients. Hepatol Res. 2002;23:62–77.

54. Pradat P, Tillmann HL, Sauleda S, Braconier JH, Saracco G, Thursz M, Goldin R, Winkler R, Alberti A, Esteban JI, et al. Long-term follow-up of the hepatitis C HENCORE cohort: response to therapy and occurrence of liver-related complications. J Viral Hepat. 2007;14:556–63.

55. Braks RE, Ganne-Carrie N, Fontaine H, Paries J, Grando-Lemaire V, Beaugrand M, Pol S, Trinchet JC. Effect of sustained virological response on long-term clinical outcome in 113 patients with compensated hepatitis C-related cirrhosis treated by interferon alpha and ribavirin. World J Gastroenterol. 2007;13:5648–53.

56. Bruno S, Stroffolini T, Colombo M, Bollani S, Benvegnù L, Mazzella G, Ascione A, Santantonio T, Piccinino F, Andreone P, et al. Sustained virological response to interferon-alpha is associated with improved outcome in HCV-related cirrhosis: a retrospective study. Hepatology. 2007;45:579–87.

57. Hasegawa E, Kobayashi M, Kawamura Y, Yatsuji H, Sezaki H, Hosaka T, Akuta N, Suzuki F, Suzuki Y, Arase Y, et al. Efficacy and anticarcinogenic activity of interferon for hepatitis C virus-related compensated cirrhosis in patients with genotype 1b low viral load or genotype 2. Hepatol Res. 2007;37:793–800.

58. Veldt BJ, Heathcote EJ, Wedemeyer H, Reichen J, Hofmann WP, Zeuzem S, Manns MP, Hansen BE, Schalm SW, Janssen HL. Sustained virologic response and clinical outcomes in patients with chronic hepatitis C and advanced fibrosis. Ann Intern Med. 2007;147:677–84.

59. Floreani A, Baldo V, Rizzotto ER, Carderi I, Baldovin T, Minola E. Pegylated interferon alpha-2b plus ribavirin for naive patients with HCV-related cirrhosis. J Clin Gastroenterol. 2008;42:734–7.

60. Kurokawa M, Hiramatsu N, Oze T, Mochizuki K, Yakushijin T, Kurashige N, Inoue Y, Igura T, Imanaka K, Yamada A, et al. Effect of interferon alpha-2b plus ribavirin therapy on incidence of hepatocellular carcinoma in patients with chronic hepatitis. Hepatol Res. 2009;39:432–8.

61. Asahina Y, Tsuchiya K, Tamaki N, Hirayama I, Tanaka T, Sato M, Yasui Y, Hosokawa T, Ueda K, Kuzuya T, et al. Effect of aging on risk for hepatocellular carcinoma in chronic hepatitis C virus infection. Hepatology. 2010;52:518–27.

62. Kawamura Y, Arase Y, Ikeda K, Hirakawa M, Hosaka T, Kobayashi M, Saitoh S, Yatsuji H, Sezaki H, Akuta N, et al. Diabetes enhances hepatocarcinogenesis in noncirrhotic, interferon-treated hepatitis C patients. Am J Med. 2010;123:951–6.e1.

63. Cardoso AC, Moucari R, Figueiredo-Mendes C, Ripault MP, Giuily N, Castelnau C, Boyer N, Asselah T, Martinot-Peignoux M, Maylin S, et al. Impact of peginterferon and ribavirin therapy on hepatocellular carcinoma: incidence and survival in hepatitis C patients with advanced fibrosis. J Hepatol. 2010;52:652–7.

64. Morgan TR, Ghany MG, Kim HY, Snow KK, Shiffman ML, De Santo JL, Lee WM, Di Bisceglie AM, Bonkovsky HL, Dienstag JL, et al. Outcome of sustained virological responders with histologically advanced chronic hepatitis C. Hepatology. 2010;52:833–44.

65. Velosa J, Serejo F, Marinho R, Nunes J, Glória H. Eradication of hepatitis C virus reduces the risk of hepatocellular carcinoma in patients with compensated cirrhosis. Dig Dis Sci. 2011;56:1853–61.

66. Iacobellis A, Perri F, Valvano MR, Caruso N, Niro GA, Andriulli A. Long-term outcome after antiviral therapy of patients with hepatitis C virus infection and decompensated cirrhosis. Clin Gastroenterol Hepatol. 2011;9:249–53.

67. Hung CH, Lee CM, Wang JH, Hu TH, Chen CH, Lin CY, Lu SN. Impact of diabetes mellitus on incidence of hepatocellular carcinoma in chronic hepatitis C patients treated with interferon-based antiviral therapy. Int J Cancer. 2011;128:2344–52.

68. Takahashi H, Mizuta T, Eguchi Y, Kawaguchi Y, Kuwashiro T, Oeda S, Isoda H, Oza N, Iwane S, Izumi K, et al. Post-challenge hyperglycemia is a significant risk factor for the development of hepatocellular carcinoma in patients with chronic hepatitis C. J Gastroenterol. 2011;46:790–8.

69. Backus LI, Boothroyd DB, Phillips BR, Belperio P, Halloran J, Mole LA. A sustained virologic response reduces risk of all-cause mortality in patients with hepatitis C. Clin Gastroenterol Hepatol. 2011;9:509–16.e1.

70. Osaki Y, Ueda Y, Marusawa H, Nakajima J, Kimura T, Kita R, Nishikawa H, Saito S, Henmi S, Sakamoto A, et al. Decrease in alpha-fetoprotein levels predicts reduced incidence of hepatocellular carcinoma in patients with hepatitis C virus infection receiving interferon therapy: a single center study. J Gastroenterol. 2012;47:444–51.

71. van der Meer AJ, Veldt BJ, Feld JJ, Wedemeyer H, Dufour JF, Lammert F, Duarte-Rojo A, Heathcote EJ, Manns MP, Kuske L, et al. Association between sustained virological response and all-cause mortality among patients with chronic hepatitis C and advanced hepatic fibrosis. JAMA. 2012;308:2584–93.

72. Alfaleh FZ, Alswat K, Helmy A, Al-hamoudi W, El-sharkawy M, Omar M, Shalaby A, Bedewi MA, Hadad Q, Ali SM, et al. The natural history and long-term outcomes in patients with chronic hepatitis C genotype 4 after interferon-based therapy. Liver Int. 2013;33:871–83.

73. Di Marco V, Calvaruso V, Ferraro D, Ferraro D, Bavetta MG, Cabibbo G, Conte E, Cammà C, Grimaudo S, Pipitone RM, et al. Effects of Viral Eradication in Patients with HCV and Cirrhosis Differ With Stage of Portal Hypertension. Gastroenterology. 2016;151:130-139.e2.

74. Ikezaki H, Nomura H, Furusyo N, Ogawa E, Kajiwara E, Takahashi K, Kawano A, Maruyama T, Tanabe Y, Satoh T, et al. Efficacy of interferon-beta plus ribavirin combination treatment on the development of hepatocellular carcinoma in Japanese patients with chronic hepatitis C. Hepatol Res. 2016;46:E174–80.

75. Arase Y, Ikeda K, Suzuki F, Suzuki Y, Saitoh S, Kobayashi M, Akuta N, Someya T, Koyama R, Hosaka T, et al. Long-term outcome after interferon therapy in elderly patients with chronic hepatitis C. Intervirology. 2007;50:16–23.

76. Innes HA, Hutchinson SJ, Allen S, Bhattacharyya D, Bramley P, Delahooke TE, Dillon JF, Forrest E, Fraser A, Gillespie R, et al. Excess liver-related morbidity of chronic hepatitis C patients, who achieve a sustained viral response, and are discharged from care. Hepatology. 2011;54:1547–58.

77. Singal AG, Dharia TD, Malet PF, Alqahtani S, Zhang S, Cuthbert JA. Long-term benefit of hepatitis C therapy in a safety net hospital system: a cross-sectional study with median 5-year follow-up. BMJ Open. 2013;3:e003231.

78. Dieperink E, Pocha C, Thuras P, Knott A, Colton S, Ho SB. All-cause mortality and liver-related outcomes following successful antiviral treatment for chronic hepatitis C. Dig Dis Sci. 2014;59:872–80.

15

Relevance of FXR-p62/SQSTM1 pathway for survival and protection of mouse hepatocytes and liver, especially with steatosis

Sanae Haga[1], Yimin[2] and Michitaka Ozaki[1*]

Abstract

Background: Liver injury and regeneration involve complicated processes and are affected by various physio-pathological conditions. Surgically, severe liver injury after surgical resection often leads to fatal liver failure, especially with some underlying pathological conditions such as steatosis. Therefore, protection from the injury of hepatocytes and liver is a serious concern in various clinical settings.

Methods: We studied the effects of the farnesoid X receptor (FXR) on cell survival and steatosis in mouse hepatocytes (AML12 mouse liver cells) and investigated their molecular mechanisms. We next studied whether or not FXR improves liver injury, regeneration and steatosis in a mouse model of partial hepatectomy (PH) with steatosis.

Results: An FXR-specific agonist, GW4064, induced expressions of the p62/SQSTM1 gene and protein in AML12 mouse liver cells. Because we previously reported p62/SQSTM1 as a key molecule for antioxidation and cell survival in hepatocytes, we next examined the activation of nuclear factor erythroid 2-related factor-2 (Nrf2) and induction of the antioxidant molecules by GW4064. GW4064 activated Nrf2 and subsequently induced antioxidant molecules (Nrf2, catalase, HO-1, and thioredoxin). We also examined expressions of pro-survival and cell protective molecules associated with p62/SQSTM1. Expectedly, GW4064 induced phosphorylation of Akt, expression of the anti-apoptotic molecules (Bcl-xL and Bcl-2), and reduced harmful hepatic molecules (Fas ligand and Fas). GW4064 promoted hepatocyte survival, which was cancelled by *p62/SQSTM1* siRNA. These findings suggest the potential relevance of the FXR-p62/SQSTM1 pathway for the survival and protection of hepatocytes. Furthermore, GW4064 induced the expression of small heterodimer partners (SHP) and suppressed liver X receptor (LXR)-induced steatosis in hepatocytes, expecting the in vivo protective effect of FXR on liver injury especially with steatosis. In the hepatectomy model of db/db mice with fatty liver, pre-treatment by GW4064 significantly reduced post-PH liver injury (serum levels of LDH, AST & ALT and histological study) and improved steatosis. The key molecules, p62/SQSTM1, Nrf2 and SHP were upregulated in fatty liver tissue by GW4064 treatment.

Conclusions: The present study is the first to demonstrate the relevance of FXR-p62/SQSTM1 and -SHP in the protection against injury of hepatocytes and post-PH liver, especially with steatosis.

Keywords: FXR, p62/SQSTM1, Nrf2, SHP, Oxidative stress, Liver injury, Steatosis

* Correspondence: ozaki-m@med.hokudai.ac.jp
[1]Department of Biological Response and Regulation, Faculty of Health Sciences, Hokkaido University, N-12, W-5, Kita-ku, Sapporo, Hokkaido 060-0812, Japan
Full list of author information is available at the end of the article

Background

Liver is injured as a result of various physio-pathological events and sequentially regenerates to quantitatively and functionally recover from loss of mass and to compensate for impaired function. Liver has the strong ability to restore lost volume and function, a phenomenon that is rarely seen in other organs [1, 2]. It is well established that normal adult hepatocytes usually are quiescent but have the potential to replicate. After surgical procedures that reduce liver mass/function and induce liver injury, such as partial hepatectomy (PH) or live-donor liver transplantation, a rapid enlargement of the residual or grafted liver commonly occurs to restore the liver mass and function [3]. However, post-PH injury of a diseased liver, for example, in cases of liver cirrhosis or steatosis, or of aged liver, leads to liver failure and is potentially fatal [4–7]. Therefore, a better understanding of the molecular mechanisms of liver injury and protection in various pathological conditions may lead to clinical benefits.

Fatty liver is a commonly encountered hepatic disorder and has various causes, such as obesity, diabetes mellitus, and alcohol consumption [7]. It is often considered a benign condition because it does not usually cause severe clinical symptoms. However, surgical resection of fatty liver and live-donor liver transplantation from a donor with a steatotic liver are problematic because steatosis often causes the remnant liver failure immediately and primary graft non-function [7]. Non-alcoholic steatohepatitis (NASH), has been focused on recently because its clinical importance has become apparent. NASH, characterized by persistent inflammation with mild liver damage, is considered to ultimately result in liver cancer through liver fibrosis and cirrhosis over many years [8, 9].

After hepatectomy, various mitotic factors and cytokines promptly activate various cellular signals and events, eventually leading to sufficient regeneration of the normal liver [1–3, 10, 11]. In the steatotic liver, modified signaling mechanisms due to adaptation to chronic metabolic abnormalities and decreased adenosine triphosphate (ATP) production have been reported as likely causes of increased mortality and impaired regeneration after hepatectomy [7, 12, 13]. Very importantly, hepatic steatosis is considered to reduce tolerance to ischemic injury and oxidative stress (OS) [7, 14].

By the way, p62/SQSTM1 is known as a specific substrate for autophagy and therefore has been used as a marker of autophagy [15, 16]. However, the biological relevance of p62/SQSTM1 was not understood until recently other than autophagy [17–22]. We previously reported that the marked reduction in p62/SQSTM1 in steatotic hepatocytes is a major cause of post-PH liver injury and is possibly involved in acute liver failure

following PH [23]. It is known that p62/SQSTM1 directly binds to Keap-1, which inhibits its binding to nuclear factor erythroid 2-related factor-2 (Nrf2) and allows Nrf2 to activate/translocate into the nucleus [18]. Because Nrf2 is a key player in the cellular antioxidant system, it upregulates major antioxidant molecules and also p62/SQSTM1, and protects cells from OS. In addition, it was reported that p62/SQSTM1 phosphorylates/activates Akt, a pro-survival molecule in neuronal cells [21], and reduces the expression of harmful molecules (Fas ligand; FasL and Fas) in liver cells [23]. These facts strongly suggest the pro-survival and anti-cytotoxic effects of p62/SQSTM1 in liver cells.

Nuclear receptors have been widely studied for their clinical relevance in various medical fields. In liver, the farnesoid X receptor (FXR) and liver X receptor (LXR) are deeply involved in glucose and lipid metabolism, and, therefore, are considered to play important physio-pathological roles in homeostasis and survival of living organisms [24–27]. Regarding FXR, it suppresses the sterol regulatory element-binding protein (SREBP)-1c /fatty acid synthase (FAS) pathway through upregulation of small heterodimer partner (SHP) [24, 25, 27]. The SHP negatively regulates the SREBP-1c/FAS pathway and inhibits production of triglycerides (TG) in hepatocytes [27]. Therefore, many clinical trials have been performed expecting the therapeutic efficacy of its agonistic compounds against non-alcoholic fatty liver disease (NAFLD) such as NASH [28]. Recently, there was evidence that FXR directly upregulates the p62/SQSTM1 gene in hepatocytes [29]. This promptly led us to the idea that FXR activates the pro-survival signals through the upregulation of p62/SQSTM1 and, at the same time, suppresses hepatic steatosis through the upregulation of SHP. If FXR improves hepatic steatosis as well as heals the injury in fatty liver or NASH, the signals of FXR-p62/SQSTM1 may play a pivotal role in maintaining liver homeostasis and protection against injury especially of fatty liver.

In this study, we report that FXR stimulus confers the pro-survival and anti-steatotic properties through induction of p62/SQSTM1 and SHP to hepatocytes, respectively, and that it suppresses post-PH liver injury effectively with reduced fat accumulation in a mouse model. The FXR and p62/SQSTM1-mediated signals of hepatocytes seem to be relevant in surviving and protecting hepatocytes in various liver conditions especially with fatty change.

Methods
Cell culture, reagents, and siRNAs
The alpha mouse liver 12 (AML12) cells, established from hepatocytes from a mouse transgenic for human

transforming growth factor-α (TGF-α), express high levels of human TGFα and lower levels of mouse TGFα (ATCC, Manassas, VA, USA). AML12 cells were maintained at 37 °C in 5.0% CO_2 in Dulbecco's Modified Eagle Medium: Nutrient Mixture F-12 (DMEM/F12) (Gibco, CA, USA) supplemented with 10% fetal bovine serum. GW4064, an agonist of FXR, and T0901317, an agonist for LXR-α, were purchased from Sigma-Aldrich Co., LLC. (St. Louis, MO, USA) and Merck Millipore Corporation (Darmstadt, Germany), respectively. Small interfering RNAs (siRNAs) for mouse *p62/SQSTM1* (sense 5′-GG AACUCGCUAUAAGUGCATT-3′, antisense 5′-UGCAC UUAUAGCGAGUUCCCA) and *GAPDH* used as the control were purchased from Ambion, Inc. (Austin, TX, USA). Transfection of siRNAs into AML12 liver cells was accomplished using Lipofectamine 2000 (Invitrogen, Rockville, MD, USA) according to the manufacturer's instructions. p62/SQSTM1 and GAPDH expressions were both evaluated by PCR and Western blot analyses.

Reverse transcription-PCR assay

First-strand cDNA synthesis used 2.5 μg of total RNA from AML12 cells, Superscript III reverse transcriptase, and oligo(dT)$_{20}$ primers (Invitrogen, Carlsbad, CA, USA), according to the manufacturer's instructions. The cDNA was amplified by PCR with specific primers for mouse p62/SQSTM1 (225 bp): sense 5′-GATGTGGAA-CATGGAGGGAAGAG-3′, antisense 5′-AGTCATCGT CTCCTCCTGAGCA-3′. PCR was performed by 27 cycles of denaturation at 94 °C for 30 s, annealing at 55 °C for 30 s, and extension at 72 °C for 30 s.

Monitoring and evaluation of cell survival, cell death and liver injury

Cells at 40–50% confluence were plated in a plate. Cell survival was determined by plating the cells in the xCELLigence System (Roche, Basel, Switzerland), which allows for automated non-invasive, real-time, and label-free monitoring of live cells in culture. For evaluation of cell death, we examined lactate dehydrogenase (LDH) release from hepatocytes into culture media. "LDH cytotoxicity detection kit" (Takara, Otsu, Japan) was used according to the manufacturer's instructions. Briefly, the LDH reaction mixture was added to the aliquot taken from the media for cell culture 72 h after the treatment with GW4064 and incubated at room temperature for 30 min. The absorbance at 490 nm was measured using a multi-well plate reader. In mouse experiments, biochemical analyses, such as for serum levels of aspartate aminotransferase (AST), alanine aminotransferase (ALT), and LDH were performed as indices of liver injury before and after PH.

Adipogenesis assay

Adipogenesis was evaluated by an "adipogenesis colorimetric/fluorometric assay kit" (BioVision, Milpitas, CA, USA) according to the manufacturer's instructions. Briefly, cultured cells or liver tissues were harvested, washed by phosphate buffered saline (PBS), and stored at −80 °C before the assay. The specimens were completely dissolved by the lipid extraction buffer provided by the manufacturer. For the TG assay, 5–50 μl of the lipid extracts was transferred to a 96-well plate and the volume was brought to 50 μl with the assay buffer. Specimens and standards were added with 2 μl of lipase, mixed, and incubated 10 min at room temperature to convert TG to glycerol and fatty acid. The samples and standards were mixed with 50 μl of the reaction mix and measured at 570 nm for the colorimetric assay. Nile red stain was used to quantify intracellular lipid accumulation in cultured cells. T0901317- and GW4064-treated AML12 cells were rinsed with PBS and stained with the lipid-specific Nile red stain (AdipoRed Assay Reagent, Lonza, Basel, Switzerland). After the incubation at room temperature for 10 min, cells were applied for the fluorescence assay with excitation at 485 nm and emission at 572 nm (expressed as relative fluorescence units, RFU).

Western blot analysis

Western blot analysis was performed with appropriate antibodies specific for Nrf2 (1:200 dilution), heme oxygenase-1 (HO-1, 1:500 dilution), manganese-dependent superoxide dismutase (Mn-SOD, 1:1000 dilution), thioredoxin (TRX, 1:500 dilution) (BD Transduction Laboratories, NJ, USA), Bcl-2 (1:200 dilution), Bcl-xL (1:200 dilution), Fas (1:200 dilution), SHP (1:100 dilution) (Santa Cruz Biotechnology Inc., Santa Cruz, CA, USA), FasL (1:200 dilution) (Abcam, Cambridge, UK), catalase (1:1000 dilution) (EMD Biosciences, Darmstadt, Germany), p62/SQSTM1 (1:1000 dilution), phospho-Akt (1:1000 dilution), and Akt (1:1000 dilution) (Cell Signaling Technology Inc., Danvers, MA, USA). Whole cell or tissue protein extracts (25 μg) were separated by 10% sodium dodecyl sulfate-poly acrylamide gel electrophoresis (SDS-PAGE) and transferred to a polyvinylidene difluoride (PVDF) membrane. After blocking in 5% skim milk-PBS with 1% Tween 20 (PBS-T), the membrane was incubated in the primary antibody diluted properly (as indicated above) in PBS-T buffer containing 2% bovine serum albumin (BSA) for overnight at 4 °C, and washed 3 times in PBS-T. The membrane was next incubated with anti-mouse or anti-rabbit secondary antibody conjugated to horseradish peroxidase (HRP) (1:5000 dilution) in a blocking buffer (5% skim milk in PBS-T) at room temperature for 1 h. The membrane was finally applied to chemiluminescent HRP detection reagent (Luminata Forte Western HRP substrate, Merck Millipore, Darmstadt, Germany) and the chemiluminescent signals were detected using a CCD imaging system (LuminoGraph, ATTO, Tokyo, Japan).

Activation assay of Nrf2 in AML12 cells

Activation of Nrf2 in AML12 cells was evaluated by immunofluorescence microscopic observation. Cells cultured on a glass bottom dish were stimulated by GW4064 and then fixed with ice-chilled methanol for 5 min and permeabilized with 0.1% Triton X-100 in PBS for 10 min at room temperature. After blocking treatment, cells were labeled with anti-Nrf2 as a primary antibody for 1 h at room temperature, followed by incubation with a secondary antibody conjugated Alexa Fluor 488 (Thermo Fisher Scientific Inc., Waltham, MA, USA). Then nuclei were counterstained with Hoechst 33342. We investigated the expression and localization of Nrf2 in AML12 cells with a fluorescent microscope (Biozero; Keyence Corp., Osaka, Japan).

Animal experiments

Male homozygous leptin receptor-deficient (db/db) mice (45–50 g body weight, 12 weeks old) were obtained from CLEA Japan (Tokyo, Japan) and used for the 2/3 PH experiment. GW4064 was administered daily intraperitoneally (5 mg/kg body weight) for 5 days (3 times before and 2 times after the surgical procedure). The mice were fasted overnight prior to the experiments and were anesthetized with 1.5–2.0% isoflurane (Forane©, Abbott, Tokyo, Japan). The laparotomy was performed by mid-abdominal incision and the median and left liver lobes were exposed. After ligating the vessels to each liver lobe with 3–0 braided silk at the base of each lobe, the median and left liver lobes were surgically resected. The mice underwent laparotomy after anesthesia, and were closed without liver lobe ligation and resection for sham operation. Mice were sacrificed for the collection of liver specimens at the indicated time points before and after hepatectomy, and the liver/body weight ratios were calculated to estimate the recovery of liver mass. The percentage of the whole liver constituted by each lobe was similar to the lean mice, and surgical resection of the middle and left liver lobes resulted in 2/3 PH. Sudan III stained lipid droplets in more than 90% of the hepatocytes in the liver of db/db mice. The animals were maintained under standard conditions and treated according to the Guidelines for the Care and Use of Laboratory Animals of Hokkaido University.

Histological analysis

Liver tissues were fixed in 10% buffered formalin, paraffin embedded, and subjected to hematoxylin and eosin staining (H & E). To visualize lipid accumulation in the liver, frozen sections of formalin-fixed liver tissue were stained with Sudan III. Briefly, the liver frozen sections (8 μm thick) were prepared on slide glasses, air-dried and rinsed with 50% ethanol. Next, the specimens were stained in Sudan III stain for 10 min at room temperature, and rinsed again to remove excess stain. Counterstain (nuclear stain) was performed with hematoxylin stain for 3 min. After washing gently several times by water, the specimens were mounted with coverslip and microscopically observed.

Statistical analysis

All results were expressed as means ± standard error of the mean (SEM). Data were compared by Fisher's test, and p values of less than 0.05 were considered to be statistically significant.

Results

GW4064, a specific agonist of FXR, induced p62/SQSTM1 in AML12 liver cells

We first attempted to confirm the expression of p62/SQSTM1 in AML12 liver cells by FXR stimulus. The expression of p62/SQSTM1 protein was observed 10 h after treatment with a specific agonist of FXR, GW4064 (1.0 μM) (Fig. 1a), and continued for at least 36 h. The protein expression of p62/SQSTM1 at 36 h after the treatment with GW4064 was observed in a dose-dependent manner in a range of 0.25 to 2.0 μM (Fig. 1b). The protein induction of p62/SQSTM1 by GW4064 (1.0 μM) was significantly reduced by siRNA of the p62/SQSTM1 gene (Fig. 1c). Furthermore, GW4064 induced the mRNA expression of p62/SQSTM1 in AML12 liver cells (Fig. 1d).

These data indicate that FXR-agonist upregulates p62/SQSTM1 gene expression and induces transcriptionally its protein expression in non-tumorous AML12 liver cells, supporting the previously reported data that the p62/SQSTM1 gene is upregulated by FXR in HepG2 cells [29].

An FXR agonist sent signals to anti-oxidant and pro-survival molecules but not mitosis-associated molecules in AML12 liver cells

Because FXR induced p62/SQSTM1 in AML12 cells (Fig. 1), we next studied the effect of the FXR-agonist on the expression of Nrf2 and its nuclear translocation (activation), and also the expression of the Nrf2-associated anti-oxidant molecules in AML12 cells. Treatment with GW4064 (1.0 μM) induced the rapid and marked translocation of Nrf2 into nuclei of AML12 liver cells (Fig. 2a). The immunocytochemical study clearly showed that the nuclear translocation of Nrf2 occurred within 8 h after the treatment with GW4064 and continued in nuclei at least 36 h. Interestingly, the nuclear translocation of Nrf2 was most evident at 1.0 μM

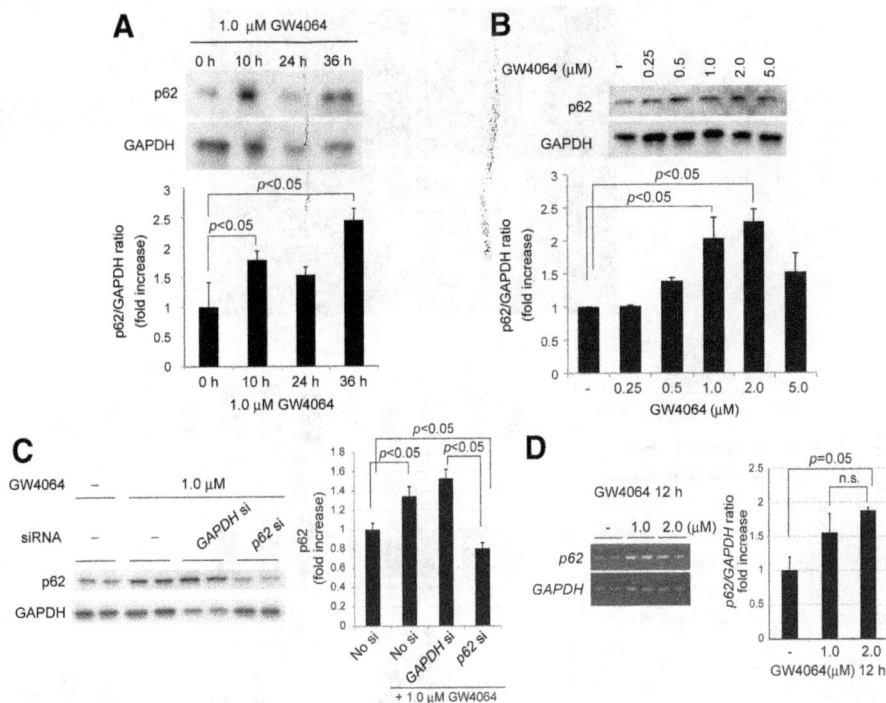

Fig. 1 FXR-agonist induced p62/SQSTM1 in AML12 liver cells. **a** GW4064 (1.0 μM), an FXR-specific agonist, expressed p62/SQSTM1 protein 10 h after administration and continued at least 36 h in AML12 liver cells. The immunoblot is a representative of the three independent experiments. **b** p62/SQSTM1 protein was expressed by GW4064 in a dose-dependent manner (0.25–5.0 μM) at 36 h after the treatment. **c** The protein induction of p62/SQSTM1 by GW4064 (1.0 μM) was cancelled by *p62/SQSTM1* siRNA (10 nM). **d** Reverse transcription–PCR analysis of the *p62/SQSTM1* gene in AML12 liver cells. GW4064 robustly upregulated the *p62/SQSTM1* gene in 1.0 and 2.0 μM of GW4064. *Each blot* represents at least three independent experiments (**a**, **b**, **c**). ImageJ software was used for quantitative analysis of western blot and reverse transcription–PCR. Data are expressed as mean ± SEM. *p* values <0.05 were considered statistically significant

(Additional file 1), though the protein was expressed more strongly at 2.0 μM (Fig. 2b). These findings indicate that GW4064 even at lower concentrations rapidly and persistently induces Nrf2 activation in AML12 liver cells. As expected, GW4064 induced significant expression of Nrf2-associated anti-oxidant-associated molecules such as Nrf2, catalase and HO-1 36 h after the treatment in AML12 liver cells (Fig. 2b). Mn-SOD and TRX were mildly induced, but not significantly. Interestingly, HO-1 was induced evidently at the low concentration of GW4064 (0.5 μM), different from other molecules.

Next, we studied the pro-survival effects of FXR on AML12 liver cells. GW4064 induced the phosphorylation of Akt (Fig. 2c). GW4064 also induced anti-apoptotic proteins such as Bcl-xL and Bcl-2 significantly at 0.5 and 1.0 μM. respectively. The protein expressions of Fas and FasL, which induce harmful effects on hepatocytes, were also evidently suppressed by GW4064 administration. Though deletion of p62/SQSTM1 clearly reduced FXR-induced phosphorylation of Akt (T308), this did not affect the protein expression of the pro-survival- and apoptosis-associated molecules examined in this study (Fig. 2d). These facts indicate that these

critical molecules for cell survival and apoptosis are not only regulated by FXR-p62/SQSTM1 pathway, but also by the mechanisms other than FXR-p62/SQSTM1.

Regarding cell cycle-associated molecules, the treatment with GW4064 did not affect phosphorylation of the signal transducer and activator of transcription 3 (STAT3) (Y705) nor protein expressions of cyclinD1 and proliferating cell nuclear antigen (PCNA) (Fig. 2e).

Activation of the FXR-p62/SQSTM1 pathway improved liver cell survival

We thereafter studied the effect of the FXR-agonist on liver cell survival and cell death by monitoring live liver cells chronologically and LDH release, respectively (Fig. 3a). We studied the pro-survival effect of GW4064 at concentrations of 0 to 5.0 μM. GW4064 prolonged cell survival significantly in 0.5–1.0 μM, showing the peak effects at 1.0 μM. In the same range of concentrations (0.5–2.0 μM), GW4064 reduced mildly but significantly LDH release (Fig. 3a). Interestingly, the most effective concentration of GW4064 for cell survival (1.0 μM) was almost coincident to that of the protein expression of p62/SQSTM1 (Fig. 1b). These facts may

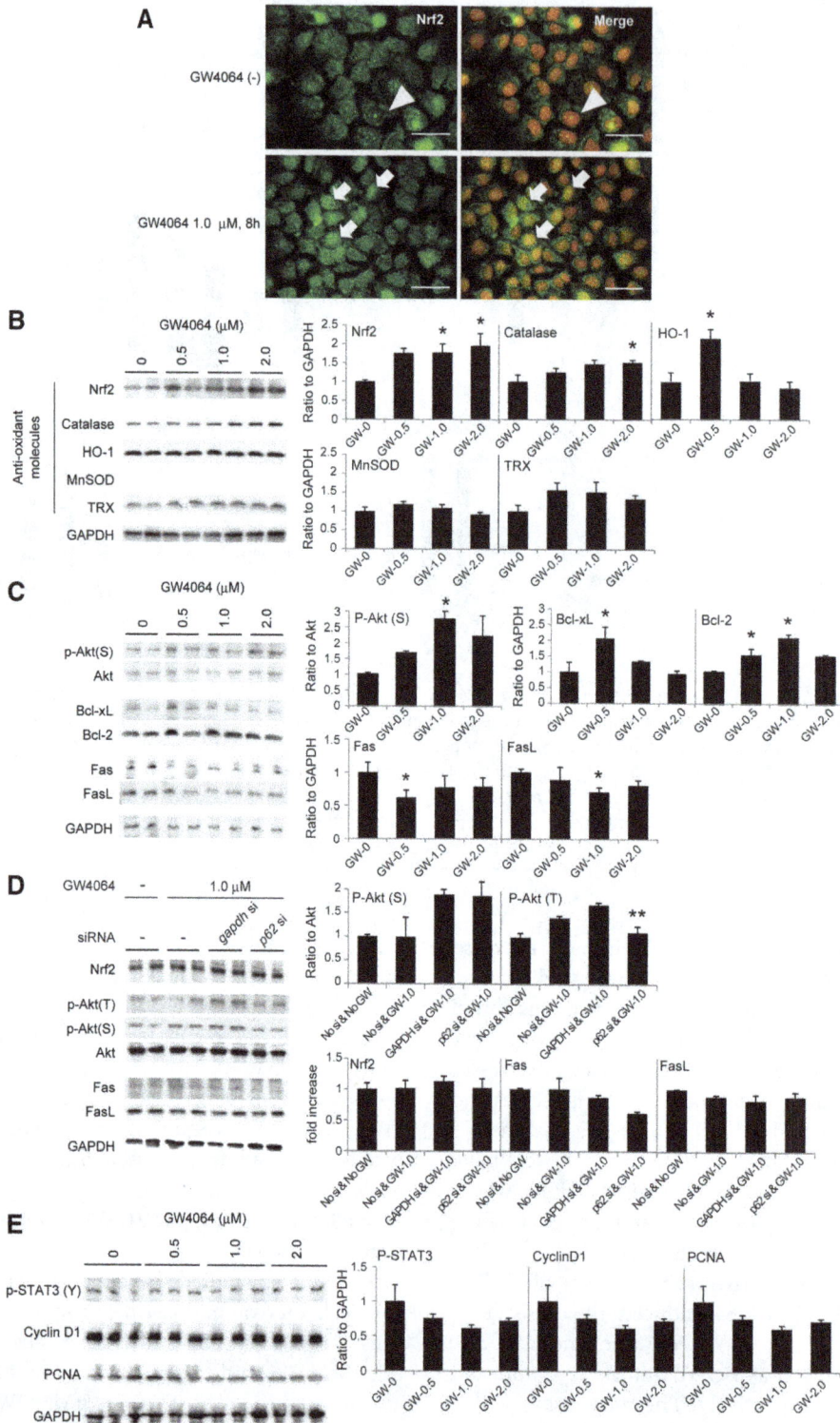

Fig. 2 (See legend on next page.)

(See figure on previous page.)

Fig. 2 FXR-agonist activated Nrf2 and induced the expressions of Nrf2 & anti-oxidant molecules in AML12 cells. **a** Nrf2 in cytosols was translocated into nuclei by GW4064 treatment (1.0 μM) in AML12 cells. Nrf2 was not stained in nuclei without GW4064 (*arrowheads*), but clearly stained in nuclei 8 h after GW4064 administration (*arrows*). 4' 6-diamidino-2-phenylindole dihydrochloride (DAPI) was used for nuclear stain in blue (*pseudo-colored red*). Scale bar, 50 μm **b** The protein expression of Nrf2 and the antioxidant molecules (catalase, heme oxygenase-1; HO-1, manganese-dependent superoxide dismutase; MnSOD, and thioredoxin; TRX) 36 h after the treatment with GW4064 (1.0 μM). **c** GW4064 induced phosphorylation of Akt and anti-apoptotic molecules (Bcl-xL and Bcl-2), and suppressed the expressions of harmful hepatic molecules such as FasL and Fas in AML12 liver cells. **d** Ablation of GW4064 by *p62/SQSTM1* siRNA reduced phosphorylation of Akt, which was induced by GW4064 in AML12 liver cells, though this does not affect the protein expressions of the other molecules. **e** GW4064 did not affect cell cycle-associated molecules. GW4064 did not phosphorylate STAT3 (Y705) nor induce cyclinD1 and PCNA. Each experiment was performed three times and representative photographs are shown. The duplicates of immunoblots are taken from the specimens of experiments performed at different times. ImageJ software was used for quantitative analysis of western blot. The quantitative analysis data are expressed as mean ± SEM. *p* values <0.05 were considered statistically significant (*: *p* < 0.05 vs GW-0 μM group; **: *p* < 0.05 vs *GAPDH* siRNA & GW-1.0 μM group)

indicate that the pro-survival effect of GW4064 mainly by protection against cell injury. This effect of GW4064 was significantly reduced by silencing the *p62/SQSTM1* gene (Fig. 3b), indicating the possible involvement of FXR in cell survival/cell protection via FXR-p62/SQSTM1-associated pathway.

FXR-agonist showed adipogenic and adipolytic effects in hepatocytes, and protected steatotic hepatocytes from injury

We studied the expression of SHP by GW4064 at the same concentrations where GW4064 showed pro-survival effects in AML12 liver cells (Fig. 4a). Though SHP was slightly expressed without GW4064 administration, its protein expression was upregulated by

GW4064 similarly at 0.5 to 2.0 μM (Fig. 4a). So, we confirmed whether GW4064 inhibits LXR-induced TG accumulation in AML12 liver cells.

GW4064 (1.0 μM and 5.0 μM), when concurrently administered with T0901317 (an LXR-agonist), effectively suppressed TG accumulation in hepatocytes (Fig. 4b). We also examined whether or not GW4064 reduces the accumulated TG in hepatocytes after the treatment with T0901317 (Fig. 4c). GW4064 reduced TG content of AML12 liver cells dose-dependently, showing the adipolytic effect on steatotic hepatocytes. In the steatotic hepatocytes, GW4064 reduced mildly but significantly LDH release from steatotic hepatocytes (cell protective effect). Though the protective effect of hepatocytes by GW4064 was not great, it showed evident adipolytic effect in the steatotic

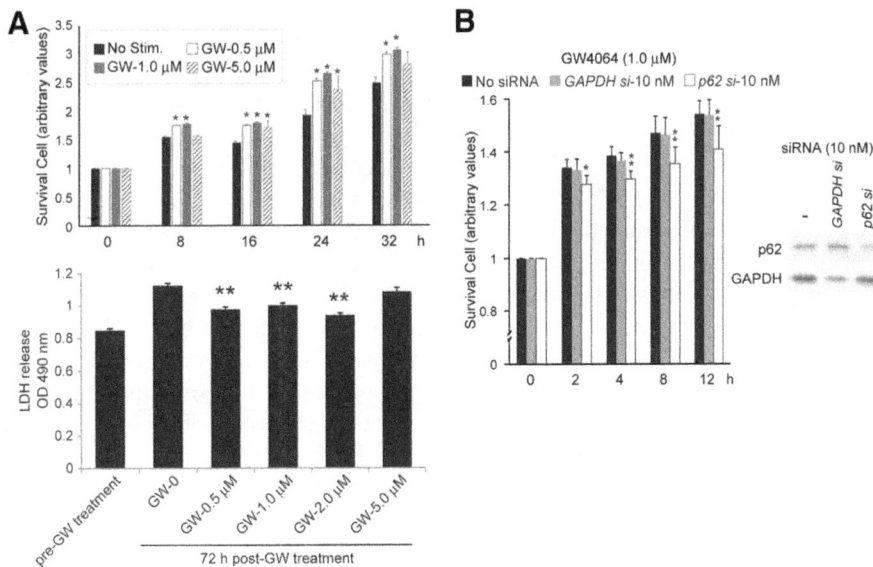

Fig. 3 FXR-agonist improved cell survival through p62/SQSTM1 in AML12 liver cells. **a** GW4064 improved cell survival significantly at 0.5, 1.0 and 5.0 μM, showing the peak effect at 1.0 μM. (*: *p* < 0.05 vs non-stimulant group) GW4064 significantly suppressed LDH release 72 h after the treatment at 0.5, 1.0 and 5.0 μM. (**: *p* < 0.05 vs GW-0 μM group) **b** Cell survival effects of GW4064 was cancelled partially but significantly by p62/SQSTM1 knockdown (10nM of siRNA of *p62/SQSTM1* gene). (* : *p* < 0.05 vs no siRNA group; **: *p* < 0.05 vs no siRNA & *GAPDH* siRNA groups) Each experimental group consisted of at least three independent experiments. Data are expressed as mean ± SEM. *p* values <0.05 were considered statistically significant

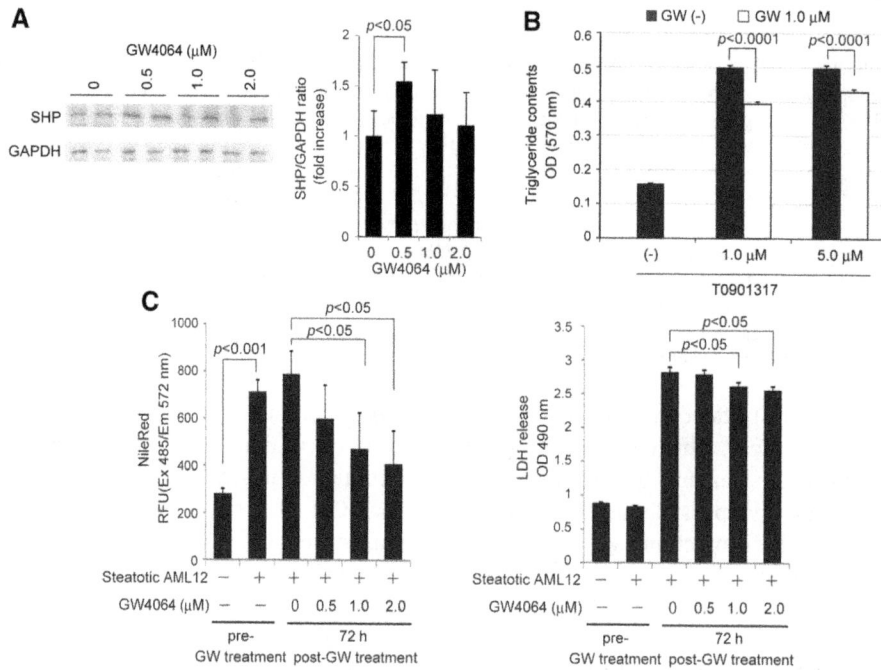

Fig. 4 FXR-agonist induced expression of SHP, showed adipogenic and adipolytic effects in hepatocytes, and protected steatotic hepatocytes. **a** Expression of SHP was induced by GW4064 (0.5 to 2.0 μM) 36 h after the treatment in AML12 liver cells. *Each blot* represents at least three independent experiments. The duplicates of immunoblots are taken from the specimens of experiments performed at different times. ImageJ software was used for quantitative analysis of western blot. **b** Steatosis was observed in AML12 liver cells by treatment with 1.0 and 5.0 μM of T0901317 (a specific agonist of LXR) for 7 days. The accumulation of TG induced by T0901317 was significantly suppressed by the concurrently administered GW4064 (1.0 μM). **c** The adipolytic and protective effects of GW4064 were evaluated by using LXR-induced steatotic hepatocytes. The treatment with T0901317 robustly reduced TG contents in a dose-dependent manner, and reduced cell death (LDH release) of the steatotic hepatocytes. Each experiment was performed three times and the data are expressed as mean ± SEM. *p* values of <0.05 were considered statistically significant

hepatocytes. These facts led us to expect the in vivo effect in a mouse model with fatty liver.

LXR-agonist improved post-PH liver injury and steatosis in db/db mice

Lastly, we examined in vivo effects of FXR by using a mouse PH model with fatty liver. We studied whether a FXR-agonist suppresses post-PH liver injury, improves steatosis and recovery in the db/db mouse. To study the injury of steatotic liver, we evaluated biochemical markers (serum levels of LDH, AST, and ALT) and histological changes. A significant improvement in liver injury was observed in the GW4064-treated mice 72 h post-PH (Fig. 5a and b). The biochemical markers in both groups (GW4064-untreated and -treated groups) similarly increased immediately after PH (24 h post-PH), possibly due to the direct mechanical injury to the liver by surgical maneuver. However, an improvement in the biochemical markers was observed in the GW4064-treated mice 72 h post-PH (Fig. 5a). Histological examination also supported the blood biochemistry data, showing that detachment of endothelial cells of central veins (arrowheads in black) and spotty cellular necrosis

and hemorrhage (arrowheads in white) were observed mainly in the liver of non-treated db/db mice, but not in the liver of the GW4064-treated mice (Fig. 5b). The mitotic hepatocytes were not particularly observed both in GW4064-treated and non-treated livers. These data and observations indicate that the treatment with GW4064 (5 mg/kg BW) suppressed post-PH liver injury, but did not affect mitotic response. Histological examination (H & E and Sudan III stains) also revealed that lipid accumulation in liver was obviously lower pre- and post-PH in the GW4064-treated mice (Fig. 5b and c). Biochemical analysis of TG contents in liver tissue also showed reduction tendency of TG in the livers of GW4064-treated mice (Fig. 5c), though the difference was not statistically significant. Serum levels of glucose and TG after PH were not affected by GW4064 treatment (Additional file 2).

Western blot analysis revealed that GW4064 induced p62/SQSTM1, Nrf2 and SHP significantly after PH (Fig. 5d). SHP protein was induced even before PH (pre-operative 3 day-administration of GW4064, 5 mg/kg) continued until 72 h post-PH. Post-PH liver mass recovery was improved slightly 24 h post-PH and more 72 h

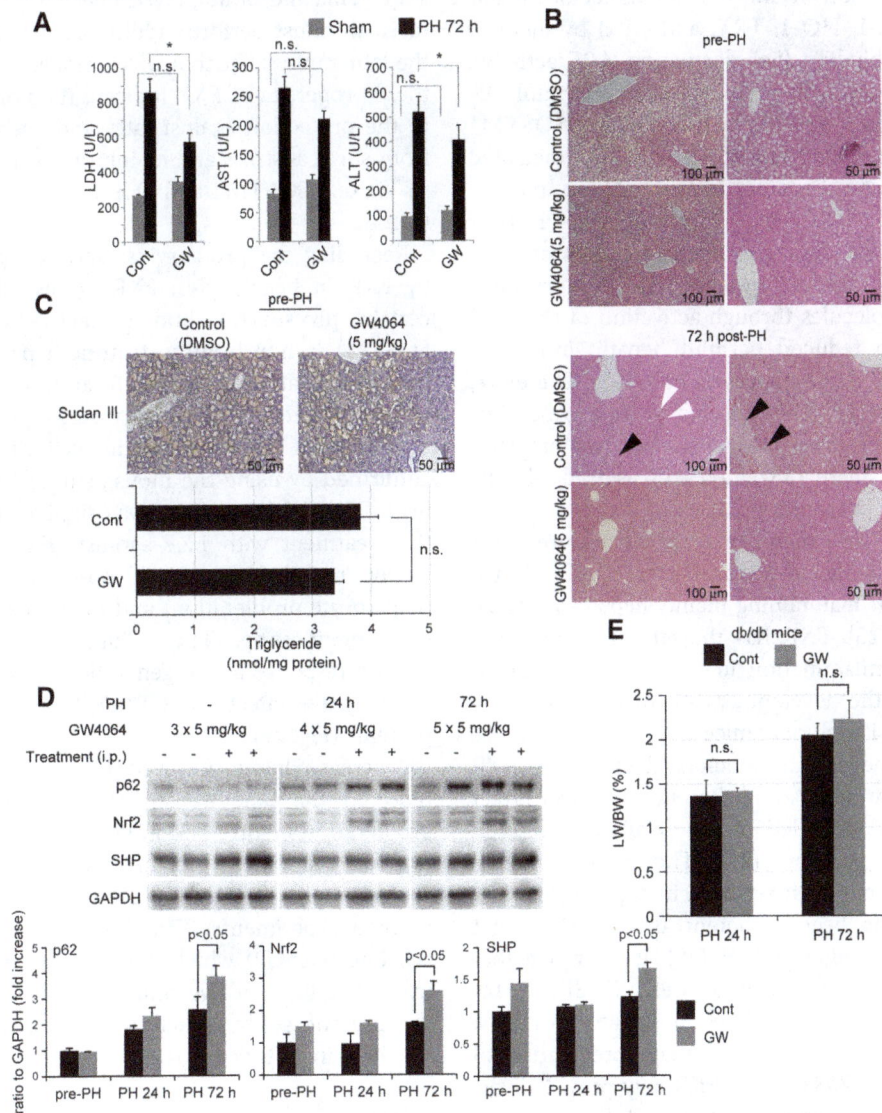

Fig. 5 FXR-agonist improved post-PH liver injury and steatosis in db/db mice. **a** Blood biochemistry data are shown. Serum levels of LDH, AST and ALT were reduced 72 h post-PH by the treatment with GW4064 (5 mg/kg BW, refer to Materials and Methods for details). **b** Hematoxylin and eosin (H & E) staining of liver tissue. *Upper panel*: The droplets of hepatocytes were obviously reduced in the GW4064-treated mice before PH. *Lower panel*: The detachment of endothelial cells (*arrowhead in black*) and spotty necrosis with hemorrhage (*arrowheads in white*) observed 72 h post-PH in control mice were not notable in the GW4064-treated mice. **c** Sudan III staining of liver tissue revealed that steatotic hepatocytes were obviously reduced in the GW4064-treated mice without PH. The content of TG was reduced in the liver treated with GW4064, but not statistically significant. **d** Western blot analysis revealed the increased expression of p62/SQSTM1, Nrf2 and SHP in the liver tissue of the GW4064-treated mice. *Each blot* represents at least three independent experiments. The duplicates of immunoblots are taken from the specimens of experiments performed at different times. ImageJ software was used for quantitative analysis of western blot. **e** Post-PH liver mass recovery was slightly improved in the GW4064-treated mice, but the difference was not statistically significant. At least four mice were used for each experiment and the representative data are shown (**a**, **b**, **c**, **e**). The data are expressed as mean ± SEM (**a**, **c**, **d**, **e**). *p* values <0.05 were considered statistically significant

post-PH by GW4064 treatment, but the difference was not statistically significant (Fig. 5e).

Discussion

Recently, p62/SQSTM1 has been considered to play major roles in the protection from injury in various organs and pathological conditions, independent of autophagy [18–23]. In liver, we previously demonstrated

that steatosis induced the reduction of p62/SQSTM1 in hepatocytes, which causes post-PH necrotic and apoptotic acute liver injury by enhancing OS and the FasL/Fas signaling pathway [23]. p62/SQSTM1 positively regulated the DNA binding activity of Nrf2 by physical association with Keap-1 and activates its transcriptional activity on *ARE*. Therefore, reduction of p62/SQSTM1 in hepatocytes, regardless of the existence of steatosis, lowered the expression of anti-oxidant molecules (catalase, MnSOD, Ref-1, HO-1, TRX, and GPx) by increasing Keap-1/Nrf2 binding (i.e., decreasing *ARE* activity), making the hepatocytes/liver susceptible to harmful OS. The increases in FasL and Fas by reduced p62/SQSTM1 led to caspase-mediated apoptosis and OS-mediated necrosis in steatotic hepatocytes/liver. These mechanisms were likely to be a main cause of post-PH fatty liver injury. On the contrary, overexpression of p62/SQSTM1 by gene transduction increased the expressions of anti-oxidant molecules through activation of the Nrf2 pathway and also reduced harmful hepatic molecules such as FasL and Fas in hepatocytes and liver. Therefore, upregulation of p62/SQSTM1 seems to be a good clinical target for liver protection, especially against fatty liver and NASH where OS and FasL/Fas undoubtedly contribute to fatty liver injury [23].

By the way, FXR is a member of the nuclear receptor superfamily and is a ligand-activated transcription factor that is essential for maintaining mainly hepato-intestinal homeostasis [24, 25]. FXR has the effects against carcinogenesis and inflammation in liver and intestine as demonstrated by the development of inflammation and tumors of FXR knock-out mice [29]. However, the mechanisms of the physio-pathological effects of FXR are not completely understood. Recently, a novel target gene of FXR was identified in the regulation of *p62/SQSTM1* gene expression [29]. The anti-adipogenic effect of FXR also has been reported in hepatocytes [30]. FXR therefore has been a potent therapeutic target against NAFLD including NASH [28]. It is known that FXR upregulates SHP, which suppresses LXR/SREBP-1c/FAS-mediated production of TG in hepatocytes [27]. This promptly led us to the idea that upregulation of liver-protective p62/SQSTM1 by FXR may provide liver-specific protection against oxidative and Fas-mediated injuries. FXR-p62/SQSTM1 may send "protective signals" to steatotic hepatocytes and fatty liver which are vulnerable to oxidative stress and Fas-mediated death signals. Here in the present study, the treatment with GW4064 reduced TG contents in hepatocytes presumably by suppressing adipogenesis and promoting adipolysis (Fig. 4b and c). FXR suppressed accumulation of TG in AML12 cells possibly by reducing its cellular production through upregulating SHP and inhibiting the SREBP-1c/FAS pathway. Regarding adipolysis by LXR, further study has to be performed to confirm this result and elucidate the underlying mechanism. Though the treatment with FXR slightly lowered hepatic TG contents in db/db mice, the defatting effect of FXR was not evident in vivo. Because the model mice used in this study were diabetic with severe fatty liver (Fig. 5c), they might have been too extreme to evaluate correctly the effect of GW4064. In order to confirm the anti-adipogenic and/or adipolytic effects of FXR on liver steatosis, we must perform additional experiments by using the other physio-pathological mouse models. However, these properties of FXR indicate the potent contribution to the protection against fatty and even non-fatty livers from surgical stress and/or injury and to improve steatosis via p62/SQSTM1 and SHP in various clinical settings (Fig. 6).

Regarding the pro-survival and cell protective effects by FXR in hepatocytes, FXR-agonist showed mild but certain pro-survival and protective effects via p62/SQSTM1 in non-healthy steatotic hepatocytes as well as healthy hepatocytes (Figs. 3 and 4c), indicating the potent protective effect in various physio-pathological conditions of liver and intestine cells. These effects were confirmed by using the mouse surgical model with fatty liver. Post-PH liver injury was significantly improved by the treatment with LXR-agonist (Fig. 5a, b). Unfortunately, it failed to induce post-PH mitotic response (hepatocyte proliferation) and to regenerate the remnant liver significantly. The failure to promote post-PH mitotic response and regeneration may be explained by the negative effects of GW4064 on mitosis-associated proteins (Fig. 2e).

Whereas, Huang, W. et al. [31] and Xie, Y. et al. [32] reported the potential effects of FXR on hepatocyte proliferation in vitro and in vivo. FXR stimulated mitotic response in the post-PH mouse liver [31] and acetaminophen-treated mouse liver [32]. Regarding the in vitro experiments, Xie, Y. et al. used human cancer cell line (HepG2) which possesses autonomic proliferative capability, and we differently used AML12 cells in the present study, which were maintained by TGF-α secreted in autocrine/paracrine fashions. They studied

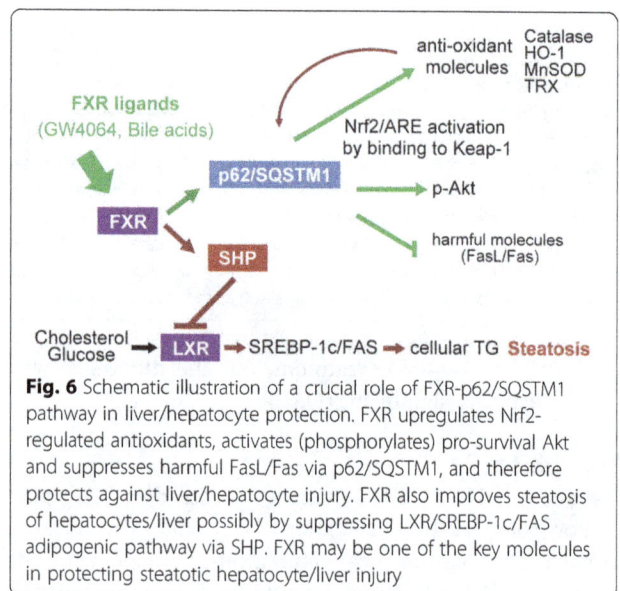

Fig. 6 Schematic illustration of a crucial role of FXR-p62/SQSTM1 pathway in liver/hepatocyte protection. FXR upregulates Nrf2-regulated antioxidants, activates (phosphorylates) pro-survival Akt and suppresses harmful FasL/Fas via p62/SQSTM1, and therefore protects against liver/hepatocyte injury. FXR also improves steatosis of hepatocytes/liver possibly by suppressing LXR/SREBP-1c/FAS adipogenic pathway via SHP. FXR may be one of the key molecules in protecting steatotic hepatocyte/liver injury

MTT assay for evaluation of live cells and BrdU incorporation for proliferation in HepG2 cells. The live cell numbers and BrdU incorporation of HepG2 cells were certainly increased by the treatment with GW4064 (1.0–5.0 μM). In the paper, they concluded that FXR may promote proliferation of HepG2 tumor cells by activating pyruvate dehydrogenate kinse4 (PDK4)-mediated metabolic reprogramming and generating glycolytic intermediates required for cell proliferation, which was not observed in healthy hepatocytes. This indicates that FXR-stimulus may promote cell proliferation, but not be a sufficient condition for non-tumorous cells. The enhancement of proliferation by GW4064 may require basically the autonomic proliferative capability of cells (such as HepG2 cells). Taken together, we think that the hepatocytes with autonomic/strong proliferative capability can be stimulated with some kinds of trigger such as "metabolic switch", whereas that of healthy hepatocytes whose proliferation is not driven autonomically/strongly cannot be stimulated by the metabolic changes alone. Similar to FXR, the association of p62/SQSTM1 with tumor have been reported [30, 33]. The anti-oxidant and pro-survival properties of p62/SQSTM1, is surely expected to prevent oxidative stress, cell death (injury) and inflammation in normal hepatocytes/liver. However, p62/SQSTM1, if accumulated excessively in cells, may contribute to oncogenesis, especially in liver.

These complicated mechanisms in FXR- and p62/SQSTM1-associated physio-pathology make it difficult to understand its role in various conditions. Therefore, it seems to be a limitation for interpretation of the physio-pathological roles of FXR and p62/SQSTM1 in the present study. In order to evaluate properly the proliferative/pro-survival and the other effects of FXR on liver physio-pathology, we must perform additional experiments using other ligands with various concentrations in healthy and non-healthy hepatocytes, and also confirm by using the other physio-pathological models.

Conclusions
This study is the first to show the critical roles of the FXR-p62/SQSTM1 pathway in the protection against post-PH liver injury and possibly the FXR-SHP pathway in the improvement of liver steatosis. Further studies are required to elucidate thoroughly the mechanisms of protection against injury in steatotic and non-steatotic liver. However, the present data provide important clues toward the development of new therapies specifically against liver injury without affecting other organs/tissues.

Additional files

Additional file 1: The nuclear translocation of Nrf2 by GW4064 (0, 0.5, 1.0 and 2.0 μM) was studied immunocytochemically in AML12 mouse liver cells.

Additional file 2: Liver X Receptor (LXR)-agonist did not affect serum levels of glucose (GLU) and triglyceride (TG) after PH in db/db mice with fatty liver. Serum levels of glucose and TG were not affected post-PH 24 and 72 h by the pre-treatment of GW4064 in db/db mice with fatty liver (5 mg/kg BW, refer to Materials and Methods in details).

Abbreviations
ALT: Alanine aminotransferase; AML12: Alpha mouse liver 12; ARE: Transcriptional activity on antioxidant response elements; AST: Aspartate aminotransferase; ATP: Abnormalities and decreased adenosine triphosphate; BSA: Bovine serum albumin; DMEM/F12: Dulbecco's modified eagle medium: nutrient mixture F-12; FAS: Fatty acid synthase; FasL: Fas ligand; FXR: Farnesoid X receptor; H & E: Hematoxylin and eosin; HO-1: Heme oxygenase-1; HRP: Horseradish peroxidase; Keap-1: Kelch like ECH-associated protein-1; LDH: Lactate dehydrogenase; LXR: Liver X receptor; Mn-SOD: Manganese-dependent superoxide dismutase; NAFLD: Non-alcoholic fatty liver disease; NASH: Non-alcoholic steatohepatitis; Nrf2: Nuclear factor erythroid 2-related factor-2; OS: Oxidative stress; PBS: Phosphate buffered saline; PCNA: Proliferating cell nuclear antigen; PH: Partial hepatectomy; PVDF: Polyvinylidene difluoride; RFU: Relative fluorescence units; SDS-PAGE: Sodium dodecyl sulfate-poly acrylamide gel electrophoresis; SEM: Standard error of the mean; SHP: Small heterodimer partners; siRNAs: Small interfering RNAs; SREBP: Sterol regulatory element-binding protein; STAT3: Signal transducer and activator of transcription 3; TG: Triglyceride; TGF-α: Transforming growth factor-α; TRX: Thioredoxin

Funding
JSPS Grants-in-Aid for Scientific Research (KAKENHI): Grant Number 23659631 (to M.O.), No.26670573 & 15H05659 (to S.H.). Research grant from The Akiyama Life Science Foundation (to S.H.). Heartfelt donation from Mr. & Mrs. Hiroyasu Fujikawa (to M.O.)

Authors' contributions
MO conceived and designed the study, performed the experiments, and analyzed the data. SH conceived the study, designed and performed the experiments, and analyzed the data. Y performed the experiments and analyzed the data. MO and SH wrote the manuscript. All authors read and approved the final manuscript.

Competing interests
The authors declare that they have no competing interests.

Consent for publication
Not applicable.

Author details
[1]Department of Biological Response and Regulation, Faculty of Health Sciences, Hokkaido University, N-12, W-5, Kita-ku, Sapporo, Hokkaido 060-0812, Japan. [2]Department of Advanced Medicine, Graduate School of Medicine, Hokkaido University, N-15, W-7, Kita-ku, Sapporo, Hokkaido 060-8638, Japan.

References

1. Fausto N. Liver regeneration: from laboratory to clinic. Liver Transpl. 2001;7: 835–44.
2. Michalopoulos GK, DeFrances MC. Liver regeneration. Science. 1997;276:60–6.
3. Fausto N. Liver regeneration. J Hepatol. 2000;32:19–31.
4. Aoyama T, Ikejima K, Kon K, Okumura K, Arai K, Watanabe S. Pioglitazone promotes survival and prevents hepatic regeneration failure after partial hepatectomy in obese and diabetic KK-A(y) mice. Hepatology. 2009;49: 1636–44.
5. Murata S, Hashimoto I, Nakano Y, Myronovych A, Watanabe M, Ohkohchi N. Single administration of thrombopoietin prevents progression of liver fibrosis and promotes liver regeneration after partial hepatectomy in cirrhotic rats. Ann Surg. 2008;248:821–8.
6. Schmucker DL. Age-related changes in liver structure and function: Implications for disease? Exp Gerontol. 2005;40:650–9.
7. Selzner M, Clavien PA. Steatotic liver in liver transplantation and surgery. Semin Liver Dis. 2001;21:105–13.
8. Brunt EM. Nonalcoholic fatty liver disease: pros and cons of histologic systems of evaluation. Int J Mol Sci. 2016;17:97.
9. Ahmed A, Wong RJ, Harrison SA. Nonalcoholic fatty liver disease review: diagnosis, treatment, and outcomes. Clin Gastroenterol Hepatol. 2015;13: 2062–70.
10. Taub R. Liver regeneration: from myth to mechanism. Nat Rev Mol Cell Biol. 2004;5:836–47.
11. Haga S, Ozaki M, Inoue H, Okamoto Y, Ogawa W, Takeda K, et al. The survival pathways phosphatidylinositol-3 kinase (PI3-K)/ phosphoinositide-dependent protein kinase 1 (PDK1)/Akt modulate liver regeneration through hepatocyte size rather than proliferation. Hepatology. 2009;49:204–14.
12. Murata H, Yagi T, Iwagaki H, Ogino T, Sadamori H, Matsukawa H, et al. Mechanism of impaired regeneration of steatotic liver in mouse partial hepatectomy model. J Gastroenterol Hepatol. 2007;22:2173–80.
13. Tanoue S, Uto H, Kumamoto R, Arima S, Hashimoto S, Nasu Y, et al. Liver regeneration after partial hepatectomy in rat is more impaired in a steatotic liver induced by dietary fructose compared to dietary fat. Biochem Biophys Res Commun. 2011;407:163–8.
14. Caraceni P, Domenicali M, Vendemiale G, Grattagliano I, Pertosa A, Nardo B, et al. The reduced tolerance of rat steatotic liver to ischemia reperfusion is associated with mitochondrial oxidative injury. J Surg Res. 2005;124:160–8.
15. Katsuragi Y, Ichimura Y, Komatsu M. p62/SQSTM1 functions as a signaling hub and an autophagy adaptor. FEBS J. 2015;282:4672–8.
16. Manley S, Williams JA, Ding WX. Role of p62/SQSTM1 in liver physiology and pathogenesis. Exp Biol Med. 2013;238:525–38.
17. Bitto A, Lerner CA, Nacarelli T, Crowe E, Torres C, Sell C. p62/SQSTM1 at the interface of aging, autophagy, and disease. Age. 2014;36:9626.
18. Komatsu M, Kurokawa H, Waguri S, Taguchi K, Kobayashi A, Ichimura Y, et al. The selective autophagy substrate p62 activates the stress responsive transcription factor Nrf2 through inactivation of Keap1. Nat Cell Biol. 2010;12:213–23.
19. Nogalska A, Terracciano C, D'Agostino C, King Engel W, Askanas V. p62/ SQSTM1 is overexpressed and prominently accumulated in inclusions of sporadic inclusion-body myositis muscle fibers, and can help differentiating it from polymyositis and dermatomyositis. Acta Neuropathol. 2009;118:407–13.
20. Liang X, Wei SQ, Lee SJ, Fung JK, Zhang M, Tanaka A, et al. p62 sequestosome 1/light chain 3b complex confers cytoprotection on lung epithelial cells after hyperoxia. Am J Respir Cell Mol Biol. 2013;48:489–96.
21. Heo SR, Han AM, Kwon YK, Joung I. p62 protects SH-SY5Y neuroblastoma cells against H_2O_2-induced injury through the PDK1/Akt pathway. Neurosci Lett. 2009;450:45–50.
22. Sun X, Ou Z, Chen R, Niu X, Chen D, Kang R, et al. Activation of the p62-Keap1-NRF2 pathway protects against ferroptosis in hepatocellular carcinoma cells. Hepatology. 2016;63:173–84.
23. Haga S, Ozawa T, Yamada Y, Morita N, Nagashima I, Inoue H, et al. p62/SQSTM1 plays a protective role in oxidative injury of steatotic liver in a mouse hepatectomy model. Antioxid Redox Signal. 2014;21: 2515–30.
24. Ding L, Pang S, Sun Y, Tian Y, Yu L, Dang N. Coordinated actions of FXR and LXR in metabolism: from pathogenesis to pharmacological targets for type 2 diabetes. Int J Endocrinol. 2014;2014:751859.
25. Calkin AC, Tontonoz P. Transcriptional integration of metabolism by the nuclear sterol-activated receptors LXR and FXR. Nat Rev Mol Cell Biol. 2012;13:213–24.
26. Kim TH, Kim H, Park JM, Im SS, Bae JS, Kim MY, et al. Interrelationship between liver X receptor alpha, sterol regulatory element-binding protein-1c, peroxisome proliferator-activated receptor gamma, and small heterodimer partner in the transcriptional regulation of glucokinase gene expression in liver. J Biol Chem. 2009;284:15071–83.
27. Watanabe M, Houten SM, Wang L, Moschetta A, Mangelsdorf DJ, Heyman RA, et al. Bile acids lower triglyceride levels via a pathway involving FXR, SHP, and SREBP-1c. J Clin Invest. 2004;113:1408–18.
28. Ali AH, Carey EJ, Lindor KD. Recent advances in the development of farnesoid X receptor agonists. Ann Transl Med. 2015;3:5.
29. Williams JA, Thomas AM, Li G, Kong B, Zhan L, Inaba Y, et al. Tissue specific induction of p62/Sqstm1 by farnesoid X receptor. PLoS One. 2012;7:e43961.
30. Taniguchi K, Yamachika S, He F, Karin M. p62/SQSTM1-Dr. Jekyll and Mr. Hyde that prevents oxidative stress but promotes liver cancer. FEBS Lett. 2016;590:2375–97.
31. Huang W, Ma K, Zhang J, Qatanani M, Cuvillier J, Liu J, et al. Nuclear receptor-dependent bile acid signaling is required for normal liver regeneration. Science. 2006;312:233–6.
32. Xie Y, Wang H, Cheng X, Wu Y, Cao L, Wu M, et al. Farnesoid X receptor activation promotes cell proliferation via PDK4-controlled metabolic reprogramming. Sci Rep. 2016;6:18751.
33. Saito T, Ichimura Y, Taguchi K, Suzuki T, Mizushima T, Takagi K, et al. p62/Sqstm1 promotes malignancy of HCV-positive hepatocellular carcinoma through Nrf2-dependent metabolic reprogramming. Nat Commun. 2016;7:12030.

16

Telbivudine versus entecavir in patients with undetectable hepatitis B virus DNA

Jihyun An[1], Young-Suk Lim[1*], Gi-Ae Kim[2], Seong-bong Han[3], Wonhee Jeong[1], Danbi Lee[1], Ju Hyun Shim[1], Han Chu Lee[1] and Yung Sang Lee[1]

Abstract

Background: Telbivudine has been suggested to induce hepatitis B surface antigen (HBsAg) decline to the similar degree as pegylated interferon. We aimed to investigate whether telbivudine could further decrease HBsAg titer in patients who maintain undetectable serum hepatitis B virus (HBV) DNA after initial entecavir treatment.

Methods: In this open-label trial, patients who had serum HBsAg and HBV DNA levels ≥1,000 IU/mL and <60 IU/mL, respectively, following entecavir (0.5 mg/day) treatment for HBeAg-positive chronic hepatitis B were randomized to either switch treatment to telbivudine (600 mg/day, $n = 47$) or continue entecavir ($n = 50$) for 48 weeks.

Results: The baseline characteristics were comparable between groups including HBsAg levels (median, 3.41 $\log_{10}$ IU/mL). All patients had undetectable HBV DNA and normal alanine aminotransferase level. At week 48, the mean change in serum HBsAg levels was not significantly different between the telbivudine and entecavir groups (-0.03 $\log_{10}$ IU/mL vs. -0.05 $\log_{10}$ IU/mL; $P = 0.57$). No patient experienced HBsAg seroclearance or HBsAg decline >0.5 $\log_{10}$ IU/mL. Eleven patients (23.4%) in the telbivudine group, but none in the entecavir group, experienced virologic breakthrough ($P < 0.001$). Seven patients (14.9%) exhibited genotypic resistance mutations (M204I +/− L180M) during the virologic breakthrough.

Conclusion: Sequential therapy with entecavir followed by telbivudine resulted in a high rate of virologic breakthrough and drug-resistance without any beneficial effect on HBsAg decline. These results do not support the use of low genetic barrier drugs as a switch treatment strategy in patients who achieve virologic response with high genetic barrier drugs.

Keywords: Hepatitis B surface antigen, HBsAg, Resistance, Virologic breakthrough, Virologic response

Background

Approximately 400 million people worldwide are chronically infected with hepatitis B virus (HBV). These patients have a substantially increased risk of cirrhosis and hepatocellular carcinoma (HCC), which are responsible for approximately 1 million deaths worldwide annually [1, 2]. The availability of potent nucleos(t)ide analogs (NUC) such as entecavir and tenofovir disoproxil fumarate (TDF) has made the suppression of serum HBV DNA to levels undetectable by polymerase chain reaction (PCR) assays achievable in most patients, with a minimal risk of drug-resistance [3, 4]. However, the eradication of HBV, which is best indicated by serum hepatitis B surface antigen (HBsAg) seroclearance, is rarely achievable with long-term NUC therapy [5–9]. The discontinuation of treatment before HBsAg seroclearance is associated with high rate of hepatitis relapse and disease progression [10, 11]. Therefore, treatments that can induce a rapid decline in HBsAg levels would have a clear advantage in reducing the treatment duration required to achieve HBsAg seroclearance.

* Correspondence: limys@amc.seoul.kr
[1]Department of Gastroenterology, Liver Center, Asan Medical Center, University of Ulsan College of Medicine, 88, Olympic-ro 43-gil, Songpa-gu, Seoul 05505, Korea
Full list of author information is available at the end of the article

Treatment with pegylated-interferon (PEG-IFN) has been reported to be associated with a greater HBsAg decline than NUC-treatment in patients with chronic HBV infection (CHB), regardless of hepatitis B envelope antigen (HBeAg) positivity [12, 13]. Interestingly, recent preliminary study demonstrated that telbivudine, a nucleoside analog, was associated with rapid HBsAg decline that was comparable to that induced by PEG-IFN in patients with HBeAg-positive CHB [14]. Although there has been no head-to-head trial comparing the induction of HBsAg decline by different NUCs, previous studies have repeatedly suggested that the decline in HBsAg may be greater during telbivudine treatment than it is with lamivudine or entecavir [12, 15–17]. Although telbivudine is associated with a relatively high rate of resistance, the risk could be reduced by profound early viral suppression to undetectable levels [18, 19].

In this randomised trial, we aimed to determine whether telbivudine induces a decline in HBsAg levels to a different degree compared with entecavir in patients with HBeAg-positive CHB, who have achieved undetectable serum HBV DNA levels by previous entecavir treatment.

Methods
Study design
This study was a randomized open-label trial (Clinical-Trials.gov ID NCT01595685; TERESA study) conducted in patients who had achieved a virologic response (serum HBV DNA <15 IU/mL) by preceding entecavir (0.5 mg once daily) treatment (Fig. 1). The patients were randomized (in a 1:1 ratio using a centralized procedure and an interactive web response system) to groups that either changed the treatment to telbivudine 600 mg once daily (Telbivudine group) or continued the entecavir treatment (Entecavir group) for 48 weeks.

The treatment assignments were generated by using a permuted block size of four after stratification based on serum HBsAg levels (1,000 – 5,000 vs. ≥5,000 IU/mL)

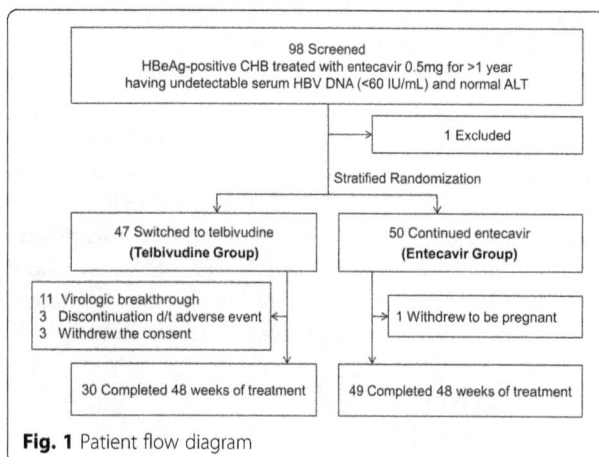

Fig. 1 Patient flow diagram

and the duration of the preceding entecavir treatment (1–2 vs. ≥2 years). There was no interruption in entecavir therapy before randomization. This study was approved by the Institutional Review Board of the Asan Medical Center, and written informed consent was obtained from all study participants.

Study subjects
The patients were enrolled between July 2012 and March 2013 at Asan Medical Center, an academic tertiary referral hospital in Korea. Patients were considered eligible for enrollment if they were positive for the HBeAg at the initiation of preceding entecavir treatment, received entecavir for more than 1 year, had undetectable serum HBV DNA levels (<60 IU/mL) on at least two occasions more than 3 months apart, and serum HBsAg levels >1,000 IU/mL at screening. Patients were required to be between 18 and 80 years old and have serum creatinine levels <1.5 mg/dL.

Patients were excluded if they met any of the following criteria: history of interferon therapy; prior exposure to oral antiviral agents other than entecavir for more than 1 week; evidence of decompensated liver disease; any malignant neoplasm; suspicion of HCC; received organ transplantation; concomitant use of immunosuppressive agent; or co-infection with hepatitis C, hepatitis D, or human immunodeficiency virus.

Efficacy and safety assessments
The primary efficacy endpoint of this study was defined as a change in serum HBsAg levels from baseline to the end of week 48. The secondary endpoints were the proportions of patients with HBsAg loss/seroconversion, HBsAg decline ≥0.5 $\log_{10}$ IU/mL, HBeAg loss/seroconversion in those who were HBeAg-positive at randomization, and the incidence of virologic breakthrough (increases in HBV DNA levels ≥1 $\log_{10}$ IU/mL from nadir in two consecutive tests). The probability of developing genotypic resistance was assessed in all patients who experienced a virologic breakthrough or had viremia (i.e., HBV DNA >60 IU/mL) by the last time point of treatment and week 48.

Routine liver biochemistry, hepatitis B serology, and serum HBV DNA measurements were assessed at week 12, 24, and 48 after randomization. During each visit, patients were evaluated for adherence to study drugs by counting the number of pills and empty blister packets returned. The adverse events (clinical and laboratory) were assessed throughout the 48 weeks.

Serum assays
The serum HBsAg levels were quantified by using the Architect assay (Abbott Laboratories, Chicago, IL, USA), which has a lower limit of detection (LLOD) of 0.05 IU/mL. Serum HBV DNA levels were measured using a

real-time PCR assay (linear dynamic detection range, 15 IU/mL to 1×10^9 IU/mL; Abbott Laboratories). Serological markers including anti-HBs, HBeAg, and anti-HBe were determined by using enzyme immunoassays (Abbott Laboratories) while resistance mutations were determined by direct sequencing of the reverse transcriptase domain (pol/RT) of the HBV polymerase gene. The HBV genotype was not determined because more than 98% of Korean patients with CHB have the HBV genotype C2 [20].

Statistical analysis

The primary dataset for the efficacy and safety analyses was defined as all randomized patients. All the analyses were performed according to the intention-to-treat principle. Patients who discontinued the study prior to week 48 were considered failures for all endpoints from the time of discontinuation. The efficacy and safety analyses were performed by comparing the originally randomized Telbivudine and Entecavir groups.

The primary efficacy endpoint was the change in serum HBsAg levels at week 48. To observe a mean difference of 0.3 $\log_{10}$ IU/mL in the HBsAg decline between the Telbivudine and Entecavir groups with a two-sided 5% significance level and taking into account a dropout rate of up to 5%, an estimated 184 patients would have to be randomly assigned to each group to achieve 80% power. However, the study recruitment was discontinued after the inclusion of 97 patients because of slow accrual and identifying the significantly higher rate of virological breakthrough in the Telbivudine group at interim analysis.

The between-group comparisons of the continuous or categorical variables were conducted by using the t-test, Chi-square test, or Fisher's exact test, as deemed appropriate. All the statistical analyses were performed by using the statistical package for the social sciences (SPSS, version 20, SPSS, Chicago, IL, USA) and R (version 3.0, http://cran.r-project.org/). A $P < 0.05$ was considered statistically significant.

Results

Baseline characteristics of patients

A total of 97 patients who had undetectable serum HBV DNA following entecavir treatment were randomly assigned to either the Telbivudine ($n = 47$) or Entecavir group ($n = 50$) as shown in Fig. 1.

Treatment groups were comparable in baseline demographic and laboratory characteristics (Table 1). The mean age was 47 years, and the population was predominantly male (69.1%). The median level of HBsAg was 3.41 $\log_{10}$ IU/mL. All patients were HBeAg-positive at the beginning of the preceding entecavir therapy; however, HBeAg positivity at randomization was 75.3%. All patients had an undetectable HBV DNA and normal alanine aminotransferase level. Thirty-four percent of the patients had cirrhosis. The median duration of prior entecavir treatment was 36 months.

Serologic responses

The mean change in serum HBsAg levels at week 48 of the treatment was not significantly different between the Telbivudine and Entecavir groups (–0.03 vs. -0.05 $\log_{10}$

Table 1 Baseline characteristics of the study patients

Characteristics	Total ($N = 97$)	Telbivudine ($n = 47$)	Entecavir ($n = 50$)
Age[a], years	47 ± 10	48 ± 11	47 ± 10
Male, n (%)	67 (69.1%)	32 (68.1%)	35 (70.0%)
HBsAg[b], $\log_{10}$ IU/mL	3.41 (3.15-3.69)	3.43 (3.17-3.84)	3.40 (3.10-3.67)
HBeAg positivity[c], n (%)	73 (75.3%)	40 (85.1%)	33 (66.0%)
HBV DNA undetectable (<60 IU/mL), n (%)	97 (100%)	47 (100%)	50 (100%)
ALT[b], IU/L	20 (16–30)	24 (16–31)	19 (14–27)
Bilirubin[b], mg/dL	1.0 (0.8-1.2)	1.0 (0.7-1.3)	1.0 (0.8-1.2)
Albumin[b], g/dL	4.4 (4.2-4.5)	4.3 (4.1-4.5)	4.4 (4.2-4.5)
INR[b]	0.98 (0.95-1.04)	0.98 (0.95-1.03)	0.98 (0.95-1.04)
Platelet[b], ×1,000/mm³	167 (134–208)	170 (129–207)	166 (137–209)
Cirrhosis[d], n (%)	33 (34.0%)	15 (31.9%)	18 (36.0%)
Creatinine[b], mg/dL	0.9 (0.7-1.0)	0.9 (0.7-1.0)	0.9 (0.8-1.0)
Creatine kinase[b], U/L	100 (77–129)	102 (81–156)	87 (72–116)
Duration of prior entecavir treatment[b], months	36 (24–46)	33 (24–42)	39 (23–47)

[a]Mean ± standard deviation (SD)
[b]median (interquartile range)
[c]HBeAg positivity at randomization. All patients were HBeAg-positive at the beginning of preceding entecavir therapy
[d]Cirrhosis was diagnosed by using ultrasonography with identification of liver surface nodularity and splenomegaly
HBsAg hepatitis B surface antigen, *HBeAg* hepatitis B envelope antigen, *HBV* hepatitis B virus, *ALT* alanine aminotransferase, *INR* international normalized ratio

IU/mL; $P = 0.57$; Table 2 and Fig. 2). No patient experienced HBsAg seroclearance or HBsAg decline >0.5 $\log_{10}$ IU/mL (Table 2). The proportion of patients who achieved HBsAg decline >0.1 $\log_{10}$ IU/mL was not significantly different between the Telbivudine and Entecavir groups (23.4% vs. 30.0%; $P = 0.46$). The proportion of HBeAg-positive patients who achieved HBeAg seroclearance was low without any significant difference between both groups at week 48 (5.0% vs. 15.2%; $P = 0.14$; Table 2). The serologic response at week 48 was not significantly different between the two groups by baseline HBeAg positivity, status of cirrhosis, and gender. An additional file showed these results in more detail [see Additional file 1].

Virologic responses

Over the 48-week treatment period, 11 patients who were all in the Telbivudine group experienced virologic breakthrough (23.4%; $P < 0.001$; Table 2). All those had good adherence to study medication (>95%). Of these patients, genotypic resistance mutations to Telbivudine (M204I +/− L180M) were detected in seven during the virologic breakthrough. The detailed characteristics of the 11 patients are shown in Additional file 1. All of the patients recovered virologic response in 12 weeks following the administration of TDF or entecavir rescue therapy.

At week 48, the proportion of patients who maintained the virologic response in the study was significantly lower in the Telbivudine group than it was in the Entecavir group (63.8% vs 98.0%; $P < 0.001$, Table 2 and Fig. 3).

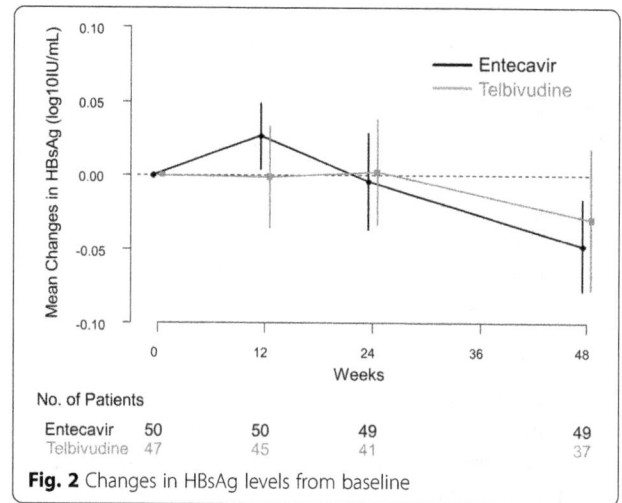

Fig. 2 Changes in HBsAg levels from baseline

Safety profiles

Three patients in the Telbivudine group discontinued the study because of headache, gastrointestinal trouble, and myopathy at week 1, 24, and 48, respectively. The symptoms improved after switching the drug to entecavir (Table 3). An elevation in serum creatine kinase (CK) levels >3 times of upper limit of normal (ULN, 250 IU/mL) was observed in three (6.4%) patients who all belonged to the Telbivudine group. A patient in the Telbivudine group experienced myopathy accompanied with elevated CK (920 IU/L) at week 48. The symptom improved and the serum CK level was normalized after the telbivudine was discontinued.

Table 2 Serological, virological, and biochemical responses at week 48

Variables	Telbivudine ($n = 47$)	Entecavir ($n = 50$)	P-value
Serologic Responses			
Change in HBsAg level from baseline[a,b], $\log_{10}$ IU/mL	−0.03 ± 0.14	−0.05 ± 0.11	0.57
HBsAg level[a, c], $\log_{10}$ IU/mL	3.37 (3.22 - 3.63)	3.39 (3.10 - 3.67)	0.65
HBsAg seroclearance, n (%)	0 (0%)	0 (0%)	NA
HBsAg level decline from baseline >0.5 $\log_{10}$ IU/mL, n (%)	0 (0%)	0 (0%)	NA
HBsAg level decline from baseline >0.1 $\log_{10}$ IU/mL, n (%)	11 (23.4%)	15 (30.0%)	0.46
HBeAg seroclearance[d], n (%)	2/40 (5.0%)	5/33 (15.2%)	0.14
HBeAg seroconversion[d], n (%)	0/40 (0%)	2/33 (6.1%)	0.11
Virologic Responses			
Virologic breakthrough, n (%)	11 (23.4%)	0 (0%)	<0.001
Genotypic resistance, n (%)	7 (14.9%)	0 (0%)	0.005
Virologic response at week 48, n (%)	30 (63.8%)	49 (98.0%)	<0.001

Missing values were considered as failure for categorical endpoints
[a]Among participants whose serum HBsAg and HBV DNA level at week 48 was available ($n = 37$ in the Telbivudine group, $n = 49$ in the Entecavir group)
[b]Mean ± standard deviation (SD)
[c]Median (interquartile range)
[d]Among HBeAg-positive patients at randomization ($n = 73$)
HBsAg hepatitis B surface antigen, HBeAg hepatitis B envelope antigen, NA not applicable

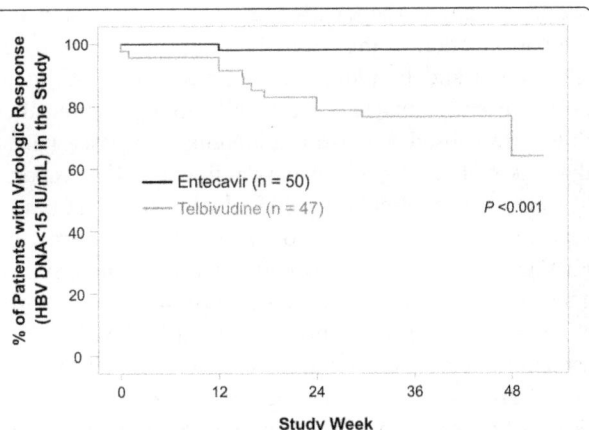

Fig. 3 The proportion of patients maintaining virologic response (HBV DNA <60 IU/mL) in the study. Patients who discontinued the study prior to week 48 for any reason were considered failures in virologic response at the time of discontinuation

Discussion

In this randomized trial, we found that in the patients with HBeAg-positive CHB, who achieved undetectable serum HBV DNA with the preceding entecavir treatment, switching the treatment to telbivudine for 48 weeks was not associated with a greater reduction in serum HBsAg levels. By contrast, telbivudine treatment was associated with a 23.4% virologic breakthrough and 14.9% genotypic resistance. None of the patients in the Entecavir group experienced virologic breakthrough or drug-resistance. Overall, the rate of maintaining virologic response was significantly lower in the Telbivudine group than that in the Entecavir group at week 48.

To date, few head-to-head randomized trials have investigated whether various NUCs induce a decline in HBsAg levels to different degrees. In HBeAg-positive patients, the rate of HBeAg seroconversion is only approximately 20–35% even after long-term treatment with a potent NUC such as entecavir or TDF [10, 21]. Furthermore, even after HBeAg-loss or -seroconversion induced by a potent NUC, the suppression of serum HBV DNA to undetectable levels is sustained only in approximately 23–37% at 24 weeks after treatment is discontinued. Therefore, HBsAg seroclearance is currently regarded as an optimal endpoint of treatment with NUC [22, 23]. In fact, our previous study demonstrated that HBsAg seroclearance achieved after NUC treatment persists in most cases and is associated with favorable clinical outcomes during long-term off-treatment follow-up [5]. However, HBsAg seroclearance is very rarely achievable, and almost life-long treatment is required in most patients. Based on HBsAg kinetics, it has been estimated that the predicted median time to HBsAg loss in patients treated with lamivudine or entecavir is more than 30–52 years [15, 24, 25]. A recent randomized trial showed that even the combination of the potent NUCs, entecavir and TDF, was not associated with greater decline in HBsAg levels compared with entecavir monotherapy through 96 weeks of treatment.

It has been suggested that the decline in HBsAg levels during lamivudine or entecavir therapy is slower and less pronounced than it is during interferon treatment, despite its higher suppression of HBV DNA [12, 15, 24]. Interestingly, experimental reports have suggested that telbivudine shares some common clinical mechanisms of action with interferon including dynamic changes in Th1/Th2 type cytokines [26]. In a trial for patients with

Table 3 Safety profiles of the study patients

Adverse event category	Telbivudine (n = 47)	Entecavir (n = 50)	P-value
Any adverse event	29 (61.7%)	29 (58.0%)	0.71
Serious adverse events[a]	2 (4.3%)	1 (2.0%)	0.52
Discontinuation due to adverse event[b]	3 (6.4%)	0	0.11
Dose reduction due to adverse event	0	0	-
Deaths	0	0	-
Serum CK >3 x ULN	3 (6.4%)	0	0.11
Myopathy	1 (2.1%)	0	0.30
HCC[c], n (%)	1 (2.1%)	0	0.30
Serum creatinine ≥0.5 mg/dL above baseline	0	0	-
eGFR <50 mL · min^{-1} · 1.73 m$^{(2)-1}$	0	0	-

[a]Telbivudine group: cholangitis with intra-hepatic duct stone, hepatocellular carcinoma; Entecavir group: scrub typhus. None was determined to be related to study drug administration
[b]By headache, gastrointestinal issues, and myopathy (n = 1 each). The symptoms improved after discontinuation of the treatment
[c]HCC was diagnosed at week 36
CK creatine kinase, ULN upper limit of normal, HCC hepatocellular carcinoma, eGFR estimated glomerular filtration rate

HBeAg-positive CHB who received telbivudine treatment for up to 3 years and maintained undetectable serum HBV DNA level, up to 71 and 57% of the patients achieved HBeAg-loss and HBeAg seroconversion, respectively [16]. Another trial consisting of treatment-naïve patients with HBeAg-positive CHB revealed that the rate of patients with rapid HBsAg decline (≥ 0.5 $\log_{10}$ IU/mL) in the telbivudine monotherapy group (41%) was comparable to that in the PEG-IFN monotherapy group (31%) [14]. An observational study in Hong Kong including various NUC-treated patients with an initial immune active phase showed a significant reduction of HBsAg only in the telbivudine treatment group [17]. Although it is well known that telbivudine is associated with a higher rate of drug-resistance, previous studies identified the association of early profound viral suppression with a very low rate of drug resistance during long-term treatment. In patients who achieved HBV DNA levels undetectable in the quantitative PCR assay at week 24, the resistance risk at week 104 was only 4% [19]. However, the results of our current study contrast strikingly with our hypothesis. Switching the treatment of patients with virologic response induced by preceding entecavir treatment to telbivudine was associated with an unacceptably high rate of virologic breakthrough and drug-resistance without any beneficial effect on the HBsAg decline. This rate of virologic breakthrough (23.4%) during the 48-week telbivudine therapy in this study was comparable to that in a previous trial, which showed a 28.8% virologic breakthrough during a 2-year telbivudine treatment regimen in patients who were HBeAg-positive [19]. This observed rate is also similar to the rate of virologic rebound (24%) observed during lamivudine treatment in patients who had achieved undetectable serum HBV DNA following the preceding entecavir treatment [27].

The majority of our study patients did not exhibit HBeAg-seroclearance after the preceding >1-year entecavir therapy, which might have hindered the observation of a decline in the HBsAg levels. The HBsAg levels have been shown to decline rapidly during the first year of treatment [28]. Moreover, in HBeAg-positive patients, the decline in serum HBsAg is mainly confined to those who experience a clearance of HBeAg by either PEG-IFN or entecavir treatment [12]. However, because a high serum HBV DNA level is a strong predictor of the development of telbivudine-resistance, comparing telbivudine and entecavir in treatment-naïve patients could not be ethically justified.

This study has several limitations that are worth mentioning. First, the small sample size and short duration may have decreased the statistical power of the study to observe the differences in the decline of HBsAg levels between the Telbivudine and Entecavir groups. Nevertheless, the significantly higher rate of virologic breakthrough in the Telbivudine group did not justify the continuation of the study. Second, this was an open-label study and blinding was not performed. Although objective endpoints (serologic and virologic determinations) were used and drug adherence was ascertained, the lack of blinding might have influenced the response of the study patients or biased the investigators in reporting the adherence and adverse events. Lastly, the HBV genotype of our study patients was not determined. This was because one of the inclusion criteria of this study was an undetectable serum HBV DNA level at screening. However, since almost all Korean patients with CHB have the C HBV genotype [29], the application of the results of this study may be limited, and not extrapolatable to patients with other HBV genotypes.

Conclusions

In conclusion, in patients who have achieved undetectable serum HBV DNA by entecavir treatment, switching the treatment to telbivudine for 48 weeks resulted in an unacceptably high rate of virologic breakthrough and drug-resistance without any beneficial effect on HBsAg decline. Prior viral suppression by entecavir did not confer any significant advantage to patients who switched to telbivudine. These results do not support the use of low genetic barrier drugs as a switch treatment strategy in patients who achieve virologic response by high genetic barrier drugs.

Abbreviations

CHB: Chronic hepatitis B; CK: Creatine kinase; HBeAg: Hepatitis B envelope antigen; HBsAg: Hepatitis B surface antigen; HBV: Hepatitis B virus; HCC: Hepatocellular carcinoma; LLOD: Lower limit of detection; NUC: Nucleos(t)ide analog; PCR: Polymerase chain reaction; PEG-IFN: Pegylated interferon; pol/RT: Polymerase/reverse transcriptase domain; TDF: Tenofovir disoproxil fumarate; ULN: Upper limit of normal

Acknowledgement

We are indebted to Dr. So-Young Park and Ms. HaYeong Koo for critically reviewing the manuscript without receiving any compensation for their work. The electronic CRF development and data management for this study were performed by using the Internet-based Clinical Research and Trial (iCReaT) management system (http://icreat.nih.go.kr), which is a data management system established by the Centers for Disease Control and Prevention, Ministry of Health and Welfare, Republic of Korea (iCReaT Study No. C120003).

Funding

This study was supported by funding from Novartis; the Korean National Health Clinical Research (NHCR) Project, Ministry of Health and Welfare (HC15C3380); the Korean Health Technology R&D Project, Ministry of Health

& Welfare (HI14C1061), Republic of Korea; and the Proteogenomic Research Program through the National Research Foundation of Korea funded by the Korea government (MSIP). Novartis was permitted to review the manuscript and suggest changes but had no role in the study design, data collection, analysis, decision to publish, or preparation of the manuscript. The final decision on content was exclusively retained by the authors. None of other funding bodies played any role in the design of the study and collection, analysis, and interpretation of data and in writing the manuscript.

Authors' contributions

Concepts and design of the study, acquisition, analysis and interpretation of the data, and drafting of the manuscript: JA, YSL; statistical analyses: SH; data acquisition: WJ; data acquisition and critically revised for manuscript for important intellectual content: GK, DL, JHS, HCL, and YSL. All authors have read and approved the final version of this manuscript.

Competing interests

YS Lim is an advisory board member of Bayer Healthcare, Bristol-Myers Squibb, and Gilead Sciences, and receives research funding from Bayer Healthcare, Bristol-Myers Squibb, Gilead Sciences, and Novartis. The other authors have nothing to disclose that would be relevant for the publication of this manuscript. The results of this study were presented in part at the Liver Meeting of the European Association for the Study of Liver, Barcelona, Spain, on April 15, 2016.

Consent for publication

Not applicable.

Author details

[1]Department of Gastroenterology, Liver Center, Asan Medical Center, University of Ulsan College of Medicine, 88, Olympic-ro 43-gil, Songpa-gu, Seoul 05505, Korea. [2]Health Screening and Promotion Center, Asan Medical Center, Seoul, Republic of Korea. [3]Department of Applied Statistics, Gachon University, Seongnam-si, Gyeonggi-do, Republic of Korea.

References

1. Perz JF, Armstrong GL, Farrington LA, Hutin YJ, Bell BP. The contributions of hepatitis B virus and hepatitis C virus infections to cirrhosis and primary liver cancer worldwide. J Hepatol. 2006;45:529–38.
2. Schiff ER. Prevention of mortality from hepatitis B and hepatitis C. Lancet. 2006;368:896–7.
3. Chang TT, Lai CL, Yoon SK, Lee SS, Coelho HS, Carrilho FJ, et al. Entecavir treatment for up to 5 years in patients with hepatitis B e antigen-positive chronic hepatitis B. Hepatology. 2010;51:422–30.
4. Kitrinos KM, Corsa A, Liu Y, Flaherty J, Snow-Lampart A, Marcellin P, et al. No detectable resistance to tenofovir disoproxil fumarate after 6 years of therapy in patients with chronic hepatitis B. Hepatology. 2014;59:434–42.
5. Kim GA, Lim YS, An J, Lee D, Shim JH, Kim KM, et al. HBsAg seroclearance after nucleoside analogue therapy in patients with chronic hepatitis B: clinical outcomes and durability. Gut. 2014;63:1325–32.
6. Chu CM, Liaw YF. HBsAg seroclearance in asymptomatic carriers of high endemic areas: appreciably high rates during a long-term follow-up. Hepatology. 2007;45:1187–92.
7. Moucari R, Korevaar A, Lada O, Martinot-Peignoux M, Boyer N, Mackiewicz V, et al. High rates of HBsAg seroconversion in HBeAg-positive chronic hepatitis B patients responding to interferon: a long-term follow-up study. J Hepatol. 2009;50:1084–92.
8. Buster EH, Flink HJ, Cakaloglu Y, Simon K, Trojan J, Tabak F, et al. Sustained HBeAg and HBsAg loss after long-term follow-up of HBeAg-positive patients treated with peginterferon alpha-2b. Gastroenterology. 2008;135:459–67.
9. Yuen MF, Wong DK, Fung J, Ip P, But D, Hung I, et al. HBsAg seroclearance in chronic hepatitis B in Asian patients: replicative level and risk of hepatocellular carcinoma. Gastroenterology. 2008;135:1192–9.
10. Gish RG, Lok AS, Chang TT, de Man RA, Gadano A, Sollano J, et al. Entecavir therapy for up to 96 weeks in patients with HBeAg-positive chronic hepatitis B. Gastroenterology. 2007;133:1437–44.
11. Seto WK, Hui AJ, Wong VW, Wong GL, Liu KS, Lai CL, et al. Treatment cessation of entecavir in Asian patients with hepatitis B e antigen negative chronic hepatitis B: a multicentre prospective study. Gut. 2015;64:667–72.
12. Reijnders JG, Rijckborst V, Sonneveld MJ, Scherbeijn SM, Boucher CA, Hansen BE, et al. Kinetics of hepatitis B surface antigen differ between treatment with peginterferon and entecavir. J Hepatol. 2011;54:449–54.
13. Marcellin P, Ahn SH, Ma X, Caruntu FA, Tak WY, Elkashab M, et al. Combination of tenofovir disoproxil fumarate and peginterferon alpha-2a increases loss of hepatitis B surface antigen in patients with chronic hepatitis B. Gastroenterology. 2016;150:134–44. e10.
14. Marcellin P, Wursthorn K, Wedemeyer H, Chuang WL, Lau G, Avila C, et al. Telbivudine plus pegylated interferon alfa-2a in a randomized study in chronic hepatitis B is associated with an unexpected high rate of peripheral neuropathy. J Hepatol. 2015;62:41–7.
15. Liaw YF. Clinical utility of hepatitis B surface antigen quantitation in patients with chronic hepatitis B: a review. Hepatology. 2011;53:2121–9.
16. Wursthorn K, Jung M, Riva A, Goodman ZD, Lopez P, Bao W, et al. Kinetics of hepatitis B surface antigen decline during 3 years of telbivudine treatment in hepatitis B e antigen-positive patients. Hepatology. 2010;52:1611–20.
17. Wong DK, Seto WK, Fung J, Ip P, Huang FY, Lai CL, et al. Reduction of hepatitis B surface antigen and covalently closed circular DNA by nucleos(t)ide analogues of different potency. Clin Gastroenterol Hepatol. 2013;11:1004–10. e1.
18. Zeuzem S, Gane E, Liaw YF, Lim SG, DiBisceglie A, Buti M, et al. Baseline characteristics and early on-treatment response predict the outcomes of 2 years of telbivudine treatment of chronic hepatitis B. J Hepatol. 2009;51:11–20.
19. Liaw YF, Gane E, Leung N, Zeuzem S, Wang Y, Lai CL, et al. 2-year GLOBE trial results: telbivudine is superior to lamivudine in patients with chronic hepatitis B. Gastroenterology. 2009;136:486–95.
20. Kim H, Jee YM, Song BC, Shin JW, Yang SH, Mun HS, et al. Molecular epidemiology of hepatitis B virus (HBV) genotypes and serotypes in patients with chronic HBV infection in Korea. Intervirology. 2007;50:52–7.
21. Heathcote EJ, Marcellin P, Buti M, Gane E, De Man RA, Krastev Z, et al. Three-year efficacy and safety of tenofovir disoproxil fumarate treatment for chronic hepatitis B. Gastroenterology. 2011;140:132–43.
22. Lok AS, McMahon BJ. Chronic hepatitis B: update 2009. Hepatology. 2009;50:661–2.
23. European Association for the Study of the Liver. EASL clinical practice guidelines: management of chronic hepatitis B virus infection. J Hepatol. 2012;57:167–85.
24. Chan HL, Thompson A, Martinot-Peignoux M, Piratvisuth T, Cornberg M, Brunetto MR, et al. Hepatitis B surface antigen quantification: why and how to use it in 2011 - a core group report. J Hepatol. 2011;55:1121–31.
25. Chevaliez S, Hezode C, Bahrami S, Grare M, Pawlotsky JM. Long-term hepatitis B surface antigen (HBsAg) kinetics during nucleoside/nucleotide analogue therapy: finite treatment duration unlikely. J Hepatol. 2013;58:676–83.
26. Chen Y, Li X, Ye B, Yang X, Wu W, Chen B, et al. Effect of telbivudine therapy on the cellular immune response in chronic hepatitis B. Antiviral Res. 2011;91:23–31.
27. Fung J, Lai CL, Yuen J, Cheng C, Wu R, Wong DK, et al. Randomized trial of lamivudine versus entecavir in entecavir-treated patients with undetectable hepatitis B virus DNA: outcome at 2 Years. Hepatology. 2011;53:1148–53.
28. Zoulim F, Carosi G, Greenbloom S, Mazur W, Nguyen T, Jeffers L, et al. Quantification of HBsAg in nucleos(t)ide-naive patients treated for chronic hepatitis B with entecavir with or without tenofovir in the BE-LOW study. J Hepatol. 2015;62:56–63.
29. Bae SH, Yoon SK, Jang JW, Kim CW, Nam SW, Choi JY, et al. Hepatitis B virus genotype C prevails among chronic carriers of the virus in Korea. J Korean Med Sci. 2005;20:816–20.

17

Influence of cirrhosis on long-term prognosis after surgery in patients with combined hepatocellular-cholangiocarcinoma

Yan-Ming Zhou[1,2†], Cheng-Jun Sui[2†], Xiao-Feng Zhang[2], Bin Li[1] and Jia-Mei Yang[2*]

Abstract

Background: Little is known about the prognostic impact of cirrhosis on long-term survival of patients with combined hepatocellular-cholangiocarcinoma (cHCC-CC) after hepatic resection. The aim of this study was to elucidate the long-term outcome of hepatectomy in cHCC-CC patients with cirrhosis.

Methods: A total of 144 patients who underwent curative hepatectomy for cHCC-CC were divided into two groups: cirrhotic group ($n = 91$) and noncirrhotic group ($n = 53$). Long-term postoperative outcomes were compared between the two groups.

Results: Patients with cirrhosis had worse preoperative liver function, higher frequency of HBV infection, and smaller tumor size in comparison to those without cirrhosis. The 5-year overall survival rate in cirrhotic group was significantly lower than that in non-cirrhotic group (34.5% versus 54.1%, $P = 0.032$). The cancer recurrence-related death rate was similar between the two groups (46.2% versus 39.6%, $P = 0.446$), while the hepatic insufficiency-related death rate was higher in cirrhotic group (12.1% versus 1.9%, $P = 0.033$). Multivariate analysis indicated that cirrhosis was an independent prognostic factor of poor overall survival (hazard ratio 2.072, 95% confidence interval 1.041–4.123; $P = 0.038$).

Conclusions: The presence of cirrhosis is significantly associated with poor prognosis in cHCC-CC patietns after surgical resection, possibly due to decreased liver function.

Keywords: Combined hepatocellular-cholangiocarcinoma, Long-term survival, Cirrhosis, Surgical resection

Background

Combined hepatocellular-cholangiocarcinoma (cHCC-CC) is a very rare entity that includes elements of both hepatocellular carcinoma (HCC) and cholangiocarcinoma (CC) and represents 0.4–14.2% of primary liver malignancies [1]. Hepatic resection affords the best chance of long-term survival with a reported 5-year overall survival (OS) rate of 23.1–54.1%. Vascular invasion, lymph node metastasis, satellite nodules, and tumor size were reported as prognostic factors [2–5].

Patients with cHCC-CC, especially in Asian countries, are frequently accompanied by liver cirrhosis, with a prevalence of 27.7–84.6% [6]. However, little is known about the prognostic significance of cirrhosis in cHCC-CC patients after surgery. In this study, we compared the long-term outcomes of hepatic resection in cHCC-CC patients with and without cirrhosis.

Methods
Patients
From February 2000 to December 2011, 151 patients with cHCC-CC who underwent curative resection at our institutes. Curative resection was defined as complete excision of the tumor with clear microscopic margin conformed by histopathological examination. Allen and Lisa [7]

* Correspondence: yjm1952@sina.cn
†Equal contributors
[2]Department of Special Treatment, Eastern Hepatobiliary Surgery Hospital, Second Military Medical University, Shanghai, China
Full list of author information is available at the end of the article

categorized cHCC-CC into three types; type A: HCC and CC exist separately (double cancer); type B: HCC and CC exist contiguously but independentlyonly; and type C: HCC and CC components show contiguity with intermingling. Histologically, only type C tumors that displayed the characteristics of a genuine mixture of both HCC and CC elements were regarded as true combined tumors [5]. Seven patients with Allen type A and B tumors were therefore excluded from the study. Finally, 144 patients were subjected to this study. Of them, 91 (63.2%) patients had cirrhosis as confirmed by histology and the remaining 53 (36.8%) patients did not have cirrhosis. Patient demographics, operative data, tumor characteristics, and follow-up findings were reviewed retrospectively. Postoperative morbidity and mortality were analyzed 90 days after operation. Liver dysfunction was defined as total bilirubin level >10 mg/dL unrelated to biliary obstruction or leak and/or the international normalized ratio >2 for more than 2 days after resection and/or clinically significant ascites/hepatic encephalopathy [8].

All patients were followed postoperatively by serum tumor marker (alpha-fetoprotein [AFP] and carbohydrate antigen 19–9 [CA 19–9]) analysis and ultrasound or computed tomography at least every 3 months in the first year after hepatectomy, and then at gradually increasing intervals. Intrahepatic recurrence was identified by new lesions on imaging with typical appearances of cHCC-CC with or without a rising serum AFP or CA 19–9 level. Determination of treatment strategy for recurrent tumors depended on the number and site of the tumors, any concurrent extrahepatic recurrence, liver function, and the general status of the patient. Re-hepatectomy and percutaneous radiofrequency ablation (PRFA) were considered as first-choice treatments. Re-hepatectomy was performed for Child A patients with solitary or multiple tumors limited in the semi-liver with sufficient liver remnant volume. PRFA was given to Child A and selected Child B patients with solitary tumor ≤3 cm located deeply in the liver parenchyma or multiple tumors (up to 3 lesions all ≤ 3 cm) in different lobes without vascular invasion or gross ascites. Transarterial chemoembolization (TACE) was considered when the above two treatments were not possible, as in patients with advanced multinodular recurrent tumors, poor liver function, and insufficient liver remnant volume. Systemic chemotherapy or conservative treatment was considered for patients with extensive systemic recurrence and/or very poor liver function or general condition.

Statistical analysis

Categorical and continuous data were compared by the χ^2 test and the Student t test, respectively. Patient OS and disease-free survival (DFS) rates were estimated using the Kaplan-Meier method, and differences between groups were compared by log-rank test. Multivariate analysis was performed by the Cox proportional hazard regression model. All statistical analyses were performed using SPSS for Windows (version 11.0; SPSS Institute, Chicago, IL, USA). $P < 0.05$ was considered statistically significant.

Results

Patient characteristics and outcomes

The clinicopathologic data of noncirrhotic and cirrhotic patients are summarized in Table 1. Cirrhotic patients had higher prevalence of men, alcohol abuse, and positive hepatitis B surface antigen (HBsAg), higher serum alanine aminotransferase (ALT) and aspartate aminotransferase (AST) levels, higher prevalence of abnormal serum AFP level, and smaller tumors than non-cirrhotic patients.

Regarding operative procedures and preoperative outcomes, less major resection (≥3 segments) was applied in cirrhotic patients. Postoperative morbidity was similar in the two groups except for the higher incidence of liver dysfunction in cirrhotic group. One patient in cirrhotic group died of hepatorenal failure resulting in a mortality rate of 1.1%, showing no statistically significant difference with 0% in non-cirrhotic group (Table 2).

The median postoperative follow-up period was 35 (range 3–127) months. The 5-year DFS rate was similar between cirrhotic and non-cirrhotic patients (29.6% versus 38.7%, $P = 0.079$). However, the 5-year OS rate and the median OS time in cirrhotic group was significantly lower than that in non-cirrhotic group, with values of 34.5% and 31 months, versus 54.1% and 63 months, respectively ($P = 0.032$) (Fig. 1).

By the time of analysis, recurrences developed in 68 cirrhotic and 35 non-cirrhotic patients with a similar frequency (75.5% versus 66.1%, $P = 0.567$). Also, there was no difference in the median time to recurrence and the pattern of recurrence between the two groups. Regarding the initial treatment for recurrences, aggressive approaches including re-hepatectomy and local ablation were applied less frequently in cirrhotic patients as compared with non-cirrhotic patients (36.8% versus 60.0%, $P = 0.025$) (Table 3).

Investigation on the cause of death showed that 56 cirrhotic patients and 23 non-cirrhotic patients died during the follow-up period in this study ($P = 0.029$). Cancer recurrence-related death was similar between cirrhotic and non-cirrhotic group (46.2% versus 39.6%, $P = 0.446$), while hepatic insufficiency-related death was more frequently observed in cirrhotic group (12.1% versus 1.9%, $P = 0.033$).

Prognostic factors for overall survival

Univariate analysis showed that factors affecting OS were maximum tumor size > 5 cm, intraoperative transfusion,

Table 1 Comparison of clinicopathologic features

Variables	Cirrhosis n = 91	Non- cirrhosis n = 53	P-value
Sex (male/female), n	89/2	46/7	0.274
Age (years; mean ± SD)	53.2 ± 9.2	52.1 ± 8.1	0.463
Overweight (BMI 25.0-29.99 kg/m²), n (%)	15 (16.5)	10 (18.9)	0.716
Obesity (BMI ≥ 30 kg/m2), n (%)	3 (3.3)	2 (3.8)	0.880
Hypertension, n (%)	12 (13.2)	6 (11.3)	0.744
Diabetes mellitus, n (%)	10 (11.0)	4 (7.5)	0.501
Hepatitis B surface antigen, n (%)	79 (63.8)	22 (37.2)	<0.001
Alcohol use, n (%)	24 (26.4)	5 (9.4)	0.015
Total bilirubin (μmol/L; mean ± SD)	17.8 ± 8.8	15.4 ± 4.1	0.090
Albumin (g/L; mean ± SD)	40.5 ± 5.3	41.2 ± 4.6	0.417
Aspartate aminotransferase (IU/L; mean ± SD)	51.2 ± 35.3	39.6 ± 22.3	0.021
Alanine aminotransferase (IU/L; mean ± SD)	54.5 ± 50.6	41.8 ± 36.7	0.043
Child-Pugh (A/B), n	85/6	53/0	0.056
Tumor diameter (cm; mean ± SD)	4.9 ± 2.5	6.7 ± 2.8	<0.001
Tumor number (St/Mt), n	82/9	46/7	0.541
Encapsulation, n (%)	34 (37.4)	15 (28.3)	0.268
Vascular invasion, n (%)	41 (45.1)	27 (50.9)	0.495
Bile duct invasion, n (%)	17 (18.7)	11(20.8)	0.762
Lymph node involvement, n (%)	12 (13.2)	8 (15.1)	0.750
Alpha-fetoprotein ≥ 20 ng/mL, n (%)	56 (61.5)	22 (41.5)	0.020
Carbohydrate antigen 19–9 ≥ 37 U/mL, n (%)	31 (34.1)	21 (39.6)	0.503
Carcinoembryogenic antigen ≥ 5 ng/mL, n (%)	7 (7.7)	3 (5.7)	0.644

BMI body mass index; St single tumor; Mt multiple tumors

cirrhosis, bile duct invasion, lymph node involvement, and vascular invasion. Multivariate analysis showed that cirrhosis was an independent prognostic factor for poor OS (hazard ratio 2.072, 95% confidence interval 1.041–4.123; P = 0.038) (Table 4).

Discussion

The reported prevalence of cirrhosis in cHCC-CC patients ranges widely from 27.7% to 84.6% worldwide based on operative findings [6]. This figure is 63.2% in

Table 2 Comparison of operative procedures and preoperative outcomes

Variables	Cirrhosis n = 91 (%)	Non- cirrhosis n = 53 (%)	P-value
Extent of resection			0.006
Major resection	21 (23.1)	24 (45.3)	
Minor resection	70 (76.9)	29 (54.7)	
Liver disfuction	31 (34.1)	7 (13.2)	0.006
Complications other than liver disfuction	34 (37.4)	18 (34.0)	0.682
Mortality	1 (1.1)	0 (0)	0.444

our cohort. The sex ratio of cHCC-CC shows a prominent male predominance, which is compatible with the findings of several previous reports [2–5]. It has been reported that this male predominance correlated with high activities of androgen axis, an oncogenic pathway involved in hepatocarcinogenesis [9]. However, further analysis of the precise mechanisms for male susceptibility to cHCC-CC is needed.

cHCC-CC is reportedly similar to HCC in terms of clinicopathologic characteristics including mean age, male/female ratio, hepatitis viral positivity, serum AFP level, and the presence of cirrhosis [1]. Some researchers from Asian institutions therefore speculated that cHCC-CC represents a variant of ordinary HCC that exhibits cholangiocellular metaplasia, rather than a true intermediate disease entity between HCC and CC [3]. As is the case with HCC, we find that hepatitis B virus (HBV) is a main etiologic factor in the development of cHCC-CC in a cirrhotic liver. Accordingly, ALT and ALT values as indicators of activity or severity of the hepatitis state were both higher in cirrhotic patients than those in non-cirrhotic patients. A comparison of the pathologic findings in resected specimens showed the tumor size was generally smaller in

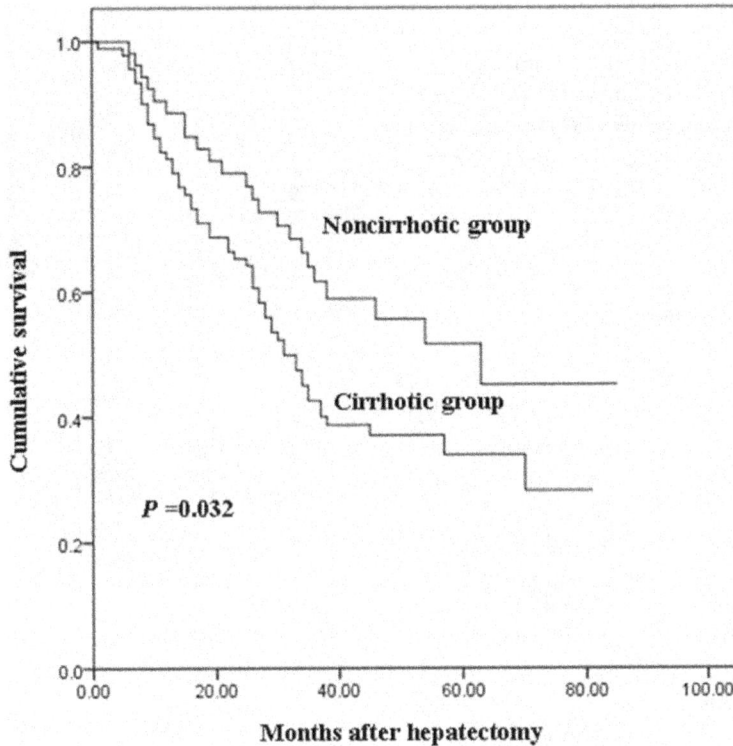

Fig. 1 Comparison of patient overall survival rates between the cirrhotic and non-cirrhotic groups

cirrhotic group. One possible explanation for this phenomenon is that cirrhotic patients generally have active liver disease and may have image-based liver screening, which enabled detection of small tumors. However, it should be acknowledged that there may be a selection bias for hepatic resection. Many cirrhotic patients were unable to undergo hepatectomy because of poor liver function reserve, and most patients with large tumors may be treated

by a nonsurgical modality such as hepatic artery embolization or conservative treatment.

As expected, cirrhotic patients had a significantly higher incidence of liver dysfunction after surgical resection. As cirrhotic patients have relatively small tumours and limited hepatic functional reserve, they usually undergo minor hepatectomy.

The negative impact of cirrhosis on long-term survival has been reported in postoperative HCC patients [10, 11], but its impact on long-term survival of cHCC-CC patients undergoing hepatectomy remains unclear. The present study is the first to present data to indicate that the cirrhosis is an independent predictor for postoperative OS of cHCC-CC patients. The 5-year OS rate was 34.5% in cirrhotic patients *versus* 54.1% in non-cirrhotic counterparts.

Table 3 Tumor recurrence data

Variables	Cirrhosis n = 68	Non- cirrhosis n = 35	P-value
Median time to recurrence, months	13	14	0.693
Recurrence type, n (%)			
Intrahepatic recurrence	42 (61.8)	24 (68.6)	0.495
Extrahepatic recurrence	19 (27.9)	8 (22.8)	0.578
Both	7 (10.3)	3 (8.6)	0.780
Treatment of recurrence, n (%)			
Aggressive approach	25 (36.8)	21 (60.0)	0.025
Rehepatectomy	3 (4.3)	5 (14.3)	0.076
Local ablation	22 (32.4)	16 (45.7)	0.183
Transarterial chemoembolization	26 (38.2)	9 (25.7)	0.204
Systemic chemotherapy	5 (7.4)	2 (5.7)	0.754
Conservative treatment	12 (17.6)	3 (8.6)	0.216

Table 4 Multivariate analysis of risk factors for poor overall survival

Variables	HR	95% CI	P-value
Maximum tumor size > 5 cm	2.115	0.901–4.960	0.085
Intraoperative transfusion	1.704	1.062–2.732	0.027
Cirrhosis	2.072	1.041–4.123	0.038
Bile duct invasion	1.662	0.614–4.511	0.317
Lymph node involvement	1.943	0.829–4.490	0.126
Vascular invasion	2.583	1.380–4.834	0.002

HR hazard ratio; *CI* confidence interval

This difference is likely attributable to more hepatic decompensation caused by ongoing cirrhosis itself in cirrhotic patients. As demonstrated in our study, hepatic insufficiency-related death accounted for 11 (12.1%) deaths in cirrhotic patients and only one (1.9%) death in non-cirrhotic patients. Difference in treatment strategies for recurrent disease may also account for differences in outcomes. Cirrhotic patients usually have impaired hepatic function after the initial hepatic resection, which limits the application of aggressive management for recurrence, which is often the leading cause for an unfavorable outcome.

Several studies have documented an association between cirrhosis and recurrence of HCC, which is likely attributable to multicentric *de novo* carcinogenesis in the remnant liver [10, 12]. However, our study failed to find such an association in cHCC-CC patients. One of the explanations for this discrepancy is that cHCC-CC with CC components exhibits a more aggressive behavior and has high probability of intrahepatic metastasis, which would overshadow the effect of cirrhotic liver related-carcinogenesis.

Theoretically, liver transplantation (LT) offers the potential benefit of resecting the entire tumor-bearing liver and eliminating cirrhosis simultaneously, and therefore it is generally believed to be an ideal approach for the treatment of cHCC-CC in cirrhotic patients. In the three cHCC-CC patients receiving LT reported by Chan et al. [13], one patient died from distant metastasis 16.5 months after operation while the other two patients survived 25 and 35 months after operation, respectively. Wu et al. [14] reported a 5-year OS rate of 39% in a case series of 21 patients with cHCC-CC treated with LT. Panjala et al. [15] reported a 5-year OS rate of 16% in their 12 cHCC-CC patients receiving LT. Employing the Surveillance, Epidemiology, and End Results database (1988–2009), Garancini et al. [16] reported a 5-year OS rate of 41.1% in 16 cHCC-CC patients receiving LT. Currently, it is difficult to assess the effectiveness of LT in the management of cHCC-CC because of insufficient data and limited evidence available.

Conclusion

This study showed that cHCC-CC patients with cirrhosis had a poorer long-term prognosis after surgical resection as compared with those without cirrhosis, possibly due to the decreased liver function.

Abbreviations
AFP: Alpha-fetoprotein; ALT: Alanine aminotransferase; AST: Aspartate aminotransferase; CC: Cholangiocarcinoma; cHCC-CC: Hepatocellular-cholangiocarcinoma; CI: Confidence interval; DFS: Disease-free surviva; HBsAg: Hepatitis B surface antigen; HBV: Hepatitis B virus; HCC: Hepatocellular carcinoma; HR: Hazard ratio; LT: Liver transplantation; OS: Overall survival; PRFA: Percutaneous radiofrequency ablation; TACE: Transarterial chemoembolization

Acknowledgements
We thank Dr. Yanfang Zhao (Department of Health Statistics, Second Military Medical University, Shanghai, China) for her critical revision of the statistical analysis section.

Funding
The design of the study and collection, analysis, and interpretation of data and in writing the manuscript for this research was mainly supported by Foundation of Health and Family Planning Commission of Fujian Province of China (Project no.2013-ZQN-JC-31) and Nature Science Foundation of Shanghai (12ZR1440000).

Authors' contributions
YZ and JY designed the study. YZ and CS supervised the study. XZ and BL collected data. YZ and JY analyzed the data and drafted the manuscript. All authors read and approved the final manuscript.

Competing interests
The authors declare that they have no conflicts of interest concerning this article.

Consent for publication
Not applicable.

Author details
[1]Department of Hepatobiliary & Pancreatovascular Surgery, First affiliated Hospital of Xiamen University, Xiamen, China. [2]Department of Special Treatment, Eastern Hepatobiliary Surgery Hospital, Second Military Medical University, Shanghai, China.

References
1. Kassahun WT, Hauss J. Management of combined hepatocellular and cholangiocarcinoma. Int J Clin Pract. 2008;62:1271–8.
2. Jarnagin WR, Weber S, Tickoo SK, Koea JB, Obiekwe S, Fong Y, et al. Combined hepatocellular and cholangiocarcinoma: demographic, clinical, and prognostic factors. Cancer. 2002;94:2040–6.
3. Yano Y, Yamamoto J, Kosuge T, Sakamoto Y, Yamasaki S, Shimada K, et al. Combined hepatocellular and cholangiocarcinoma: a clinicopathologic study of 26 resected cases. Jpn J Clin Oncol. 2003;33:283–7.
4. Lee SD, Park SJ, Han SS, Kim SH, Kim YK, Lee SA, et al. Clinicopathological features and prognosis of combined hepatocellular carcinoma and cholangiocarcinoma after surgery. Hepatobiliary Pancreat Dis Int. 2014;13:594–601.
5. Tang D, Nagano H, Nakamura M, Wada H, Marubashi S, Miyamoto A, et al. Clinical and pathological features of Allen's type C classification of resected combined hepatocellular and cholangiocarcinoma: a comparative study with hepatocellular carcinoma and cholangiocellular carcinoma. J Gastrointest Surg. 2006;10:987–98.
6. Zhou YM, Zhang XF, Wu LP, Sui CJ, Yang JM. Risk factors for combined hepatocellular-cholangiocarcinoma: a hospital-based case–control study. World J Gastroenterol. 2014;20:12615–20.
7. Allen RA, Lisa JR. Combined liver and bile duct carcinoma. Am J Pathol. 1949;25:647–55.
8. Vauthey JN, Pawlik TM, Abdalla EK, Arens JF, Nemr RA, Wei SH, et al. Is extended hepatectomy for hepatobiliary malignancy justified? Ann Surg. 2004;239:722–30.

9. Wang SH, Yeh SH, Lin WH, Yeh KH, Yuan Q, Xia NS, et al. Estrogen receptor α represses transcription of HBV genes via interaction with hepatocyte nuclear factor 4α. Gastroenterology. 2012;142:989–98.

10. Sasaki Y, Imaoka S, Masutani S, Ohashi I, Ishikawa O, Koyama H, Iwanaga T. Influence of coexisting cirrhosis on long-term prognosis after surgery in patients with hepatocellular carcinoma. Surgery. 1992;112:515–21.

11. Zhou Y, Lei X, Wu L, Wu X, Xu D, Li B. Outcomes of hepatectomy for noncirrhotic hepatocellular carcinoma: a systematic review. Surg Oncol. 2014;23:236–42.

12. Imamura H, Matsuyama Y, Tanaka E, Ohkubo T, Hasegawa K, Miyagawa S, et al. Risk factors contributing to early and late phase intrahepatic recurrence of hepatocellular carcinoma after hepatectomy. J Hepatol. 2003;38:200–7.

13. Chan AC, Lo CM, Ng IO, Fan ST. Liver transplantation for combined hepatocellular cholangiocarcinoma. Asian J Surg. 2007;30:143–6.

14. Wu D, Shen ZY, Zhang YM, Wang J, Zheng H, Deng YL, et al. Effect of liver transplantation in combined hepatocellular and cholangiocellular carcinoma: a case series. BMC Cancer. 2015;15:232.

15. Panjala C, Senecal DL, Bridges MD, Kim GP, Nakhleh RE, Nguyen JH, et al. The diagnostic conundrum and liver transplantation outcome for combined hepatocellular-cholangiocarcinoma. Am J Transplant. 2010;10:1263–7.

16. Garancini M, Goffredo P, Pagni F, Romano F, Roman S, Sosa JA, et al. Combined hepatocellular-cholangiocarcinoma: a population-level analysis of an uncommon primary liver tumor. Liver Transpl. 2014;20:952–9.

18

"Non alcoholic fatty liver disease and eNOS dysfunction in humans"

Marcello Persico[1]*[iD], Mario Masarone[1], Antonio Damato[2], Mariateresa Ambrosio[2], Alessandro Federico[3], Valerio Rosato[4], Tommaso Bucci[1], Albino Carrizzo[2] and Carmine Vecchione[5]

Abstract

Background: NAFLD is associated to Insulin Resistance (IR). IR is responsible for Endothelial Dysfunction (ED) through the impairment of eNOS function. Although eNOS derangement has been demonstrated in experimental models, no studies have directly shown that eNOS dysfunction is associated with NAFLD in humans. The aim of this study is to investigate eNOS function in NAFLD patients.

Methods: Fifty-four NAFLD patients were consecutively enrolled. All patients underwent clinical and laboratory evaluation and liver biopsy. Patients were divided into two groups by the presence of NAFL or NASH. We measured vascular reactivity induced by patients' platelets on isolated mice aorta rings. Immunoblot assays for platelet-derived phosphorylated-eNOS (p-eNOS) and immunohistochemistry for hepatic p-eNOS have been performed to evaluate eNOS function in platelets and liver specimens. Flow-mediated-dilation (FMD) was also performed. Data were compared with healthy controls.

Results: Twenty-one (38, 8%) patients had NAFL and 33 (61, 7%) NASH. No differences were found between groups and controls except for HOMA and insulin ($p < 0.0001$). Vascular reactivity demonstrated a reduced function induced from NAFLD platelets as compared with controls ($p < 0.001$), associated with an impaired p-eNOS in both platelets and liver ($p < 0.001$). NAFL showed a higher impairment of eNOS phosphorylation in comparison to NASH ($p < 0.01$). In contrast with what observed in vitro, the vascular response by FMD was worse in NASH as compared with NAFL.

Conclusions: Our data showed, for the first time in humans, that NAFLD patients show a marked eNOS dysfunction, which may contribute to a higher CV risk. eNOS dysfunction observed in platelets and liver tissue didn't match with FMD.

Keywords: Non-alcoholic fatty liver disease, Endothelial dysfunction, Metabolic syndrome, Insulin resistance

Background

Non-Alcoholic Fatty Liver Disease (NAFLD) is represented by two clinical features: Non-Alcoholic Fatty Liver (NAFL) (namely "steatosis"), and Non-Alcoholic-Steato-Hepatitis (NASH) (namely: "steatohepatitis"). NAFLD is a unique "challenge" for the hepatologists and has increased worldwide in the last few years, due to the changes in dietary habits and increased sedentary lifestyle. Consequently NAFLD can be considered one of the most frequent liver diseases in the world [1]. It is generally considered a "benign disease" with low rates of progression to fibrosis, cirrhosis and hepatocellular carcinoma (HCC) [2]. Nevertheless, because of the high number of affected patients, the prevalence of related cirrhosis gradually increased, and actually it represents the third cause of liver transplantation in the USA. Moreover, even if the incidence of HCC in NAFLD patients is lower than that in HCV/HBV cirrhotic patients, the absolute burden of NASH-related HCC is higher, due to the higher number of patients with NAFLD [3]. It is very likely that the importance of this disease will continue to increase in the future, when the new therapies and prevention programs for hepatitis C and B will further reduce the size of viral infections of the liver. For these reasons, to recognize the mechanisms underlying its onset and progression is very important. Even if a lot of insights on this topic have been postulated

* Correspondence: mpersico@unisa.it
[1]Internal Medicine and Hepatology Unit, PO G. Da Procida—AOU- San Giovanni e Ruggi D'Aragona, University of Salerno, Via Salvatore Calenda 162, CAP: 84126 Salerno, Italy
Full list of author information is available at the end of the article

in the last few years, many aspects of the pathophysiological mechanisms underlying this disease remain to be explored. The hypothesis, risen from recent papers on animal experimental models, that found a possible linkage among microvascular abnormalities in the fatty liver, the lipid accumulation into the hepatocytes, and the fibrosis [4–6], seems to be of interest. In particular, it has been postulated that in NAFLD may be present an endothelial dysfunction that could be one of the earliest factors associated to fat accumulation and liver damage [7–9]. This finding is not totally surprising if we consider that, since its discovery, NAFLD has been widely associated to cardio-metabolic syndrome and its components: hepatic and systemic insulin resistance (IR), dyslipidemia, visceral obesity, hypertension, impaired fasting glucose, [10] and increased stroke risk [11]. Although a large number of insights on the linkage between IR and liver damage are yet unknown, what we know is that IR per se is responsible for endothelial dysfunction, for example via the imbalance of the enzymatic system of Nitric Oxide production (NO) [12]. In fact, insulin was proven to induce endothelial Nitric Oxide Synthase (eNOS) activation, resulting in vasodilation and vascular protection [13]. When IR appears, it can also lead to endothelial dysfunction, through the impairment of NO production and the inhibition of insulin-induced vasorelaxation [14], and eNOS function impairment has been widely associated to it [15]. Moreover, it was demonstrated that endothelial dysfunction with impaired NO production is involved in the progression of advanced liver diseases such as cirrhosis [16, 17], and it is associated with increased vascular resistance (resulting in portal hypertension) and hepatic stellate activation in the liver (resulting in fibrosis) [18]. All together these evidence led to consider the possibility, subsequently confirmed, that this mechanism already acts in earlier stages of murine experimental models of NAFLD-related liver damage [7–9]. Nevertheless, to our knowledge, no experimental studies have confirmed these findings on human models of NAFLD.

Flow-mediated vasodilation (FMD) of the brachial artery by means of ultrasonography [19] is a well known test to assess systemic endothelial function in humans [20, 21] and its significant clinical value is based on the assumption that the vasodilatory capacity of a vessel during post-ischemic hyperemia depends on a preserved NO synthesis and release [19]. In noncirrhotic subjects, cardiovascular risk factors impair FMD due to the oxidative stress-induced systemic endothelial dysfunction [22, 23].

The aim the of the present study is to try to demonstrate that eNOS derangement together with FMD impairment are associated with NAFLD.

Methods

Fifty-four consecutive patients (38 males, 16 females), coming from January 2014 to April 2015 to our tertiary center of Hepatology for the evaluation of their liver disease by liver biopsy, were enrolled in the present prospective case-control study. Inclusion criteria were histological diagnosis of non alcoholic steatosis (NAFL) and/or steatohepatitis (NASH). Exclusion criteria were the presence of any other concomitant liver disease: viral infections (HCV, HBV, HIV), autoimmunity, drug hepatitis, unsafe alcohol consumption (more than 20gr/day) or neoplastic diseases. The control group consisted of healthy volunteers matched for age and sex with the study population was recruited by a local blood bank.

Patients were divided into two groups according to the liver biopsy results: 1) simple steatosis (NAFL), 2) steatohepatitis (NASH). The results obtained in the individual groups were compared between each other and with the control group. NASH patients were also stratified by fibrosis degree at liver biopsy.

Clinical evaluation: Of each patient (and control) clinical history with alcohol consumption and smoking habits registration, physical examination, arterial pressure, waist circumference, body mass index (BMI), blood glucose, total and fractioned cholesterol, triglycerides, AST, ALT, GGT, ALP, complete blood count, metabolic syndrome evaluation by NCEP-ATPIII criteria were recorded [24].

Liver disease assessment: An abdomen ultrasound examination with the evaluation of the liver echo pattern of liver steatosis was performed by a skilled ultrasonographist at the time of enrollment [25]. On the basis of the clinical status of the patient and the good clinical practice behaviour, liver tissue samples were collected by performing a hepatic percutaneous biopsy with Surecut 17G needles, via the intercostal route using an echo-guided method. Liver specimens were used for histological examination if they were at least 1.5-cm long and contained >5 portal spaces. Biopsies were evaluated by using both the Kleiner score [26] for necroinflammation grading and fibrosis staging and the Brunt score [27] for the presence and extent of steatosis by a skilled pathologist. Each patient, and control, was included in the study after signing a written informed consent.

Ethics statement: The present study was approved by our local ethical committees (Ethical Committee of Istituto Neurologico Mediterraneo IRCCS Neuromed for experimental animals and Ethical Committee Campania Sud for patients and control subjects). The study protocol is in accordance with the ethical guidelines of the 1975 Declaration of Helsinki. All animals received humane care according to the criteria outlined in the "Guide for the Care and Use of Laboratory Animals" prepared by the National Academy of Sciences and published by the National Institutes of Health (NIH publication 86-23 revised 1985).

Evaluation of vasorelaxation activity inhibition

Platelet isolation and isolated vessel study: The assessment of the eNOS function was performed by evaluating vasorelaxation activity induced on isolated mice vessels by platelet-rich plasma (PRP) obtained by peripheral blood samples of patients and controls, activated with insulin. The response to vasodilator supernatants obtained through the stimulation of platelets with insulin was examined after achieving a preconstricted tone with increasing doses of phenylephrine on isolate mice aorta rings. These were mounted between stainless steel triangles. The whole method has been already described by our group in a study on another patients' setting [28].

Immunoblotting

After the isolation, platelets were solubilized in lysis buffer. Then, the supernatants were used to perform immunoblot analysis with anti-phospho-eNOS S1177 (Cell Signaling, rabbit polyclonal antibody 1:800); anti-total-eNOS (Cell Signaling, mouse mAb 1:1000), anti-iNOS (BD Laboratories cod.610599 mAb 1:800), anti-pAkt (Thr 308, Santa Cruz sc-135650 mAb 1:800), anti-Akt (Santa Cruz sc-56878 mAb 1:800) and β-actin (Cell Signaling, mouse mAb 1:2000). The whole method has been previously described [28].

Immunohistochemistry for hepatic eNOS

Sections of liver tissue were immunostained with p-eNOS serin 1177 antibody (abcam ab75639). Briefly, 3-L thick slices of formalin-fixed, paraffin-embedded liver were mounted on slides. The slides were deparaffinized, followed by suppression of endogenous peroxidase activity by immersion in PBS containing 2% H_2O_2 for 30 min. Nonspecific binding was blocked with 10% horse serum in PBS at room temperature for 1 h. The sections were washed in PBS with 0.05% Tween-20 thrice for 2 min each time, followed by incubation overnight at 4 °C with mouse anti-p-eNOS antibody [1:50] in PBS containing 4% horse serum. The sections were washed in PBS twice for 2 min each time, followed by incubation for 1 h at room temperature with biotinylated goat anti-mouse IgG [1:200] in PBS containing 1.5% horse serum. Then, the slides were incubated with avidin-biotin peroxidase conjugate for 30 min at room temperature; the coloured reaction product was developed by incubation for 7 min with 0.05% diaminobenzidine in 0.01% H_2O_2 in PBS. Negative controls were carried out under the same conditions by using mouse IgG instead of p-eNOS antibody.

FMD of brachial artery by ultrasound

FMD measurements were performed by a single operator trained in this method, holding an intra-observer variability less than 5%. The technique was carried out following the published guidelines [29]. In particular, patients, after a fasting of at least 8 h, were examined after a 20 min rest in a quiet and darkened room. They were instructed of avoiding smoking, drinking coffee and/or alcohol, and eating high-fatty food within the previous 12 h. A standard cuff was positioned around the right arm, 2 in. below the antecubital fossa, with the patient in the supine position.

To acquire images of the right brachial artery, a 10-MHz linear probe connected to a Hi Vision Preirus ultrasound system (Hitachi Hi Vision Preirus, Hitachi Medical Corporation, Tokyo, Japan) was used. Baseline images were obtained for 2 min, then the right brachial artery was occluded by inflating the cuff to above 250 mmHg, and kept inflated for 5 min. Subsequently, the cuff was deflated and images of the right brachial artery were captured. FMD was calculated with the following formula: (maximum diameter-baseline diameter)/baseline diameter) × 100 [30].

Statistical analysis

Statistical analyses were performed by using the Statistical Program for Social Sciences (SPSS®) ver.16.0 for Macintosh® (SPSS Inc., Chicago, Illinois, USA). Student *t*-test and Mann-Whitney *U* test were performed to compare continuous variables, chi-square with Yates correction or Fisher-exact test to compare categorical variables. Univariate and multivariate analyses were performed to test independent variables affecting the endothelial dysfunction, by performing ANOVA, linear regressions and binary logistic regressions, where applicable. Statistical significance was defined when "$p < 0.05$" in a "two-tailed" test with a 95% Confidence Interval.

Sample size calculation: in order to find an adequate sample size, we performed an interim analysis on the first 18 patients (10 NASH and 8 NAFLD) and enrolled controls, that we used as "calibration set". The sample size was calculated on the basis of the results of vasorelaxation experiment. The number needed to elicit a statistical difference between NAFL and NASH patients, with a power of 0.9 and an alpha error of 0.01 in a two sided test with 95% CI, was of 20 subjects per arm. We decided to include all the 54 cases enrolled in the present study to further improve the reliability of our results.

Results

Of the 54 patients 21 (38, 8%) had NAFL and 33 (61, 7%) had NASH according to histological diagnosis. No statistically significant differences were found between the two groups for age, sex, BMI, ALT, prevalence of hypertension, diabetes, dyslipidemia, obesity and metabolic syndrome. The only statistical difference was found in HOMA score and insulin levels ($p < 0.001$ both), see Table 1. Six patients in NASH group at liver biopsy were found to have the histological features of cirrhosis. Due to the fact that liver cirrhosis may represent perse a cause of endothelial derangement [31], we performed the vasoreactivity and NOS evaluations with and without the samples derived from cirrhotic patients, and we did not find any significant difference in the results of the various experiments. The data here presented belong to the non-cirrhotic patients.

Histological evaluation

As reported in methods, the diagnosis of NAFL or NASH was performed by applying the Kleiner score to the collected liver samples [26]. In particular, a patient was defined to have NASH instead of simple NAFL if its "NAFLD Activity Score" was ≥ 5, see Table 2.

Vasorelaxation induced by platelet-supernatant is altered in steatosis/steatohepatitis

The supernatant from stimulated human platelets induced a rapid dose-dependent relaxation of mice aorta rings and was abolished by NOS inhibitor, L-NAME (data not shown), clearly demonstrating the involvement of NO signalling in supernatant vascular action. Interestingly, our data demonstrate that the vasorelaxant effect, induced from platelet supernatants, was markedly reduced in NASH/NAFL patients when compared to control subjects. Moreover, the vasorelaxation induced from platelet supernatants from NAFL patients was significantly reduced if compared to that obtained from NASH subjects (Fig. 1).

Platelet eNOS-phosphorylation is impaired in steatosis/steatohepatitis

Levels of eNOS phosphorylation (p-eNOS) decreased in platelets of NASH patients compared to platelets of control subjects. Interestingly, in platelets of NAFL subjects there is an important impairment of eNOS phosphorylation both versus control subjects and versus NASH patients. Conversely, eNOS expression did not change among all the groups. In addition, no changes in the levels of β-actin were observed between all the groups, whereas levels of Akt phosphorylation (pAkt) decreased as much as eNOS levels (Fig. 2). These results reproduce and confirm those found on vasorelaxation inhibitory mechanism (see Fig. 1).

To evaluate the involvement of iNOS in our results, we performed its expression in our platelet samples. Our data revealed an absence of iNOS expression in our experimental conditions.

In agreement, It has been demonstrated that iNOS expression is absent in platelets [32]. By contrast, iNOS expression was enhanced after LPS treatment in mice vessels (see Fig. 2), as previously demonstrated [9].

eNOS phosphorylation is reduced in liver from steatosis/steatohepatitis

Immunohistochemical data showed that liver samples collected from health control subjects, showed a marked staining for p-eNOS in S1177 compared to liver samples obtained from both NASH and NAFL subjects. Interestingly, the pattern of phosphorylated eNOS levels is equivalent to that found, using western blot analyses, in platelets from the same subjects (Fig. 3).

Table 1 Clinical characteristics of our study population and controls

Variable	Controls n: 15	Overall NAFLD n: 54	p	NAFL n: 21	NASH n: 33	p
Age	45,55 ± 10,24	49,89 ± 1,05	0.176	48,58 ± 10,874	50.27 ± 10.254	0.566
Sex M/F	10/5 [66,7%/32,3%]	38/16 [70,4%/27,8%]	0.784	14/7 [66,7%/33,3%]	24/9 [72,7%/27,3%]	0.634
BMI	22,91 ± 2,76	30,17 ± 3,86	<0.001	29,51 ± 3,31	30,6 ± 4,21	0.320
Hypertension	0	21 [38,9%]	0.005	7 [33,3%]	14 [42,4%]	0.521
Diabetes	0	11 [22,2%]	0.057	4 [19,0%]	7 [21,2%]	0.847
Dyslipidemia	0	35 [64,8%]	<0.001	16 [76,2%]	19 [57,6%]	0.163
Obesity	3 [20,00%]	29 [53,7%]	0.021	12 [57,1%]	17 [51,5%]	0.686
Insulin	–	17,65 ± 5,95	–	14,08 ± 2,06	21,18 ± 6,98	<0.001
HOMA	–	4,36 ± 1,72	–	3,10 ± 0,08	5,24 ± 1,58	<0.001
Metabolic Syndrome	0	19 [35,2%]	0.007	7 [33,3%]	12 [36,4%]	0.820
Cirrhosis	0	6 [11,1%]	0.177	0	6 [18,2%]	0.077
ALT	26,44 ± 9,56	67,56 ± 44,37	<0.001	66,00 ± 43,65	68,33 ± 46,64	0.085

Table 2 Histological scores [mean ± SD] according to Kleiner score in NAFLD patients

	Overall	NAFL	NASH	p	95% CI
Steatosis [0–3]	1.8 ± 0.9	1.4 ± 0.7	2,1 ± 1.1	0.0122	−1.241/−0.159
Lobular Inflammation [0–2]	1.9 ± 1.0	0.9 ± 0.7	2.2 ± 1.2	0.0001	−1.881/−0.719
Hepatocellular Ballooning [0–2]	1.16 ± 0.7	0.7 ± 0.2	1.9 ± 1.1	0.0001	−1.688/−0.712
Fibrosis [0–4]	1.9 ± 0.9	0.5 ± 1.0	2.9 ± 0.9	0.0001	−2.926/−1.874
NAS*mean ± SD (median/range)	4.7 ± 0.9 (4.5/2–11)	3.6 ± 1.2 (3.0/2–4)	6.9 ± 1.4 (6.5/5–11)	0.0001	−2.252/−1.348

*NAFLD activity score: in parenthesis median and range

Flow-mediated dilation (FMD) of the brachial artery by ultrasound

FMD resulted lower, although not significant ($p = 0.534$), in NAFL patients if compared to controls and differed between NAFL and NASH, showing a statistically significant FMD decrease ($10.72 ± 0.89$ vs $4.34 ± 1.5$ P <0.0001) in NASH patients (Fig. 4). This, apparently, seems to contradict data reproduced by platelet supernatant evoked vasorelaxation on mice aorta rings (see Fig. 1) and possible interpretation of discrepancy will be reported in discussion.

Discussion

The present study shows, for the first time in humans, that an impaired eNOS function may be present in NAFL and NASH. This could lead to a worse NO production and an impairment of platelet-mediated vasorelaxation induction. A novel "dynamic" method, already proven to be an affordable and reliable tool to investigate vascular and platelet eNOS function [33, 34], was therefore used. Data here reported show that platelet-mediated vasorelaxation effect is repressed in NAFL and NASH patients. Since this effect is suppressed by NOS

inhibitors (i.e. L-NAME), it is clear that NO signalling is involved in platelet-mediated vascular activity. This novel approach may represent a reliable tool, available to study the endothelial function in NAFLD patients. In particular, it has the benefit of being substantially constituted by a simple blood sample analysis that can be easily repeated, and might be easily used to assess the course of the disease and/or the results of eventual therapies.

The association between eNOS impairment and vascular reactivity seems to be related to the significantly reduced functional fraction of eNOS, the Serine-1177 phosphorylated-eNOS, either in platelets derived by peripheral blood samples and in liver tissue specimens of NAFL and NASH patients, if compared to healthy controls. This is in line with previous studies conducted on murine experimental models of NAFL, in which e-NOS dysfunction was also hypothesized [7, 8]. Thus, eNOS derangement, leading to NO reduction and, consequently, to endothelial dysfunction, might represent one of the main pathophysiological mechanisms involved in the liver damage by fat accumulation. In this regard, recent studies, both in humans and animal

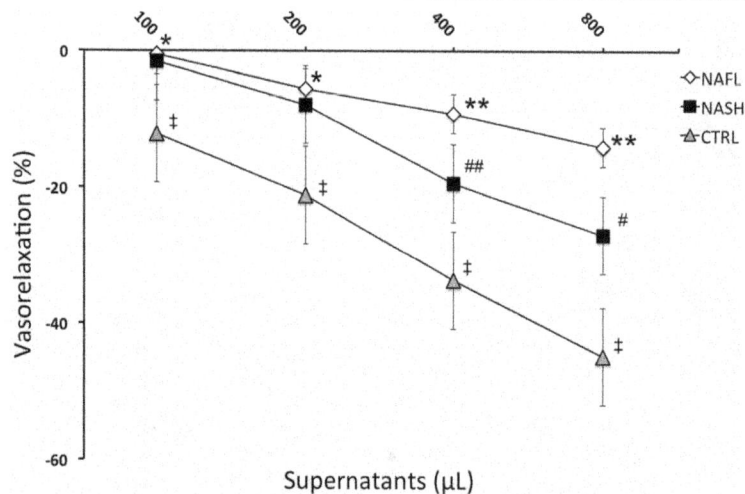

Fig. 1 Dose-response curves of phenylephrine-precontracted aorta rings to supernatants derived from stimulated platelets isolated from NASH, Steatosis patients ("NAFL") or Control subjects. Steatosis vs. controls:*, $p < 0.05$; **, $p < 0.001$; NASH vs. Steatosis: #, $p < 0.05$; ##, $p < 0,001$; NASH vs. controls: ‡, $p < 0.05$

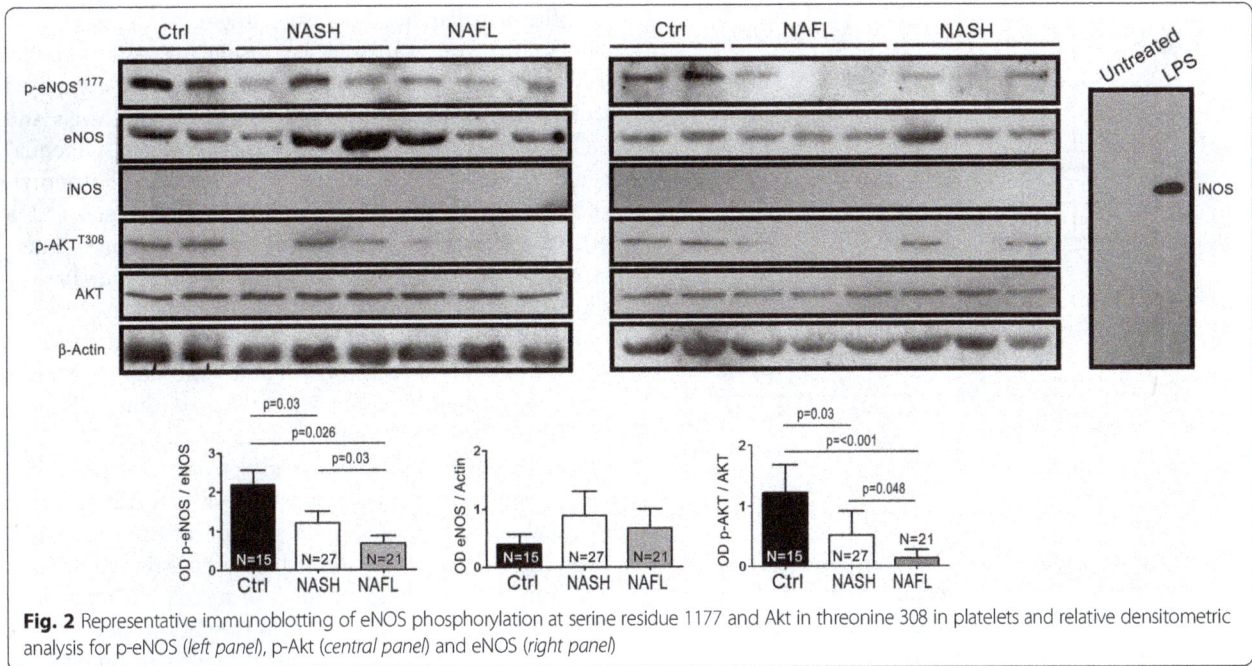

Fig. 2 Representative immunoblotting of eNOS phosphorylation at serine residue 1177 and Akt in threonine 308 in platelets and relative densitometric analysis for p-eNOS (*left panel*), p-Akt (*central panel*) and eNOS (*right panel*)

models of NASH, demonstrated derangements in microvascular functionality of the liver tissue [4, 5]. Moreover, a sinusoidal dysfunction associated with lipid accumulation in hepatocytes together with collagen deposition in the space of Disse was also highlighted [5]. Furthermore, in human liver specimens, iNOS expression, measured by immunohistochemistry, was correlated to the histological activity index and fibrosis in chronic viral hepatitis [35].

One of the main mechanisms promoting NO production through the activation of eNOS is the insulin signaling pathway [11, 12]. Insulin Resistance [IR], widely demonstrated in NAFLD, might be the main trigger of eNOS dysfunction that, therefore, might play a crucial role in the onset of NAFLD. Liver sinusoidal endothelial cells act in the same way of the other common endothelial cells. Their function is crucial to defend the tissue from inflammation and fibrosis [36, 37], therefore an impairment of their activity may promote, or worsen, the inflammatory state,

known as "low-grade inflammation", which underlies NAFLD onset and progression [38]. This seems to be supported by the fact that liver endothelial dysfunction is significantly associated to advanced liver diseases (of every etiology) and portal hypertension [39–41].

In this way, liver eNOS dysfunction might be one of the earliest "triggers" of liver damage and an important responsible for fibrosis progression.

It has been largely demonstrated in various experimental studies that the endothelial damage and derangement of endothelial regulatory mechanisms represent the pathophysiological basis of cardiovascular disease (CVD), and probably, in this regard, eNOS and iNOS are the most important elements. It is known that NAFLD may represent an independent risk factor for CVD as demonstrated in several studies, also when adjusting for the "classical" CVD risk factors, such as hypertension, dyslipidemia, obesity, and diabetes [42–45]. Moreover, a wide variety of

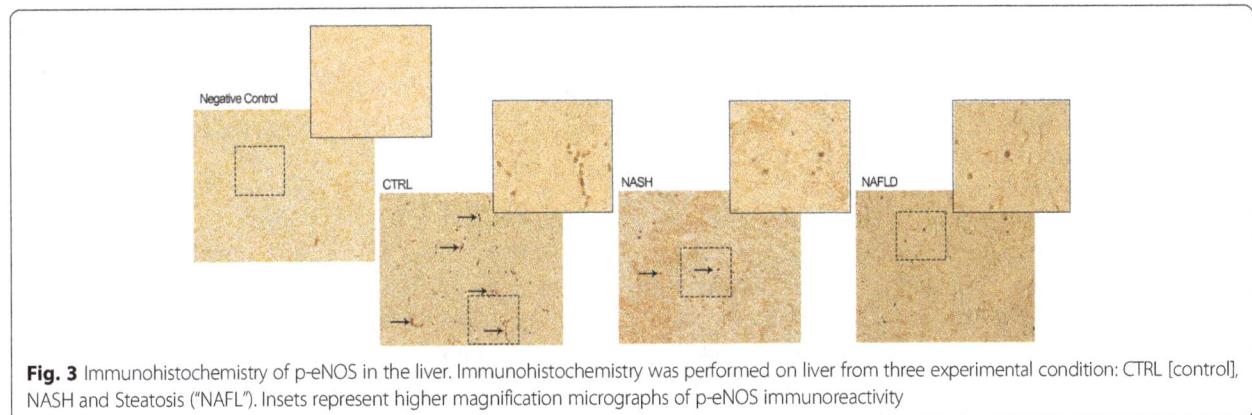

Fig. 3 Immunohistochemistry of p-eNOS in the liver. Immunohistochemistry was performed on liver from three experimental condition: CTRL [control], NASH and Steatosis ("NAFL"). Insets represent higher magnification micrographs of p-eNOS immunoreactivity

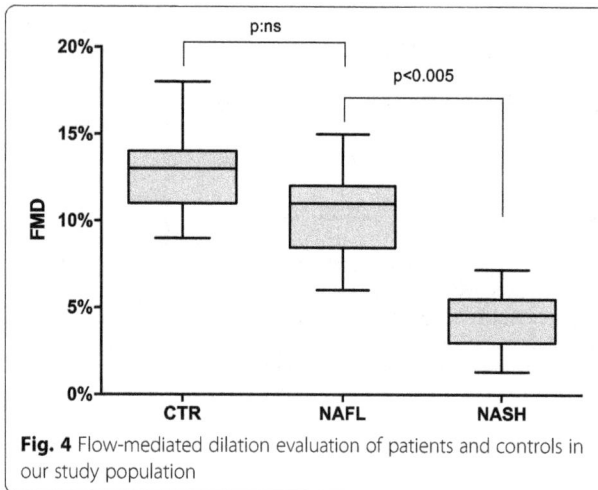

Fig. 4 Flow-mediated dilation evaluation of patients and controls in our study population

papers demonstrated that NAFLD is associated with indirect markers of microvascular dysfunction [46–49]. Here-reported eNOS dysfunction in NAFLD patients might represent a significant contribution on the comprehension of the pathophysiological linkage between NAFLD and CVD.

Another point raised by our results which deserves a discussion is that the simple steatosis (NAFL), which represents the early stage of the disease, seems to be associated to a worse eNOS impairment compared to steatohepatitis (NASH). This was confirmed both by the dynamic evaluation on mice aorta rings, on which a more intense inhibition of the vasorelaxation was found in NAFL, and by Immunoblot assays, in which it was clearly demonstrated that NAFL patients had significantly lower levels of s1177-p-eNOS if compared to both NASH and healthy controls. Finally, the immunohistochemical evaluation of p-eNOS on the liver tissue samples confirmed this trend. On the other hand, clinical evaluation of endothelial dysfunction, measured via FMD, has shown to be worse in NASH than NAFL patients, confirming a worse endothelial dysfunction and, therefore, a higher risk of cardiovascular disease in NASH subjects which has already been largely reported [22, 23]. This apparent discrepancy between the confirmation of a higher cardiovascular risk derived from a worse endothelial reactivity "in-vivo", and a "less-worse" eNOS function in NASH patients, is not explained by any pharmacological influence that may have altered the results. In fact, even if it is known that some drugs, such as insulin sensitizer metformin [50–52], PPAR-gamma agonists thiazoledinediones [53] calcium channel blockers [54], ACE inhibitors and ARBs [55] may have a positive effect on eNOS expression, no differences were found in the use of these drugs between NAFL and NASH patients in our population. Therefore, if we can reasonably exclude any pharmacological interference, a plausible

hypothesis explaining our results might be represented by the fact that, due to the worse insulin resistance, NASH subjects have a higher circulating insulin level if compared to NAFL patients, as demonstrated by insulin levels and HOMA scores (see Table 1). This "hyper-insulinemia" could lead to a "partial recovery" of the eNOS phosphorylation which, in turn, may explain the slightly better eNOS activity of NASH patients compared to NAFL ones. Interestingly, this last hypothesis is supported by our finding showing that Akt impairment is more evident in NAFL as compared to NASH. Another possible speculation could concern the fact that in a chronic disease such as NASH, a large amount of cytokines are released. Some of them (ie. VEGF, TNF-alpha and TGF-beta) were proven to have effects on eNOS expression and activity [55]. In such a "signaling storm" a mechanism of positive feedback could be postulated, and lead to a partial recovery of eNOS phosphorylation. Moreover, it has to be pointed out that not even the histological finding of a cirrhosis influenced these results: even if we presented the data without the six NASH patients with histological diagnosis of fibrosis, we carried out also the experiments including these samples, and nothing changed in terms of statistical significance. Finally, the discrepancy between clinical and laboratory results may also be explained by the higher redox status in NASH. In fact, the presence of inflammatory status leads to ROS production that reduces both bioavailability and NO production. In particular, superoxide anion $(O2-)$ can blind NO, producing peroxynitrite $(ONOO-)$, an highly toxic reactive oxygen species, and can interact with tetra-hydro-bio-pterin determining the decoupling of eNOS. These speculative interpretations need to be warranted by further studies, currently performed in our lab. However, the mechanisms underlying the endothelial dysfunction, here reported, support the idea that the endothelial dysfunction might play a crucial role in the pathological "first hit", responsible for fat accumulation in NAFLD, apparently dissociated by the following chronic inflammatory process that per se might beresponsible for the evolution, through fibrosis, to more severe steatohepatitis. Sophisticated and intriguing hypotheses of pathophysiological mechanism (s) modifying the endothelial function in NAFL and NASH patients represent the main message of the present study NASH patients have a higher cardiovascular risk, as documented by FMD measurements.

Study limitations

The present study has some limitations. Firstly, the present data need to be validated on larger series. Then, it is already well known that vascular dysfunction involves not only eNOS, but also the inducible isoform of Nitric Oxide Synthase (iNOS) which was not present in the human platelets evaluated, and it may be investigated in future studies using another experimental model. Finally, these data should be investigated together with the evaluation of direct markers of liver inflammation and fibrosis (such as TNF-alpha, TGF-beta and collagenase) in order to find any supposed direct correlation between endothelial dysfunction and liver disease progression.

Conclusions

Data here reported support the idea that IR-associated eNOS dysfunction may represent a peculiar and essential mechanism of liver damage in NAFLD, that might also represent a pathological linkage between NAFLD and CVD. Moreover, supporting the pathogenic hypothesis of "multiple parallel hits", data here reported seem to demonstrate that eNOS dysfunction might be regarded as an essential pathophysiological feature of the "first hits" of the chronic progressive process of NAFLD/NASH.

Abbreviations
ED: Endothelial dysfunction; eNOS: Endothelial nitric oxyde synthase; HOMA: Homeostasis Model Assessment; iNOS: Inducible nitric oxyde synthase; IR: Insulin resistance; NAFL: Non alcoholic fatty liver; NAFLD: Non alcoholic fatty liver disease; NAS: NAFLD Activity score; NASH: Non alcoholic steato-hepatitis; NO: Nitric oxyde

Acknowledgements
We thank Dr. Maddalena Farina (Second cycle degree in Linguistics and Translation for Special Purposes) for her English assistance.

Funding
This paper didn't receive any financial support to declare.

Authors' contributions
MP and MM: equally participated in study conception and design, data analysis and interpretation, article drafting and revised it critically for important intellectual content, and gave final approval. AD, MA, AF, TB, VR, AC and CV: participated in study conception and design, data interpretation, article drafting and revised it critically for important intellectual content, and gave final approval. All authors read and approved the final manuscript.

Competing interests
The authors declare that they don't have any conflict of interest to declare regarding this paper.

Consent for publication
No identifying images or other personal or clinical details of participants that compromise anonymity were included in the present paper. Every patient, and control, gave written consent to publish their anonymized data upon signing the informed consent.

Ethics approval and consent to participate
Every patient, and control, signed a written informed consent prior to participate the present study. The present study was approved by our local ethical committees (Ethical Committee of Istituto Neurologico Mediterraneo IRCCS Neuromed for experimental animals and Ethical Committee Campania Sud for patients and control subjects). The study protocol is in compliance with the ethical guidelines of the 1975 Declaration of Helsinki. All animals received humane care according to the criteria outlined in the "Guide for the Care and Use of Laboratory Animals" prepared by the National Academy of Sciences and published by the National Institutes of Health (NIH publication 86-23 revised 1985).

Author details
[1]Internal Medicine and Hepatology Unit, PO G. Da Procida—AOU- San Giovanni e Ruggi D'Aragona, University of Salerno, Via Salvatore Calenda 162, CAP: 84126 Salerno, Italy. [2]Vascular Physiopathology Unit IRCCS, INM Neuromed, Pozzilli, IS, Italy. [3]Hepato-Gastroenterology Division, University of Campania "L. Vanvitelli", Naples, Italy. [4]Internal Medicine and Hepatology Department, University of Campania "L. Vanvitelli", Naples, Italy. [5]Department of Medicine and Surgery, University of Salerno, Salerno, Italy.

References
1. Chalasani N, Younossi Z, Lavine JE, Diehl AM, Brunt EM, Cusi K, Charlton M, Sanyal AJ. The diagnosis and management of non-alcoholic fatty liver disease: practice Guideline by the American Association for the Study of Liver Diseases, American College of Gastroenterology, and the American Gastroenterological Association. Hepatology. 2012;55(6):2005–23.
2. Matteoni CA, Younossi ZM, Gramlich T, Boparai N, Liu YC, McCullough AJ. Nonalcoholic fatty liver disease: a spectrum of clinical and pathological severity. Gastroenterology. 1999;116(6):1413–9.
3. White DL, Kanwal F, El-Serag HB. Association between nonalcoholic fatty liver disease and risk for hepatocellular cancer, based on systematic review. Clin Gastroenterol Hepatol. 2012;10(12):1342–59. e1342.
4. McCuskey RS, Ito Y, Robertson GR, McCuskey MK, Perry M, Farrell GC. Hepatic microvascular dysfunction during evolution of dietary steatohepatitis in mice. Hepatology. 2004;40(2):386–93.
5. Seifalian AM, Chidambaram V, Rolles K, Davidson BR. In vivo demonstration of impaired microcirculation in steatotic human liver grafts. Liver Transpl Surg. 1998;4(1):71–7.
6. Kondo K, Sugioka T, Tsukada K, Aizawa M, Takizawa M, Shimizu K, Morimoto M, Suematsu M, Goda N. Fenofibrate, a peroxisome proliferator-activated receptor alpha agonist, improves hepatic microcirculatory patency and oxygen availability in a high-fat-diet-induced fatty liver in mice. Adv Exp Med Biol. 2010;662:77–82.
7. Pasarín M, Abraldes JG, Rodríguez-Vilarrupla A, La Mura V, García-Pagán JC, Bosch J. Insulin resistance and liver microcirculation in a rat model of early NAFLD. J Hepatol. 2011;55(5):1095–102.
8. Pasarín M, La Mura V, Gracia-Sancho J, García-Calderó H, Rodríguez-Vilarrupla A, García-Pagán JC, Bosch J, Abraldes JG. Sinusoidal endothelial dysfunction precedes inflammation and fibrosis in a model of NAFLD. Plos One. 2012;7(4):e32785.
9. La Mura V, Pasarín M, Rodriguez-Vilarrupla A, García-Pagán JC, Bosch J, Abraldes JG. Liver sinusoidal endothelial dysfunction after LPS administration: a role for inducible-nitric oxide synthase. J Hepatol. 2014;61(6):1321–7.
10. Perlemuter G, Bigorgne A, Cassard-Doulcier AM, Naveau S. Nonalcoholic fatty liver disease: from pathogenesis to patient care. Nat Clin Pract Endocrinol Metab. 2007;3(6):458–69.
11. Santoliquido A, Di Campli C, Miele L, Gabrieli ML, Forgione A, Zocco MA, Lupascu A, Di Giorgio A, Flore R, Pola P, et al. Hepatic steatosis and vascular disease. Eur Rev Med Pharmacol Sci. 2005;9(5):269–71.
12. Kim JA, Montagnani M, Koh KK, Quon MJ. Reciprocal relationships between insulin resistance and endothelial dysfunction: molecular and pathophysiological mechanisms. Circulation. 2006;113(15):1888–904.
13. Steinberg HO, Brechtel G, Johnson A, Fineberg N, Baron AD. Insulin-mediated skeletal muscle vasodilation is nitric oxide dependent. A novel action of insulin to increase nitric oxide release. J Clin Invest. 1994;94(3):1172–9.
14. Zeng G, Quon MJ. Insulin-stimulated production of nitric oxide is inhibited by wortmannin. Direct measurement in vascular endothelial cells. J Clin Invest. 1996;98(4):894–8.
15. Duncan ER, Crossey PA, Walker S, Anilkumar N, Poston L, Douglas G, Ezzat VA, Wheatcroft SB, Shah AM, Kearney MT, et al. Effect of endothelium-specific insulin resistance on endothelial function in vivo. Diabetes. 2008; 57(12):3307–14.
16. Gupta TK, Toruner M, Chung MK, Groszmann RJ. Endothelial dysfunction and decreased production of nitric oxide in the intrahepatic microcirculation of cirrhotic rats. Hepatology. 1998;28(4):926–31.
17. Rockey DC, Chung JJ. Reduced nitric oxide production by endothelial cells in cirrhotic rat liver: endothelial dysfunction in portal hypertension. Gastroenterology. 1998;114(2):344–51.

18. Deleve LD, Wang X, Guo Y. Sinusoidal endothelial cells prevent rat stellate cell activation and promote reversion to quiescence. Hepatology. 2008;48(3):920–30.

19. Faulx MD, Wright AT, Hoit BD. Detection of endothelial dysfunction with brachial artery ultrasound scanning. Am Heart J. 2003;145(6):943–51.

20. Celermajer DS, Sorensen KE, Gooch VM, Spiegelhalter DJ, Miller OI, Sullivan ID, Lloyd JK, Deanfield JE. Non-invasive detection of endothelial dysfunction in children and adults at risk of atherosclerosis. Lancet. 1992;340(8828):1111–5.

21. Cazzaniga M, Salerno F, Visentin S, Cirello I, Donarini C, Cugno M. Increased flow-mediated vasodilation in cirrhotic patients with ascites: relationship with renal resistive index. Liver Int. 2008;28(10):1396–401.

22. Heitzer T, Schlinzig T, Krohn K, Meinertz T, Münzel T. Endothelial dysfunction, oxidative stress, and risk of cardiovascular events in patients with coronary artery disease. Circulation. 2001;104(22):2673–8.

23. Pastori D, Loffredo L, Perri L, Baratta F, Scardella L, Polimeni L, Pani A, Brancorsini M, Albanese F, Catasca E, et al. Relation of nonalcoholic fatty liver disease and Framingham Risk Score to flow-mediated dilation in patients with cardiometabolic risk factors. Am J Cardiol. 2015;115(10):1402–6.

24. Expert Panel on Detection Ea, and Treatment of High Blood Cholesterol in Adults. Executive Summary of The Third Report of The National Cholesterol Education Program (NCEP) Expert Panel on Detection, Evaluation, And Treatment of High Blood Cholesterol In Adults (Adult Treatment Panel III). JAMA. 2001;285(19):2486–97.

25. Palmentieri B, de Sio I, La Mura V, Masarone M, Vecchione R, Bruno S, Torella R, Persico M. The role of bright liver echo pattern on ultrasound B-mode examination in the diagnosis of liver steatosis. Dig Liver Dis. 2006;38(7):485–9.

26. Kleiner DE, Brunt EM, Van Natta M, Behling C, Contos MJ, Cummings OW, Ferrell LD, Liu YC, Torbenson MS, Unalp-Arida A, et al. Design and validation of a histological scoring system for nonalcoholic fatty liver disease. Hepatology. 2005;41(6):1313–21.

27. Brunt EM, Janney CG, Di Bisceglie AM, Neuschwander-Tetri BA, Bacon BR. Nonalcoholic steatohepatitis: a proposal for grading and staging the histological lesions. Am J Gastroenterol. 1999;94(9):2467–74.

28. Carrizzo A, Di Pardo A, Maglione V, Damato A, Amico E, Formisano L, Vecchione C, Squitieri F. Nitric oxide dysregulation in platelets from patients with advanced Huntington disease. Plos One. 2014;9(2):e89745.

29. Thijssen DH, Black MA, Pyke KE, Padilla J, Atkinson G, Harris RA, Parker B, Widlansky ME, Tschakovsky ME, Green DJ. Assessment of flow-mediated dilation in humans: a methodological and physiological guideline. Am J Physiol Heart Circ Physiol. 2011;300(1):H2–H12.

30. Neunteufl T, Heher S, Katzenschlager R, Wölfl G, Kostner K, Maurer G, Weidinger F. Late prognostic value of flow-mediated dilation in the brachial artery of patients with chest pain. Am J Cardiol. 2000;86(2):207–10.

31. Iwakiri Y. Endothelial dysfunction in the regulation of cirrhosis and portal hypertension. Liver Int. 2012;32(2):199–213.

32. Bohmer A, Gambaryan S, Tsikas D. Human blood platelets lack nitric oxide synthase activity. Platelets. 2015;26(6):583–8.

33. Gentile MT, Vecchione C, Marino G, Aretini A, Di Pardo A, Antenucci G, Maffei A, Cifelli G, Iorio L, Landolfi A, et al. Resistin impairs insulin-evoked vasodilation. Diabetes. 2008;57(3):577–83.

34. Vecchione C, Brandes RP. Withdrawal of 3-hydroxy-3-methylglutaryl coenzyme A reductase inhibitors elicits oxidative stress and induces endothelial dysfunction in mice. Circ Res. 2002;91(2):173–9.

35. Atik E, Onlen Y, Savas L, Doran F. Inducible nitric oxide synthase and histopathological correlation in chronic viral hepatitis. Int J Infect Dis. 2008;12(1):12–5.

36. Failli P, Defranco RM, Caligiuri A, Gentilini A, Romanelli RG, Marra F, Batignani G, Guerra CT, Laffi G, Gentilini P, et al. Nitrovasodilators inhibit platelet-derived growth factor-induced proliferation and migration of activated human hepatic stellate cells. Gastroenterology. 2000;119(2):479–92.

37. Langer DA, Das A, Semela D, Kang-Decker N, Hendrickson H, Bronk SF, Katusic ZS, Gores GJ, Shah VH. Nitric oxide promotes caspase-independent hepatic stellate cell apoptosis through the generation of reactive oxygen species. Hepatology. 2008;47(6):1983–93.

38. Iwakiri Y, Grisham M, Shah V. Vascular biology and pathobiology of the liver: report of a single-topic symposium. Hepatology. 2008;47(5):1754–63.

39. Wiest R, Groszmann RJ. The paradox of nitric oxide in cirrhosis and portal hypertension: too much, not enough. Hepatology. 2002;35(2):478–91.

40. Graupera M, García-Pagán JC, Parés M, Abraldes JG, Roselló J, Bosch J, Rodés J. Cyclooxygenase-1 inhibition corrects endothelial dysfunction in cirrhotic rat livers. J Hepatol. 2003;39(4):515–21.

41. Gracia-Sancho J, Laviña B, Rodríguez-Vilarrupla A, García-Calderó H, Fernández M, Bosch J, García-Pagán JC. Increased oxidative stress in cirrhotic rat livers: a potential mechanism contributing to reduced nitric oxide bioavailability. Hepatology. 2008;47(4):1248–56.

42. Laviña B, Gracia-Sancho J, Rodríguez-Vilarrupla A, Chu Y, Heistad DD, Bosch J, García-Pagán JC. Superoxide dismutase gene transfer reduces portal pressure in CCl4 cirrhotic rats with portal hypertension. Gut. 2009; 58(1):118–25.

43. Kim D, Choi SY, Park EH, Lee W, Kang JH, Kim W, Kim YJ, Yoon JH, Jeong SH, Lee DH, et al. Nonalcoholic fatty liver disease is associated with coronary artery calcification. Hepatology. 2012;56(2):605–13.

44. Wong VW, Wong GL, Yip GW, Lo AO, Limquiaco J, Chu WC, Chim AM, Yu CM, Yu J, Chan FK, et al. Coronary artery disease and cardiovascular outcomes in patients with non-alcoholic fatty liver disease. Gut. 2011;60(12):1721–7.

45. Targher G, Bertolini L, Padovani R, Rodella S, Tessari R, Zenari L, Day C, Arcaro G. Prevalence of nonalcoholic fatty liver disease and its association with cardiovascular disease among type 2 diabetic patients. Diabetes Care. 2007;30(5):1212–8.

46. Boddi M, Tarquini R, Chiostri M, Marra F, Valente S, Giglioli C, Gensini GF, Abbate R. Nonalcoholic fatty liver in nondiabetic patients with acute coronary syndromes. Eur J Clin Invest. 2013;43(5):429–38.

47. Villanova N, Moscatiello S, Ramilli S, Bugianesi E, Magalotti D, Vanni E, Zoli M, Marchesini G. Endothelial dysfunction and cardiovascular risk profile in nonalcoholic fatty liver disease. Hepatology. 2005;42(2):473–80.

48. Brea A, Mosquera D, Martín E, Arizti A, Cordero JL, Ros E. Nonalcoholic fatty liver disease is associated with carotid atherosclerosis: a case-control study. Arterioscler Thromb Vasc Biol. 2005;25(5):1045–50.

49. Goland S, Shimoni S, Zornitzki T, Knobler H, Azoulai O, Lutaty G, Melzer E, Orr A, Caspi A, Malnick S. Cardiac abnormalities as a new manifestation of nonalcoholic fatty liver disease: echocardiographic and tissue Doppler imaging assessment. J Clin Gastroenterol. 2006;40(10):949–55.

50. Long MT, Wang N, Larson MG, Mitchell GF, Palmisano J, Vasan RS, Hoffmann U, Speliotes EK, Vita JA, Benjamin EJ, et al. Nonalcoholic fatty liver disease and vascular function: cross-sectional analysis in the Framingham heart study. Arterioscler Thromb Vasc Biol. 2015;35(5):1284–91.

51. Mather KJ, Verma S, Anderson TJ. Improved endothelial function with metformin in type 2 diabetes mellitus. J Am Coll Cardiol. 2001;37(5):1344–50.

52. Katakam PV, Ujhelyi MR, Hoenig M, Miller AW. Metformin improves vascular function in insulin-resistant rats. Hypertension. 2000;35(1 Pt 1):108–12.

53. Cho DH, Choi YJ, Jo SA, Jo I. Nitric oxide production and regulation of endothelial nitric-oxide synthase phosphorylation by prolonged treatment with troglitazone: evidence for involvement of peroxisome proliferator-activated receptor (PPAR) gamma-dependent and PPARgamma-independent signaling pathways. J Biol Chem. 2004;279(4):2499–506.

54. Ding Y, Vaziri ND. Calcium channel blockade enhances nitric oxide synthase expression by cultured endothelial cells. Hypertension. 1998;32(4):718–23.

55. Varin R, Mulder P, Tamion F, Richard V, Henry JP, Lallemand F, Lerebours G, Thuillez C. Improvement of endothelial function by chronic angiotensin-converting enzyme inhibition in heart failure : role of nitric oxide, prostanoids, oxidant stress, and bradykinin. Circulation. 2000;102(3):351–6.

19

Development of a novel mouse model of hepatocellular carcinoma with nonalcoholic steatohepatitis using a high-fat, choline-deficient diet and intraperitoneal injection of diethylnitrosamine

Norihiro Kishida[1], Sachiko Matsuda[1,2], Osamu Itano[1*], Masahiro Shinoda[1], Minoru Kitago[1], Hiroshi Yagi[1], Yuta Abe[1], Taizo Hibi[1], Yohei Masugi[3], Koichi Aiura[4], Michiie Sakamoto[3] and Yuko Kitagawa[1]

Abstract

Background: The incidence of hepatocellular carcinoma with nonalcoholic steatohepatitis is increasing, and its clinicopathological features are well established. Several animal models of nonalcoholic steatohepatitis have been developed to facilitate its study; however, few fully recapitulate all its clinical features, which include insulin resistance, inflammation, fibrosis, and carcinogenesis. Moreover, these models require a relatively long time to produce hepatocellular carcinoma reliably. The aim of this study was to develop a mouse model of hepatocellular carcinoma with nonalcoholic steatohepatitis that develops quickly and reflects all clinically relevant features.

Methods: Three-week-old C57BL/6J male mice were fed either a standard diet (MF) or a choline-deficient, high-fat diet (HFCD). The mice in the MF + diethylnitrosamine (DEN) and HFCD + DEN groups received a one-time intraperitoneal injection of DEN at the start of the respective feeding protocols.

Results: The mice in the HFCD and HFCD + DEN groups developed obesity early in the experiment and insulin resistance after 12 weeks. Triglyceride levels peaked at 8 weeks for all four groups and decreased thereafter. Alanine aminotransferase levels increased every 4 weeks, with the HFCD and HFCD + DEN groups showing remarkably high levels; the HFCD + DEN group presented the highest incidence of nonalcoholic steatohepatitis. The levels of fibrosis and steatosis varied, but they tended to increase every 4 weeks in the HFCD and HFCD + DEN groups. Computed tomography scans indicated that all the HFCD + DEN mice developed hepatic tumors from 20 weeks, some of which were glutamine synthetase-positive.

Conclusions: The nonalcoholic steatohepatitis-hepatocellular carcinoma model we describe here is simple to establish, results in rapid tumor formation, and recapitulates most of the key features of nonalcoholic steatohepatitis. It could therefore facilitate further studies of the development, oncogenic potential, diagnosis, and treatment of this condition.

Keywords: Nonalcoholic steatohepatitis, Hepatocellular carcinoma, Diethylnitrosamine, High-fat choline-deficient diet, Mouse model

* Correspondence: laplivertiger@gmail.com
[1]Department of Surgery, School of Medicine, Keio University, 35 Shinanomachi, Shinjuku-ku, Tokyo 160-8582, Japan
Full list of author information is available at the end of the article

Background

Worldwide, hepatocellular carcinoma (HCC) is the fifth-most common cancer in men and seventh-most common in women, and its incidence has continuously increased in recent years [1]. The major risk factors for HCC are infection with hepatitis B and C viruses; however, the incidence of viral-related HCC has decreased owing to improvements in the management and treatment of viral infections. Meanwhile, the frequency of non-viral HCC—related to alcohol consumption and other factors—has gradually increased. Nonalcoholic fatty liver disease (NAFLD), which is a hepatic manifestation of metabolic syndrome, is one of the most common causes of chronic liver disease and liver cirrhosis in the world [2, 3]. NAFLD ranges from simple steatosis to nonalcoholic steatohepatitis (NASH) associated with inflammation, fibrosis, and carcinogenesis [4]. In accordance with multiple-hit theory, metabolic syndrome, genetic factors, oxidative stress, inflammatory cytokines, endotoxins, and insulin resistance have been shown to be involved in NASH development and the progression of NASH-HCC [5]. A number of studies describing the natural history of NASH have found liver failure and HCC to be the major causes of death [6–12].

Various genetic and dietary NASH animal models exist. For example, PTEN knockout mice undergo carcinogenesis, and exhibit steatohepatitis, but not obesity, dyslipidemia, or insulin resistance [13]. ob/ob mice are diabetic owing to a defect in the leptin gene and genetically obese; db/db mice have a defective leptin receptor gene [14, 15]. Dietary models include a high-fat diet (HFD) model [16], a high-fat, choline-deficient diet model (HFCD) [17, 18], a methionine- and choline-deficient diet (MCD) model [19, 20]. These models require a relatively long period—usually about 1 year—to produce HCC [17]. A 16-week NASH-HCC mouse model based on an HFD combined with low-dose streptozotocin (STZ) has been reported [21]; however, those mice were not insulin resistant, because they exhibited a lack of insulin secretion. The liver carcinogenicity of diethylnitrosamine (DEN) has been reported [22–24], and DEN has been added to the rat NASH-HCC model in combination with an HFD [25–27]. A few models exhibit all the associated clinical features of NASH-HCC, such as insulin resistance, inflammation, fibrosis, and carcinogenesis, such as a high-fat and fructose diet model [28]. Recent genetic and dietary NASH-HCC models have included MUP-uPA transgenic mice with HFD [29] and melanocortin 4 receptor (MC4R) knockout mice with HFD [30].

Since there is no effective treatment or chemoprevention for HCC related to NASH, a mouse model with the same clinical features as human NASH is needed. In this study, by feeding C57BL/6 mice an HFCD combined with DEN exposure, we developed a novel experimental NASH-HCC mouse model that exhibits all the relevant clinical features by 20 weeks, including insulin resistance, inflammation, fibrosis, and carcinogenesis.

Methods

Animals

Three-week-old male C57Bl/6J mice were purchased from Oriental Yeast (Tokyo, Japan), housed in a temperature-, humidity-, and ventilation-controlled vivarium, and kept on a 12-h light/dark cycle under specific pathogen-free conditions. For the DEN intraperitoneal (i.p.) experiment, the mice were randomly divided into two groups: the standard diet (MF) group, which was fed an MF (11.4 % fat, 25.7 % protein, 62.9 % carbohydrate, total calories 359 kcal/100 g; purchased from Oriental Yeast); and the HFCD group, which was fed an HFCD (58.0 % fat, 16.4 % protein, 25.5 % carbohydrate, total calories 556 kcal/100 g; purchased from Oriental Yeast) [17]. The two groups were further divided into two subgroups, one of which was treated with DEN. The MF + DEN and HFCD + DEN subgroups received a one-time i.p. injection of 25 mg/kg DEN at the start of the respective feeding protocols. Food and water were given ad libitum. Five mice from each group were sacrificed every 4 weeks, and their body weights and liver weights measured. An overview of the experimental protocol appears in Fig. 1.

All procedures for animal experimentation were in accordance with the Helsinki Declaration of 1975 and Institutional Guidelines on Animal Experimentation at Keio University. This study was approved by the Keio University Institutional Animal Care and Use Committee (Approval number: 08073).

Measurement of biological parameters

Serum levels of fasting blood sugar (FBS), alanine aminotransferase (ALT), and triglyceride (TG) were measured using a Fuji Dri-Chem 3500 analyzer (Fuji Film Co. Ltd, Tokyo, Japan). Insulin levels were determined using a mouse insulin enzyme-linked immunoassay kit (Morinaga Institute of Biological Science, Inc. Yokohama, Japan). The quantitative insulin sensitivity check index was calculated as 1/log (fasting insulin) + log (fasting glucose). Interleukin (IL)-6, tumor necrosis factor (TNF)-alpha, leptin, adiponectin, and C-reactive protein (CRP) levels were measured using Procarta Multiplex Immunoassays (Affymetrix eBioscience, San Diego, CA, USA). Serum amyloid A (SAA) was determined using the PHASE RANGE Mouse SAA ELISA kit (Tridelta Development Ltd., Kildare, Ireland).

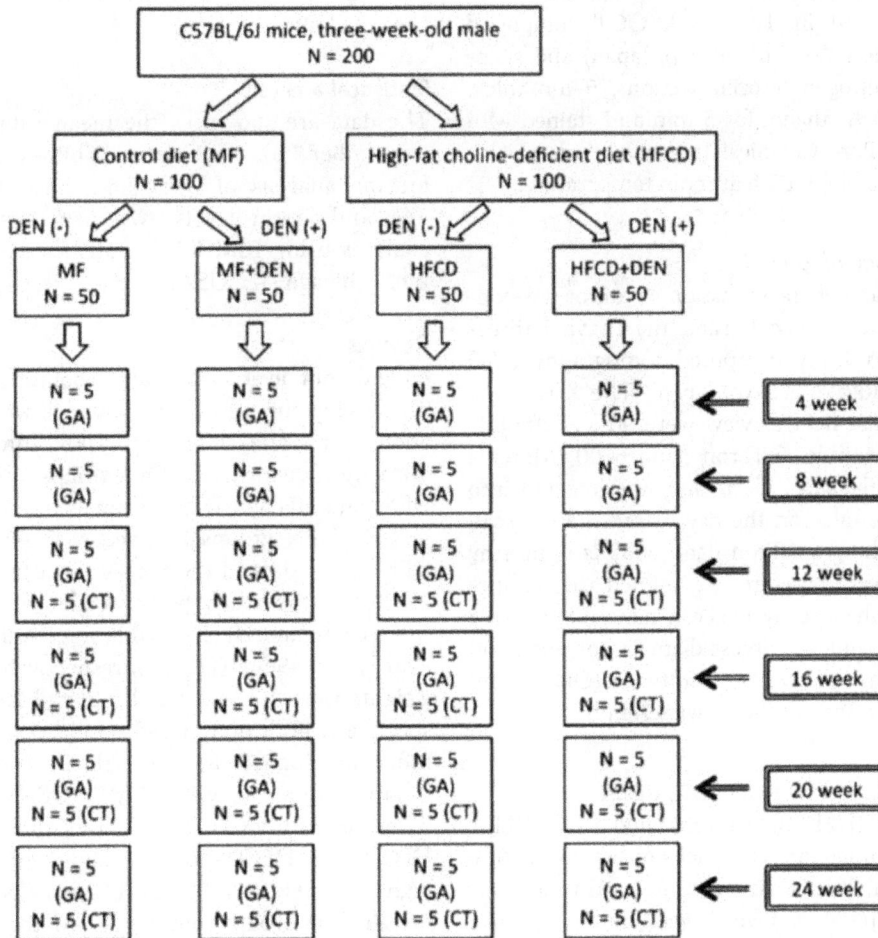

Fig. 1 Overview of the experimental design, showing intraperitoneal diethylnitrosamine (DEN) administration. N, number; GA, general assessment; CT, computed tomography scanning

Insulin tolerance test

To assess insulin resistance, we performed an insulin tolerance test. Mice were injected with 1 U/kg of insulin (Humulin R; Eli Lilly Japan, Kobe, Japan), and blood glucose was measured using an Accu-Chek meter (Roche Diagnostics Japan, Tokyo, Japan) every 20 min up to 120 min. The ratio was calculated using the pre-injection value as a standard.

Histological analysis

Liver tissue was assessed grossly, and samples were fixed in 10 % formaldehyde and processed for hematoxylin-eosin staining. Variables were blindly scored by two experienced hepatopathologists using a modified scoring system adapted from the NAFLD activity score (NAS): macrosteatosis (0–3); lobular inflammatory changes (0–3); hepatocyte ballooning (0–2); and fibrosis scored as portal and perivenular (stage 0–4).

Immunohistochemical detection of F4/80 (a macrophage marker) was performed as follows. Paraffin sections were deparaffinized in xylene, hydrated in a gradient of ethanol, and incubated with proteinase K for 10 min at room temperature for antigen retrieval. The sections were then incubated with a primary rat anti-mouse F4/80 antibody (T-2006; BMA Biomedicals, Augst, Switzerland) overnight at 4 °C, followed by incubation with Histofine Simple Stain mouse MAX-PO (Rat) (Nichirei Bioscience, Tokyo, Japan) for 30 min. Staining was detected using diaminobenzidine tetrahydrochloride. Three light microscopy images at 100 times magnification were taken of each slide to determine the ratio of F4/80-positive cells (macrophages) to hepatocyte nuclei.

Immunostaining for glutamine synthetase (GS) was performed by the Stelic Institute & Co., Inc. (Tokyo, Japan). Sirius red staining was performed using Van Gieson's stain solution and Sirius red solution from Muto Pure Chemicals Co., Ltd. (Tokyo, Japan). The degree of liver fibrosis was assessed using Histoquest (Tissue Gnostics, Vienna, Austria) using the three images of each slide described above. The caudate liver lobes were embedded in Tissue-Tek OCT compound (Sakura Finetechnical Co., Ltd., Tokyo, Japan) and snap-frozen in liquid nitrogen. Frozen sections, 5 μm thick, were fixed with 50 % ethanol for 5 min and stained with Sudan III (Wako Pure Chemical Industries Ltd., Osaka, Japan) in 55 % ethanol for 1.5 h at room temperature.

X-ray computed tomography

For the detection and characterization of tumor development, the mice were imaged using the in vivo three-dimensional micro X-ray computed tomography (CT) system R-mCT2 (Rigaku, Tokyo, Japan). The X-ray tube voltage, current, and field of view were 90 kV, 200 μA, and 30 mm, respectively. ExiTron nano 6000 (Miltenyi Biotec, Bergisch Gladbach, Germany) was injected into the tail vein of the mice on the day before the CT scan at a dose of 10 mL/kg. ExiTron nano 6000 is uptake by Kupffer cells in liver, therefore, we defined the nodules which were not enhanced by ExiTron nano 6000. Using 512 CT image of samples, largest diameter of node and numbers were measured by Osirix software (OnDemand software, Cybermed Inc., Bernex, Switzerland).

Comparison of HFCD + DEN and HFD32 + DEN

High Fat Diet 32 (HFD32) was obtained from CLEA Japan, Inc. (Tokyo, Japan). This diet consists of 32.0 % fat, 25.5 % protein, 29.4 % carbohydrate, and total calories of 507.6 kcal/100 g. Five 3-week-old male mice were fed HFD32 and received a one-time i.p. injection of 25 mg/kg DEN at the start of the feeding protocol. After 4 weeks, liver tissue was taken and snap-frozen in liquid nitrogen.

RNA was extracted from frozen liver tissue after 4 weeks of MF, HFCD + DEN, and HFD32 + DEN using the RNeasy Mini Kit (Qiagen, Hilden, Germany). Genome-wide mRNA expression levels were determined using the Superprint G3 Mouse GE microarray kit 8 x 60 k Ver 2.0, which contains 27,122 genes (G4858A#074809, Agilent Technologies, South Queensferry, UK). All microarray data of the HFCD + DEN mice and HFD32 + DEN mice were normalized with data of the MF mice using GeneSpring GX Ver 13.1 software (Agilent Technologies); the threshold was set at more than twofold changes. We analyzed the data by means of Qiagen's Ingenuity Pathway Analysis (IPA) software Ver 1.0 (Qiagen, Hilden, Germany) for functional analysis. Molecules from the dataset that exceeded the twofold cutoff and were associated with biological function or diseases in the Ingenuity Knowledge Base were considered for analysis. The right-tailed Fisher's exact test was used to calculate a p value to determine the probability that each biological

function or disease assigned to that dataset was due to chance alone.

Statistical analysis

The data are shown as the mean ± standard deviation or number (%). The Mann–Whitney U test was used for the analysis of body and liver weight and ALT, TG, and leptin levels. We performed all statistical analyses using IBM SPSS Statistics 21 software (SPSS, Inc., Chicago, IL, USA).

Results

Body weight, liver weight, and laboratory findings

To develop the NASH-HCC model, we used a combination of an HFCD and i.p. DEN administration. The mice were divided into four groups: MF; HFCD; MF + DEN; and HFCD + DEN. Animals in the MF + DEN and HFCD + DEN groups received a single i.p. injection of DEN at the start of the respective feeding protocols. At 24 weeks, the mean body weights of the MF, HFCD, MF + DEN, and HFCD + DEN mice were 31.7 g, 54.5 g, 32.6 g, and 49.5 g (Fig. 2a), respectively; the mean liver weights were 1.2 g, 4.0 g, 1.3 g, and 2.9 g (Fig. 2b), respectively. Both body weight and liver weight were significantly higher in the HFCD and HFCD + DEN groups than in the MF and MF + DEN groups.

Plasma ALT levels increased every 4 weeks, with the HFCD and HFCD + DEN groups showing remarkably high levels (Fig. 2c). Plasma TG levels peaked at 8 weeks for all four groups and decreased thereafter (Fig. 2d). There were significant differences in TG levels between the MF and HFCD + DEN groups at 16 and 20 weeks. Plasma leptin levels increased from 20 weeks in the HFCD and HFCD + DEN groups (Fig. 2e). Plasma adiponectin levels decreased from 20 weeks in the HFCD and HFCD + DEN groups (Fig. 2f).

The levels of other biomarkers, such as FBS, CRP, IL-6, and TNF-alpha, are shown in Table 1. CRP levels increased from 20 weeks in the HFCD and HFCD + DEN groups, though there was no significant difference. However, compared with the MF group, serum levels of TNF-alpha were higher in the HFCD group at 4 and 8 weeks and in the HFCD + DEN group at 8 weeks. Serum levels of IL-6 tended to be higher in the HFCD and HFCD + DEN groups; however, at 16 weeks, only the HFCD group exhibited significantly different levels compared with the MF group.

Insulin resistance

Insulin resistance was calculated using the quantitative insulin sensitivity check index. All mice in the HFCD and HFCD + DEN groups had developed insulin resistance at 12 weeks, whereas animals in the MF and MF + DEN groups had developed insulin resistance at 24 weeks

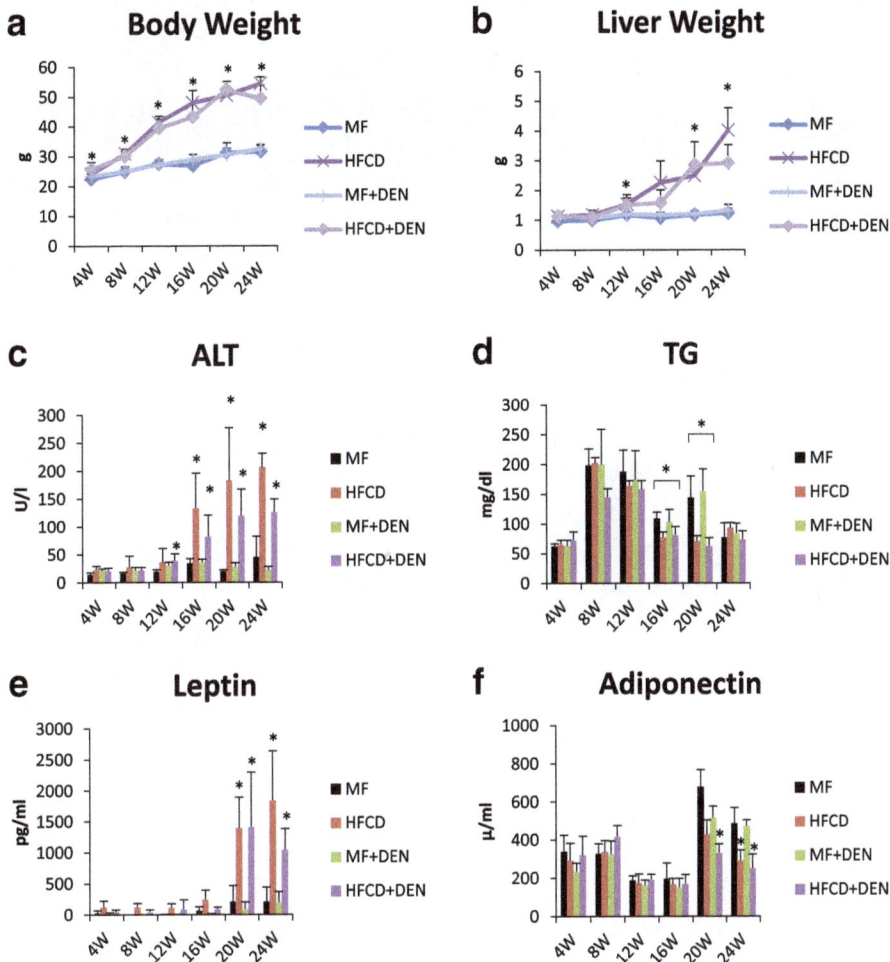

Fig. 2 Body and liver weights and laboratory findings: **a** body weight; **b** liver weight; **c** plasma alanine aminotransferase (ALT); **d** plasma triglycerides (TG); **e** plasma leptin; and **f** adiponectin. The data are shown as the mean + standard deviation. * $p < 0.05$ indicates a significant difference between the standard diet (MF) group and the other groups for each month. HFCD, high-fat choline-deficient diet; DEN, diethylnitrosamine

(Table 2). To confirm the development of insulin resistance, we performed an insulin tolerance test. There was a significant difference in insulin resistance between the MF and HFCD + DEN groups at 80 and 100 min. There was also a significant difference in insulin resistance between the MF and HFCD groups at 80, 100, and 120 min (Fig. 3).

Histological findings of non-tumor tissue

Liver specimens were evaluated using hematoxylin-eosin staining. At 12 weeks, mice in the HFCD and HFCD + DEN groups evidenced fat accumulation, lobular inflammation, and hepatocyte ballooning, which are characteristic of NASH. These changes were more evident in specimens from the HFCD + DEN group than in those from the HFCD group (Fig. 4a). We observed no apparent pathological findings, including fatty degeneration or necroinflammatory changes in hepatocytes in the hematoxylin–eosin-stained tissue of MF or MF +

DEN mice. Sudan III staining revealed remarkable macrovesicular fat accumulation in both the HFCD and HFCD + DEN groups at 12 weeks; microvesicular fat accumulation was evident in the MF group—and to a lesser extent in the MF + DEN group (Fig. 4b). Lipogranuloma (Fig. 4c), Mallory-Denk bodies (Fig. 4d), and hepatocyte ballooning (Fig. 4e), which are characteristic of NASH, were observed in the HFCD + DEN mice from 16 weeks after feeding.

NAS is an established scoring system for assessing the severity of NASH. In the NAS system, a score of 3–5 represents possible or borderline NASH; a score greater than 5 indicates definite NASH. The NAS was possible or borderline from 16 weeks and definite from 20 weeks in the HFCD mice; it was possible or borderline from 12 weeks and definite from 16 weeks in the HFCD + DEN group (Table 3).

To evaluate inflammation, we undertook immunohistochemical detection of macrophages with F4/80 antibody

Table 1 Summary of laboratory findings for FBS, CRP, IL-6, TNF-alpha, and adiponectin levels

	Week	MF	HFCD	MF + DEN	HFCD + DEN
FBS (mg/dl)	4	211.3 ± 41.7	297.5 ± 24.6	191.0 ± 11.2	282.3 ± 26.5
	8	149.6 ± 30.9	174.2 ± 32.9	177.0 ± 64.9	167.6 ± 31.3
	12	167.6 ± 41.6	241.6 ± 32.4	152.0 ± 24.2	273.4 ± 31.5
	16	109.8 ± 11.4	245.0 ± 46.4	112.8 ± 8.7	189.8 ± 52.5
	20	188.4 ± 14.6	263.2 ± 36.0	172.0 ± 36.7	242.0 ± 14.4
	24	165.2 ± 23.9	265.2 ± 6.5	205.3 ± 32.5	249.4 ± 24.2
CRP (ng/ml)	4	4552.6 ± 2533.3	3756.8 ± 1366.4	4284.9 ± 2261.0	4915.4 ± 1697.0
	8	5803.1 ± 1368.7	13324.9 ± 7100.6	5837.7 ± 2422.0	6568.3 ± 3827.0
	12	2412.0 ± 211.8	2505.3 ± 517.7	2465.9 ± 170.5	2427.1 ± 337.3
	16	2080.4 ± 756.5	3065.7 ± 1047.4	2801.3 ± 457.0	3002.1 ± 599.5
	20	2125.1 ± 306.9	3170.3 ± 711.8	2185.4 ± 256.3	3293.4 ± 416.6
	24	2227.6 ± 613.8	3143.3 ± 393.3	2044.0 ± 349.9	3686,7 ± 481.2
IL-6 (pg/ml)	4	0.2 ± 0.3	1.3 ± 1.5	0.3 ± 0.5	0.9 ± 1.3
	8	0.5 ± 0.5	1.8 ± 1.5	0.6 ± 0.7	0.9 ± 1.2
	12	0.8 ± 0.5	1.1 ± 0.7	1.1 ± 0.8	2.0 ± 1.5
	16	1.3 ± 0.6	2.9 ± 1.2	1.2 ± 0.8	0.9 ± 0.2
	20	1.6 ± 1.2	1.3 ± 0.8	1.4 ± 0.9	1.6 ± 0.9
	24	2.1 ± 1.3	4.2 ± 1.8	2.2 ± 4.5	1.6 ± 0.3
TNF-alpha (pg/ml)	4	N.D.	20.7 ± 28.9	N.D.	6.2 ± 12.0
	8	1.8 ± 3.9	270.9 ± 297.5	5.0 ± 7.1	134.6 ± 153.7
	12	2.2 ± 2.8	0.4 ± 0.9	0.9 ± 2.0	1.9 ± 3.1
	16	0.1 ± 0.1	3.4 ± 4.8	0.1 ± 0.3	N.D.
	20	1.2 ± 1.6	2.0 ± 2.2	1.4 ± 1.4	1.4 ± 1.3
	24	3.8 ± 6.4	5.8 ± 3.0	3.5 ± 5.2	0.5 ± 1.2

The data are shown as the mean ± standard deviation. Each group contained five mice. *FBS* fasting blood sugar, *CRP* C-reactive protein, *IL* interleukin, *TNF*-alpha tumor necrosis factor-alpha

and SAA measurement. Representative images of macrophages in the perivenular zone at 4 weeks in the MF and HFCD + DEN mice are presented in Fig. 5a, b. The ratio of F4/80-positive cells (macrophages) to hepatocyte nuclei was higher in the HFCD and HFCD + DEN groups than in the other two groups from 4 weeks (Fig. 5c). SAA was significantly higher after 20 weeks in the HFCD + DEN mice and at 24 weeks in the HFCD mice (Fig. 5d). Fibrosis was more conspicuous in the HFCD and HFCD + DEN mice than in the other two groups (Fig. 5e). The area of fibrosis increased dramatically from 12 weeks in the HFCD + DEN mice and from 16 weeks in the HFCD group (Fig. 5f).

CT scans and immunohistochemistry of hepatic tumors

To evaluate tumor development, we performed a CT scan every 4 weeks from week 12. The largest liver mass had a maximum diameter of 13 mm at 24 weeks in the HFCD + DEN group (Fig. 6a, b). Small nodules were typically seen in the liver macroscopically and by CT scan at 24 weeks (Fig. 6c–e). Positive findings were evident in 20 % and 100 % of the HFCD + DEN mice at 16 weeks and 20 weeks, respectively. Only one mouse had positive findings in the HFCD group at 20 weeks and one mouse in the MF + DEN group at 24 weeks. In the HFCD + DEN group, there were on average eight tumors at 24 weeks, with an average size of 2.9 mm (Table 4). To confirm malignancy, we immunostained the tumors to detect GS. GS-positive HCC was found in some specimens (Fig. 6f, g), although not all tumors were stained.

Comparison of HFCD + DEN and HFD32 + DEN

To determine why HFCD + DEN promoted cancer development, we performed RNA microarray analysis. For this, we used HFD32, which is a widely employed high-fat diet. Principal component analysis provides a way of identifying predominant gene expression patterns. Surprisingly, the general expression of HFCD + DEN was closer to MF than to HFD32 + DEN (Fig. 7a). Clustering analysis and gene ontology analysis indicated that

Table 2 Insulin resistance calculated using the quantitative insulin sensitivity check index

	4 W	8 W	12 W	16 W	20 W	24 W
MF	N.D.	**0.227**	**0.139**	N.D.	N.D.	0.413
	0.064	N.D.	0.348	N.D.	0.445	**0.12**
	N.D.	0.381	**0.193**	N.D.	N.D.	**0.249**
	N.D.	N.D.	0.416	0.315	N.D.	0.777
	N.D.	N.D.	0.672	N.D.	N.D.	**0.083**
HFCD	N.D.	**0.22**	**0.089**	**0.058**	**0.026**	**0.045**
	0.2002	**0.206**	**0.047**	**0.034**	**0.026**	**0.025**
	0.3954	**0.168**	**0.067**	**0.034**	**0.057**	**0.025**
	0.0705	N.D.	**0.081**	**0.027**	**0.034**	**0.018**
	0.1384	N.D.	**0.046**	**0.079**	**0.037**	**0.030**
MF + DEN	1.047	N.D.	0.579	N.D.	N.D.	**0.2916**
	N.D.	N.D.	N.D.	N.D.	N.D.	**0.116**
	N.D.	0.916	N.D.	0.642	N.D.	**0.131**
	N.D.	0.916	N.D.	N.D.	N.D.	**0.153**
	N.D.	0.159	N.D.	9.101	**0.245**	N.D.
HFCD + DEN	1.047	**0.0808**	**0.016**	**0.072**	**0.033**	**0.026**
	N.D.	**0.1167**	**0.031**	**0.054**	**0.063**	**0.020**
	0.1026	0.377	**0.030**	**0.025**	**0.069**	**0.034**
	0.0826	0.315	**0.048**	0.314	**0.201**	**0.031**
	0.172	**0.173**	**0.036**	**0.022**	**0.055**	**0.037**

The quantitative insulin sensitivity check index = 1/log (fasting insulin) + log (fasting glucose). A value < 0.3 indicates insulin resistance; values from 0.348 to 0.430 are normal, and values ≥ 3.0 indicate high insulin sensitivity (type 1 diabetes mellitus). Index values < 0.3 (insulin resistance) are in bold. Each group contained five mice. *W* weeks, *MF* standard diet, *HFCD* high-fat choline-deficient diet, *DEN* diethylnitrosamine, *N.D* not determined

probably as a result of hepatitis, HFCD + DEN and HFD32 commonly changed the expression gene related to defense response and immune response. Functional analysis extracted 13 genes from HFCD + DEN and 163 from HFD32 + DEN related to HCC: HFCD + DEN and HFD32 + DEN were found to have six genes in common. As seen in the heat map in Fig. 7b and Additional file 1, expression of Histone cluster 1, H3c (Hist1h3c), histone cluster 1, H3g (Hist1h3g), Mitochondrial transcription termination factor 2 (Mterf2), ArfGAP with SH3 domain, ankyrin repeat and PH domain 2 (Asap2), and Hair growth associated (Hr) showed an increase in both the HFCD + DEN and HFD32 + DEN groups. Expression of Retinoblastoma binding protein 6 (Rbbp6) in HFCD + DEN presented a slight decrease, though it was a large decrease in HFD32 + DEN.

Discussion

It has been reported that the development and progression of NASH-HCC follows a multiple-hit pathway, which includes metabolic syndrome, genetic factors, oxidative stress, inflammatory cytokine release, endotoxins, and insulin resistance [5]. Previous NASH models have combined two or more of these hits by using a special diet with a chemical agent [21, 27] or specific genetic changes [14, 20]. However, these demand relatively long periods before the onset of HCC. NASH models based only on an HFCD require considerably longer periods—usually more than 1 year—to reliably produce carcinoma [17]. By combining an HFCD with a chemical agent, DEN, our model resulted in

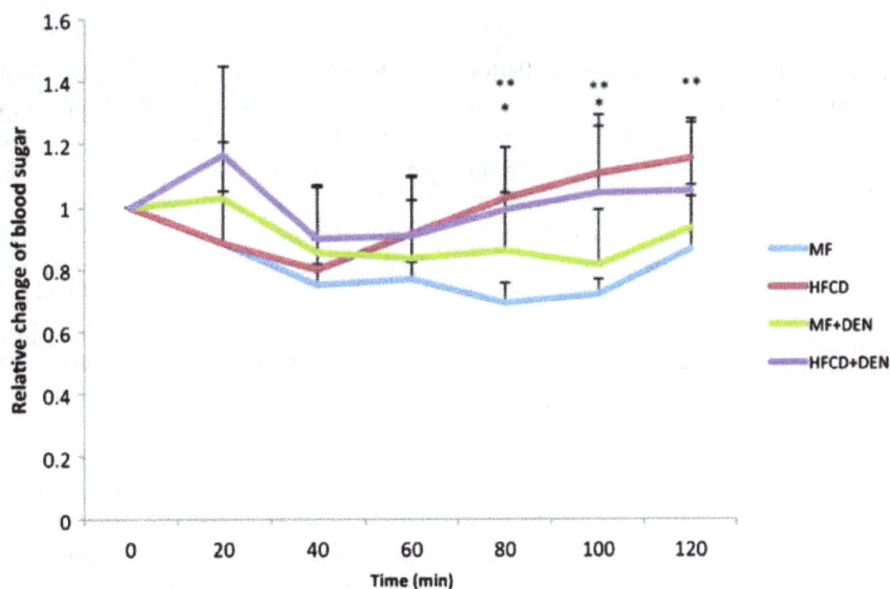

Fig. 3 Insulin tolerance test at 12 weeks. The data appear as the mean + standard deviation. * $p < 0.05$ indicates a significant difference between the standard diet (MF) group and the high-fat, choline-deficient diet (HFCD) + diethylnitrosamine (DEN) group. ** $p < 0.05$ indicates a significant difference between the MF and HFCD groups

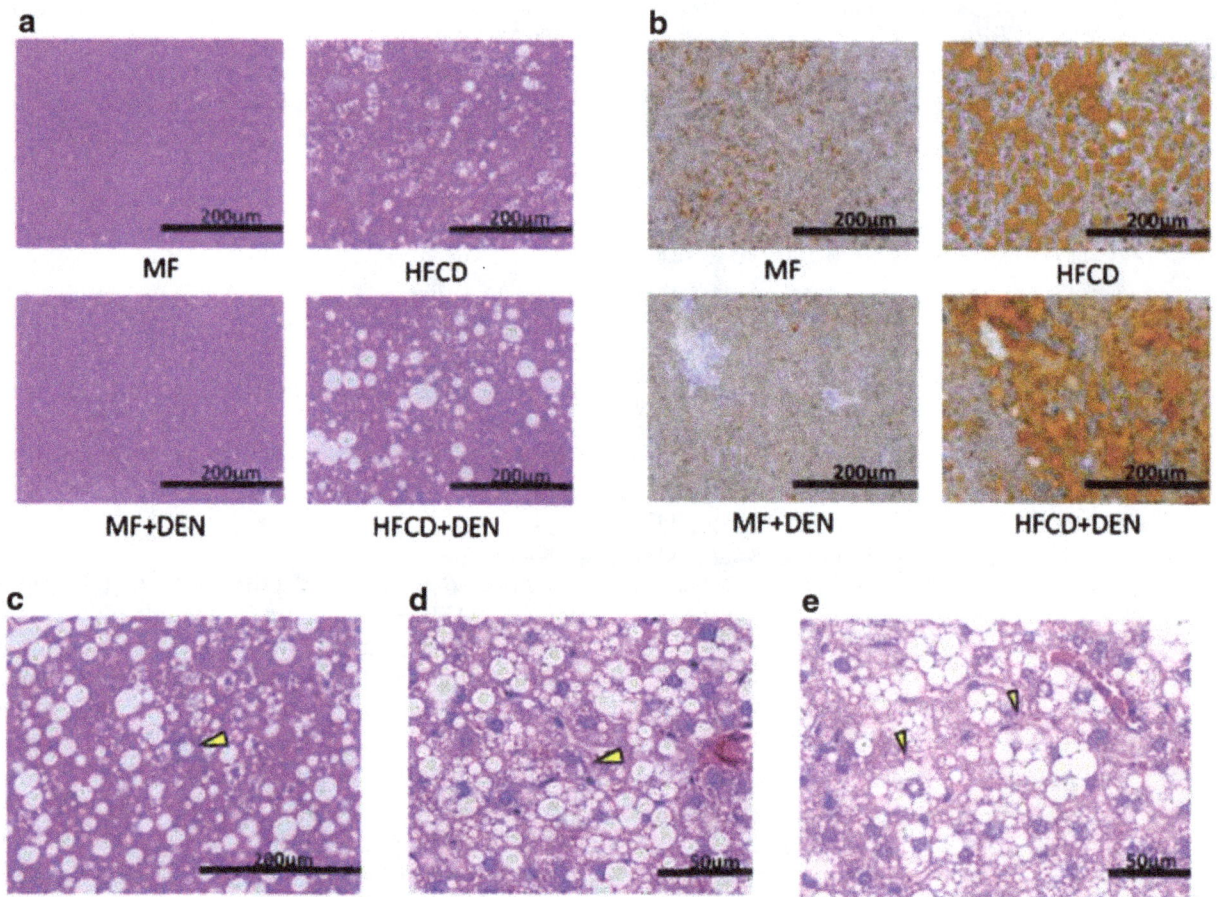

Fig. 4 Representative images of stained liver sections: **a** 12 weeks with hematoxylin-eosin staining; **b** 12 weeks with Sudan staining; **c–e** 16 weeks in HFCD + DEN mice with hematoxylin-eosin staining. The original magnification is × 200 (**a–c**) and × 400 (**d**). Lipogranuloma (**c**), a Mallory-Denk body (**d**), and hepatocyte ballooning (**e**) are indicated by yellow arrowheads. MF, standard diet; HFCD, high-fat choline-deficient diet; DEN, diethylnitrosamine

carcinoma within 20 weeks. DEN increases oxidative stress [31], which is one of the most important factors in the development and progression of NASH since it stimulates Kupffer cells [32]. Mice in the HFCD + DEN group showed elevated SAA levels, a higher NAS, and earlier fibrosis than those in the HFCD group. We also demonstrated that our NASH mouse model—based on an HFCD combined with i.p. injection of DEN—stimulated insulin resistance, fibrosis, and HCC within 20 weeks (Fig. 8).

The MCD model is one of the best-known NASH animal models [19, 20]. Choline deficiency causes Cyp2E1 upregulation with increased reactive oxygen species formation, lipid peroxidation, and mitochondrial dysfunction [27]; methionine deficiency exacerbates hepatic injury associated with oxidative and endoplasmic reticulum stress [33]. Although MCD mice develop steatohepatitis, fibrosis, and carcinogenesis, both body weight and insulin resistance tend to decrease because of reduced food intake and increased basal metabolism. The MCD model thus reflects a different pathophysiology than human NASH with respect to metabolic syndrome.

Few reported NASH-HCC models have fully incorporated all the clinical changes associated with that disease [28–30]. In our HFCD + DEN model, tumor initiation is basically dependent on a chemical carcinogen, which is artificial compared with the above spontaneous HCC

Table 3 Nonalcoholic fatty liver disease activity score (NAS)

	Week	MF	HFCD	MF + DEN	HFCD + DEN
NAS	4	0	0.6 ± 0.9	0.6 ± 0.6	1.3 ± 0.5
	8	0	0.8 ± 0.8	0.4 ± 0.6	1.2 ± 1.6
	12	0	2.6 ± 1.7	1 ± 0	3 ± 2.0
	16	0.2 ± 0.5	4.6 ± 2.2	1 ± 0	5.2 ± 1.3
	20	0	5.2 ± 0.5	1 ± 0	5.4 ± 0.6
	24	0	6.2 ± 0.8	1 ± 0	5.6 ± 0.6

Each group contained five mice. *MF* standard diet, *HFCD* high-fat choline-deficient diet, *DEN* diethylnitrosamine

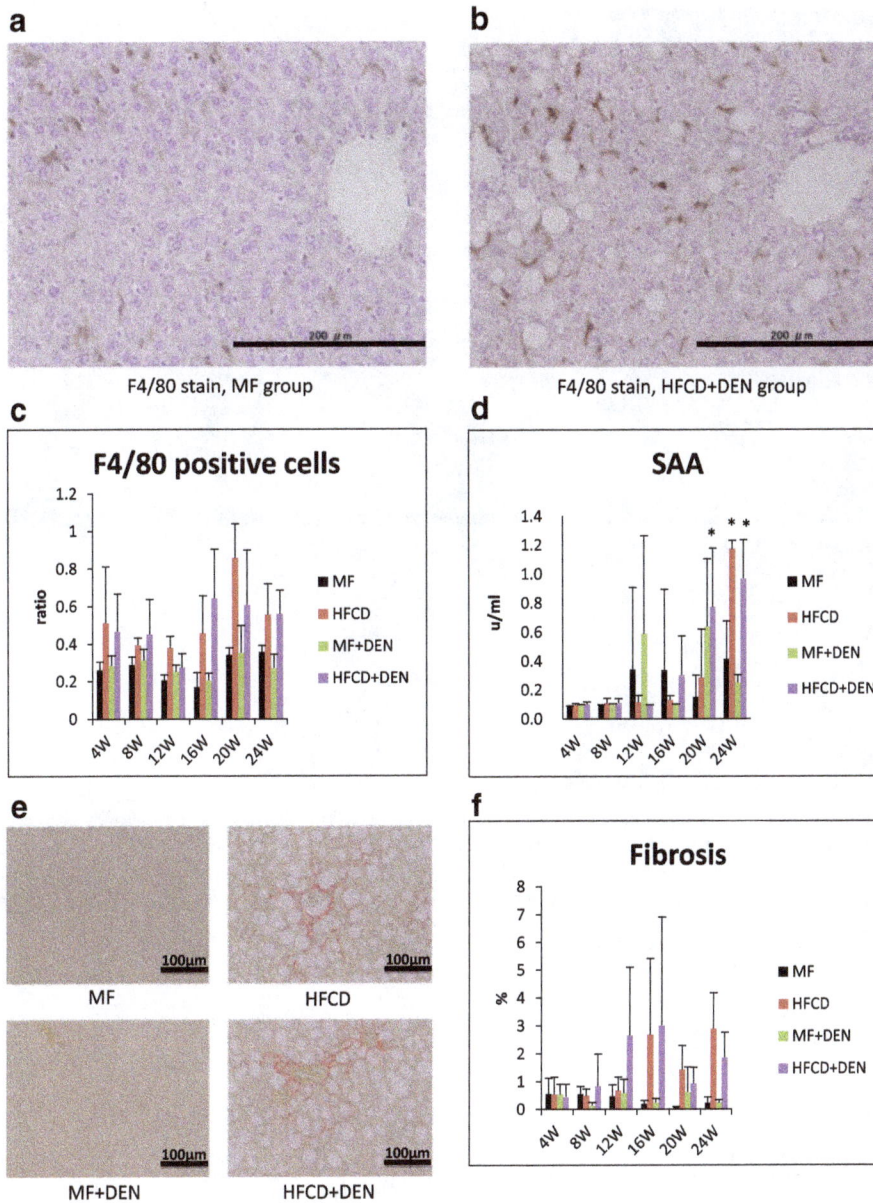

Fig. 5 Immunohistochemistry with F4/80 antibody (×200 original magnification) at 4 weeks: **a** standard diet (MF) group; **b** high-fat, choline-deficient diet (HFCD) + diethylnitrosamine (DEN) group; **c** the ratio of F4/80-positive cells (macrophages) to hepatocyte nuclei; **d** serum amyloid A (SAA) immunostaining; **e** representative images of liver sections stained with Sirius red at 24 weeks; and **f** proportion of fibrotic area measured using Histoquest. The data are shown as the mean + standard deviation

models. Thus, the HFCD + DEN model cannot assess the initiation step of NASH-HCC. However, the time to HCC development in our HFCD + DEN model is 20 weeks. This is the shortest among comparable models—the high-fat and fructose diet model, MUP-uPA transgenic mice with HFD, and MC4R knockout mice with HFD, which have 48, 32, and 48 weeks, respectively. Therefore, the HFCD + DEN model may be appropriate to assess how the NASH environment promotes HCC.

Our functional analysis extracted 13 genes from HFCD + DEN and 163 from HFD32 + DEN related to HCC. Expression of Rbbp6 in HFCD + DEN and HFD32 + DEN decreased (Fig. 7b). Rbbp6 is known to interact with MDM2, and it enhanced the affinity of MDM2 for p53, which led to the ubiquitination and degradation of p53 and repression of p53-dependent gene transcription. It would be interesting to explore in detail the differences in the cancer development mechanisms among those models. One limitation with this analysis is that the samples covered only a 4-week duration. We were thus unable to observe the long-term effects of gene expression. Further investigation is required to clarify this matter.

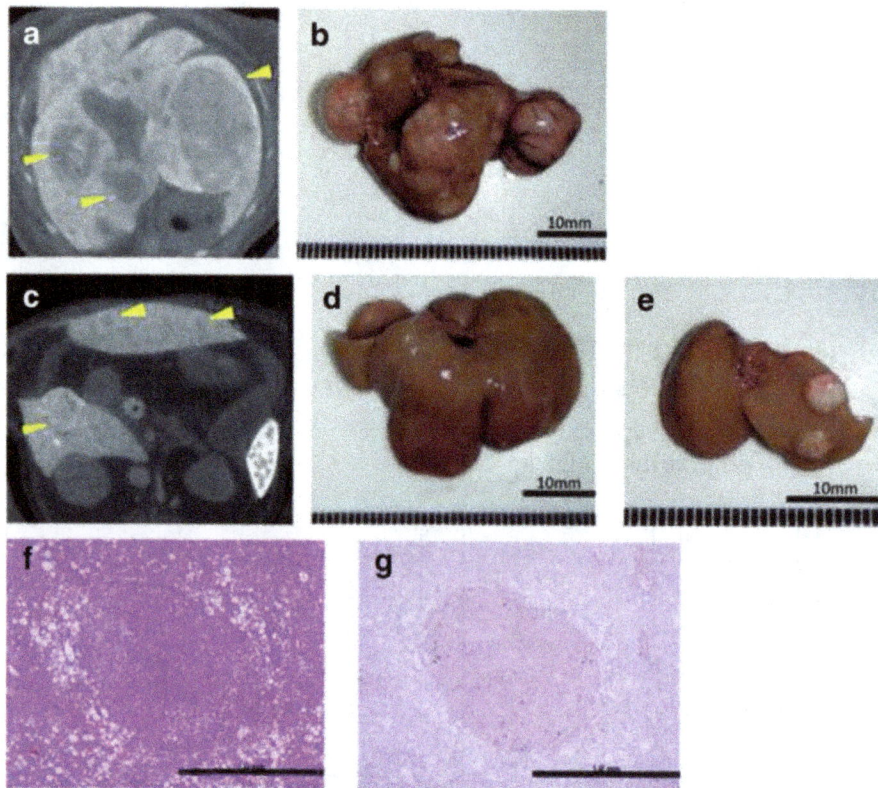

Fig. 6 Computed tomography scans and immunohistochemistry of hepatic tumors in the high-fat, choline-deficient (HFCD) + diethylnitrosamine (DEN) group at 24 weeks: **a**, **c** computed tomography findings; **b–e** macroscopic views. The image in **a** is a section of the whole liver depicted in **b**; the image in **c** is a section of the whole liver shown in **d**; and the image in panel **e** depicts the right and left medial lobes of the whole liver in panel **d**. The lesions are indicated by yellow arrowheads. **f** Hematoxylin-eosin staining of the liver tumor. **g** Immunohistochemical staining for glutamine synthetase

Table 4 Summary of computed tomography findings, rate of positive findings, tumor number, and tumor size from 12 to 24 weeks

	Week	MF	HFCD	MF + DEN	HFCD + DEN
Mice with positive findings, n (%)	12	0	0	0	0
	16	0	0	0	1/5 (20 %)
	20	0	1/5 (20 %)	0	**5/5 (100 %)**
	24	0	0	1/5 (20 %)	**5/5 (100 %)**
Tumor number	12	0	0	0	0
	16	0	0	0	5
	20	0	6	0	10.0 ± 5.4
	24	0	0	1	8.8 ± 5.4
Tumor size (mm)	12				
	16				0.6 ± 0.4
	20		0.8 ± 0.2		1.6 ± 0.8
	24			2.2	2.9 ± 2.8

Data are shown as the mean ± standard deviation. Data in bold indicate a significant difference ($p < 0.05$) between the standard diet (MF) group and the other groups for each month. *HFCD* high-fat choline-deficient diet, *DEN* diethylnitrosamine

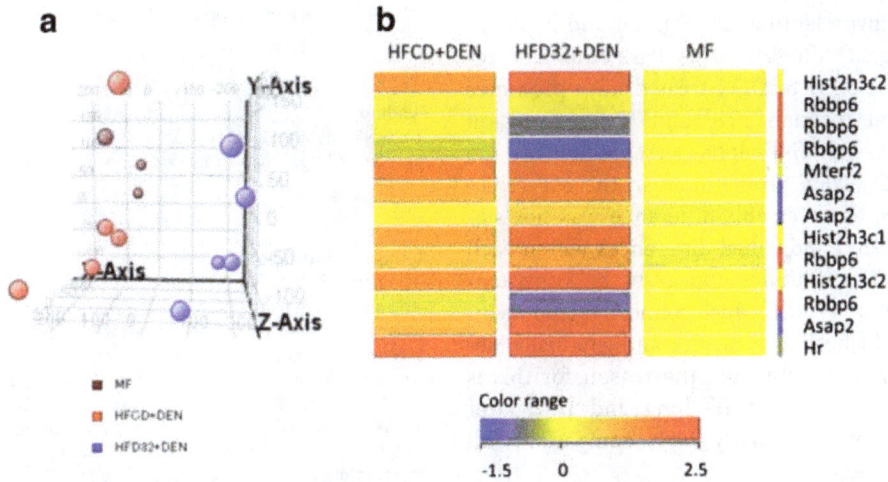

Fig. 7 Expression of MF, HFCD + DEN, and HFD32. **a** Principal component analysis of MF (brawn), HFCD + DEN (red), and HFD32 + DEN (blue). MF group contained three mice. HFCD + DEN and HFD32 + DEN group contained five mice. **b** Heat map of HCC-related genes common to both HFCD + DEN and HFD32 + DEN. DEN, diethylnitrosamine; standard diet (MF); HFCD, high-fat, choline-deficient diet; HFD32, high-fat diet

Insulin resistance is another essential feature of NASH, which is a hepatic manifestation of metabolic syndrome [34], and insulin resistance plays an important role in exacerbation of NASH. A number of NASH models with diabetes mellitus, such as the KK-A^y mouse on the MCD diet and mice fed an HFD combined with STZ, have been reported [20, 21]. The KK-A^y mouse is a genetically engineered diabetes mellitus model with insulin resistance, but it is unclear whether it exhibits carcinogenesis. STZ destroys the insulin-producing beta cells of the pancreas; therefore, mice receiving STZ develop type 1 diabetes mellitus owing to a lack of insulin secretion rather than through the de novo development of insulin resistance. In our study, most mice exhibited insulin resistance after 12 weeks (Table 2, Fig. 3).

Although a few mice in our model developed liver cirrhosis, we believe this model will be beneficial for studying NASH-HCC. Clinically, it is unclear whether cirrhosis is a prerequisite for the development of HCC in patients with NASH. Cirrhosis and advanced fibrosis appear to be the predominant risk factors for HCC development; however, 28 % of NASH-associated HCC cases have less advanced forms of fibrosis (stage 1 or 2), and fibrosis is more frequent in men [7].

Based on CT findings, all mice in the HFCD + DEN group, but no animals in the HFCD group, had liver tumors at 20 weeks (Table 4). Histologically, focal nodular hyperplasia and dysplasia were also present. Consistent with these findings, our immunohistochemistry results showed both GS-positive HCC (Fig. 6g) and GS-negative tumors.

Leptin is a peptide hormone produced by adipocytes and is involved in appetite control and energy expenditure [35]. Obese patients often have leptin resistance and high serum levels of leptin, which exacerbate obesity and hypertension owing to a sustained increase in sympathetic nerve activity. Hyperleptinemia is also related to hyper-responsiveness to low-dose endotoxin, which is

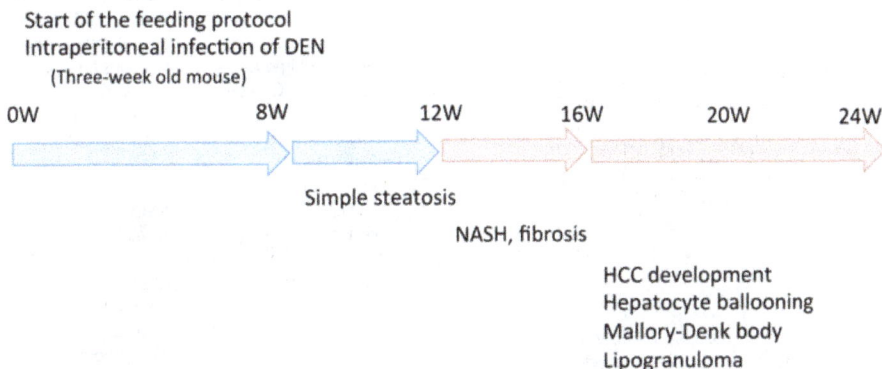

Fig. 8 Summary of the experimental model. DEN, diethylnitrosamine; HCC, hepatocellular carcinoma; NASH, nonalcoholic steatohepatitis

associated with NASH progression [36]. The mice in our model developed hyperleptinemia (Fig. 2e) and hypoadiponectinemia (Fig. 2f) after 20 weeks. Park et al. have reported that feeding HFD to DEN-treated mice promotes HCC development through TNF and IL-6 expression [37]. Serum levels of TNF-alpha were higher in the HFCD and HFCD + DEN groups than in the MF group at 4 and 8 weeks; however, this difference was not significant owing to large individual differences within each group (Table 1). Our findings appear to be consistent with those of another report, which found the adipocytokine level to be highest at 8 weeks and gradually decreased thereafter [21]. Although, the reason for this is unknown, serum levels of TNF-alpha and IL-6 after 12 weeks were not particularly high compared with those in the MF group.

Wolf et al. recently reported that long-term feeding an HFCD diet to mice can induce HCC, which depends on intrahepatic CD8+ T cells and NKT cells [38]. In our microarray analysis results, many genes known to affect the immune response exceeded the twofold cutoff.

A mouse model that bears the same clinical features as human NASH-HCC can be used for research into the treatment and chemoprevention of HCC resulting from NASH. One advantage of a mouse model is that a smaller drug amount is needed than with a rat model. Mice also have shorter generation times than rats. They are thus an efficient model for appropriate research by drug therapies. The most important advantage of a murine model is the anatomical and genetic similarity of mice to humans.

Conclusion

The NASH-HCC model we describe here is simple to establish, results in rapid tumor formation, and recapitulates most of the key features of NASH. It could therefore facilitate further studies into the development, oncogenic potential, diagnosis, and treatment of this condition.

Abbreviations

ALT, alanine aminotransferase; CRP, C-reactive protein; CT, computed tomography; DEN, diethylnitrosamine; FBS, fasting blood sugar; GS, glutamine synthetase; HCC, hepatocellular carcinoma; HFCD, high-fat, choline-deficient diet; HFD, high-fat diet; IL, interleukin; i.p, intraperitoneal; MCD, methionine- and choline-deficient diet; MF, standard diet; NAFLD, nonalcoholic fatty liver disease; NAS, NAFLD activity score; NASH, nonalcoholic steatohepatitis; SAA, serum amyloid A; TG, triglyceride; TNF, tumor necrosis factor

Acknowledgements

The authors thank Ms. Y. Nakamura, Ms. M. Matsuda, Ms. S. Matsuda, Ms. Y. Takagi, and Dr. S. Akimoto for their continued technical support. We are grateful to the Collaborative Research Resources, School of Medicine, Keio University for technical support and reagents.

Funding

This work was supported by a Grant-in Aid of Scientific Research C from Japan and Chugai Pharmaceutical as Endowed Research Chair.

Authors' contributions

NK conceived, designed, and performed the experiments, analyzed the data, and wrote the manuscript. SM conceived, designed, and performed the experiments, analyzed the data, and wrote the manuscript. OI conceived, designed, and performed the experiments, analyzed the data, and wrote the manuscript. MS analyzed the data. MK analyzed the data. HY analyzed the data. YA analyzed the data. TH analyzed the data. YM analyzed the data. MS analyzed the data. YK contributed reagents, materials, and analytical tools. KA contributed reagents, materials, and analytical tools. All authors read and approved the final version of the manuscript.

Competing interests

The authors have no potential conflicts of interest to disclose.

Consent for publication

Not applicable.

Author details

[1]Department of Surgery, School of Medicine, Keio University, 35 Shinanomachi, Shinjuku-ku, Tokyo 160-8582, Japan. [2]Chugai Pharmaceutical Endowed Research Chair in Molecular Targeted Therapy of Gastrointestinal Cancer, School of Medicine, Keio University, Tokyo, Japan. [3]Department of Pathology, School of Medicine, Keio University, Tokyo, Japan. [4]Department of Surgery, Kawasaki Municipal Hospital, Kawasaki-ku, Japan.

References

1. El-Serag HB. Hepatocellular carcinoma. N Engl J Med. 2011;365:1118–27.
2. Amarapurkar DN, Hashimoto E, Lesmana LA, Sollano JD, Chen PJ, Goh KL. How common is non-alcoholic fatty liver disease in the Asia-Pacific region and are there local differences? J Gastroenterol Hepatol. 2007;22:788–93.
3. Chitturi S, Farrell GC, Hashimoto E, Saibara T, Lau GK, Sollano JD. Non-alcoholic fatty liver disease in the Asia-Pacific region: definitions and overview of proposed guidelines. J Gastroenterol Hepatol. 2007;22:778–87.
4. Yasui K, Hashimoto E, Tokushige K, Koike K, Shima T, Kanbara Y, et al. Clinical and pathological progression of non-alcoholic steatohepatitis to hepatocellular carcinoma. Hepatol Res. 2012;42:767–73.
5. Polyzos SA, Kountouras J, Zavos C, Deretzi G. Nonalcoholic fatty liver disease: multimodal treatment options for a pathogenetically multiple-hit disease. J Clin Gastroenterol. 2012;46:272–84.
6. Okanoue T, Umemura A, Yasui K, Itoh Y. Nonalcoholic fatty liver disease and nonalcoholic steatohepatitis in Japan. J Gastroenterol Hepatol. 2011;26 Suppl 1:153–62.
7. Yasui K, Hashimoto E, Komorizono Y, Koike K, Arii S, Imai Y, et al. Characteristics of patients with nonalcoholic steatohepatitis who develop hepatocellular carcinoma. Clin Gastroenterol Hepatol. 2011;9:428–33. quiz e450.
8. Hashimoto E, Yatsuji S, Tobari M, Taniai M, Torii N, Tokushige K, et al. Hepatocellular carcinoma in patients with nonalcoholic steatohepatitis. J Gastroenterol. 2009;44 Suppl 19:89–95.
9. Yatsuji S, Hashimoto E, Tobari M, Taniai M, Tokushige K, Shiratori K. Clinical features and outcomes of cirrhosis due to non-alcoholic

steatohepatitis compared with cirrhosis caused by chronic hepatitis C. J Gastroenterol Hepatol. 2009;24:248–54.

10. Shimada M, Hashimoto E, Taniai M, Hasegawa K, Okuda H, Hayashi N, et al. Hepatocellular carcinoma in patients with non-alcoholic steatohepatitis. J Hepatol. 2002;37:154–60.

11. Marrero JA, Fontana RJ, Su GL, Conjeevaram HS, Emick DM, Lok AS. NAFLD may be a common underlying liver disease in patients with hepatocellular carcinoma in the United States. Hepatology. 2002;36:1349–54.

12. Bugianesi E, Leone N, Vanni E, Marchesini G, Brunello F, Carucci P, et al. Expanding the natural history of nonalcoholic steatohepatitis: from cryptogenic cirrhosis to hepatocellular carcinoma. Gastroenterology. 2002; 123:134–40.

13. Horie Y, Suzuki A, Kataoka E, Sasaki T, Hamada K, Sasaki J, et al. Hepatocyte-specific Pten deficiency results in steatohepatitis and hepatocellular carcinomas. J Clin Invest. 2004;113:1774–83.

14. Anstee QM, Goldin RD. Mouse models in non-alcoholic fatty liver disease and steatohepatitis research. Int J Exp Pathol. 2006;87:1–16.

15. Sahai A, Malladi P, Pan X, Paul R, Melin-Aldana H, Green RM, et al. Obese and diabetic db/db mice develop marked liver fibrosis in a model of nonalcoholic steatohepatitis: role of short-form leptin receptors and osteopontin. Am J Physiol Gastrointest Liver Physiol. 2004;287:G1035–43.

16. Deng QG, She H, Cheng JH, French SW, Koop DR, Xiong S, et al. Steatohepatitis induced by intragastric overfeeding in mice. Hepatology. 2005;42:905–14.

17. Hill-Baskin AE, Markiewski MM, Buchner DA, Shao H, DeSantis D, Hsiao G, et al. Diet-induced hepatocellular carcinoma in genetically predisposed mice. Hum Mol Genet. 2009;18:2975–88.

18. Raubenheimer PJ, Nyirenda MJ, Walker BR. A choline-deficient diet exacerbates fatty liver but attenuates insulin resistance and glucose intolerance in mice fed a high-fat diet. Diabetes. 2006;55:2015–20.

19. Weltman MD, Farrell GC, Liddle C. Increased hepatocyte CYP2E1 expression in a rat nutritional model of hepatic steatosis with inflammation. Gastroenterology. 1996;111:d1645–53.

20. Okumura K, Ikejima K, Kon K, Abe W, Yamashina S, Enomoto N, et al. Exacerbation of dietary steatohepatitis and fibrosis in obese, diabetic KK-A(y) mice. Hepatol Res. 2006;36:217–28.

21. Fujii M, Shibazaki Y, Wakamatsu K, Honda Y, Kawauchi Y, Suzuki K, et al. A murine model for non-alcoholic steatohepatitis showing evidence of association between diabetes and hepatocellular carcinoma. Med Mol Morphol. 2013;46:141–52.

22. Gans JH. Diethylnitrosamine-induced changes in mouse liver morphology and function. Proc Soc Exp Biol Med. 1976;153:116–20.

23. Travis CC, McClain TW, Birkner PD. Diethylnitrosamine-induced hepatocarcinogenesis in rats: a theoretical study. Toxicol Appl Pharmacol. 1991;109:289–304.

24. He XY, Smith GJ, Enno A, Nicholson RC. Short-term diethylnitrosamine-induced oval cell responses in three strains of mice. Pathology. 1994;26:154–60.

25. Onishi M, Sokuza Y, Nishikawa T, Mori C, Uwataki K, Honoki K, et al. Different mutation patterns of mitochondrial DNA displacement-loop in hepatocellular carcinomas induced by N-nitrosodiethylamine and a choline-deficient l-amino acid-defined diet in rats. Biochem Biophys Res Commun. 2007;362:183–7.

26. Shimizu K, Onishi M, Sugata E, Sokuza Y, Mori C, Nishikawa T, et al. Disturbance of DNA methylation patterns in the early phase of hepatocarcinogenesis induced by a choline-deficient L-amino acid-defined diet in rats. Cancer Sci. 2007;98:1318–22.

27. de Lima VM, Oliveira CP, Alves VA, Chammas MC, Oliveira EP, Stefano JT, et al. A rodent model of NASH with cirrhosis, oval cell proliferation and hepatocellular carcinoma. J Hepatol. 2008;49:1055–61.

28. Dowman JK, Hopkins LJ, Reynolds GM, Nikolaou N, Armstrong MJ, Shaw JC, et al. Development of hepatocellular carcinoma in a murine model of nonalcoholic steatohepatitis induced by use of a high-fat/fructose diet and sedentary lifestyle. Am J Pathol. 2014;184:1550–61.

29. Nakagawa H, Umemura A, Taniguchi K, Font-Burgada J, Dhar D, Ogata H, et al. ER stress cooperates with hypernutrition to trigger TNF-dependent spontaneous HCC development. Cancer Cell. 2014;26:331–43.

30. Itoh M, Suganami T, Nakagawa N, Tanaka M, Yamamoto Y, Kamei Y, et al. Melanocortin 4 receptor-deficient mice as a novel mouse model of nonalcoholic steatohepatitis. Am J Pathol. 2011;179:2454–63.

31. Paula Santos N, Colaco A, da Costa RM G, Manuel Oliveira M, Peixoto F, Alexandra Oliveira P. N-diethylnitrosamine mouse hepatotoxicity: Time-related effects on histology and oxidative stress. Exp Toxicol Pathol. 2014; 66(9-10):429–36.

32. Teufelhofer O, Parzefall W, Kainzbauer E, Ferk F, Freiler C, Knasmuller S, et al. Superoxide generation from Kupffer cells contributes to hepatocarcinogenesis: studies on NADPH oxidase knockout mice. Carcinogenesis. 2005;26:319–29.

33. Donnelly KL, Smith CI, Schwarzenberg SJ, Jessurun J, Boldt MD, Parks EJ. Sources of fatty acids stored in liver and secreted via lipoproteins in patients with nonalcoholic fatty liver disease. J Clin Invest. 2005;115:1343–51.

34. Chitturi S, Abeygunasekera S, Farrell GC, Holmes-Walker J, Hui JM, Fung C, et al. NASH and insulin resistance: Insulin hypersecretion and specific association with the insulin resistance syndrome. Hepatology. 2002;35:373–9.

35. Brennan AM, Mantzoros CS. Drug Insight: the role of leptin in human physiology and pathophysiology–emerging clinical applications. Nat Clin Pract Endocrinol Metab. 2006;2:318–27.

36. Imajo K, Fujita K, Yoneda M, Nozaki Y, Ogawa Y, Shinohara Y, et al. Hyperresponsivity to low-dose endotoxin during progression to nonalcoholic steatohepatitis is regulated by leptin-mediated signaling. Cell Metab. 2012;16:44–54.

37. Park EJ, Lee JH, Yu GY, He G, Ali SR, Holzer RG, et al. Dietary and genetic obesity promote liver inflammation and tumorigenesis by enhancing IL-6 and TNF expression. Cell. 2010;140:197–208.

38. Wolf MJ, Adili A, Piotrowitz K, Abdullah Z, Boege Y, Stemmer K, et al. Metabolic activation of intrahepatic CD8+ T cells and NKT cells causes nonalcoholic steatohepatitis and liver cancer via cross-talk with hepatocytes. Cancer Cell. 2014;26:549–64.

20

Comparative experimental investigation on the efficacy of mono- and multiprobiotic strains in non-alcoholic fatty liver disease prevention

Nazarii Kobyliak[1][*] (iD), Tetyana Falalyeyeva[2], Oleksandr Virchenko[2], Galyna Mykhalchyshyn[1], Petro Bodnar[1], Mykola Spivak[3], Dmytro Yankovsky[4], Tetyana Beregova[2] and Lyudmyla Ostapchenko[2]

Abstract

Background: To investigate the efficacy of different probiotic strains, their combinations and forms (alive or lyophilized) in nonalcoholic fatty liver disease (NAFLD) prevention.

Methods: In this study, 70 rats have been used divided into 7 groups of 10 animals in each: I – intact rats, II-VII – rats with monosodium glutamate (MSG)-induced NAFLD. Rats with NAFLD were untreated (group II, MSG-obesity group) and treated with probiotics (groups III–VII). In order to develop NAFLD, newborn rats of groups II–VII were injected with a solution of monosodium glutamate (MSG) (4 mg/g) subcutaneously (s.c.) at 2nd,4th, 6th, 8th,10th postnatal day. The groups III–V received lyophilized monoprobiotics *B. animalis VKL*, *B. animalis VKB*, *L.casei IMVB-7280*, respectively. The group VI received 2.5 ml/kg of an aqueous solution of a mixture of the three probiotic strains (2:1:1 *Lactobacillus casei IMVB-7280, Bifidobacterium animalis VKL, Bifidobacterium animalis VKB*) at a dose of 50 mg/kg (5×10^9 CFU/kg) (g) (intragastrically). The group VII was treated with multiprobiotic "Symbiter" containing biomass of 14 alive probiotic strains (*Lactobacillus + Lactococcus* (6×10^{10} CFU/g), *Bifidobacterium* (1×10^{10}/g), *Propionibacterium* (3×10^{10}/g), *Acetobacter* (1×10^6/g)) at a dose of 140 mg/kg (1.4×10^{10} CFU/kg). The treatment with probiotics was started at the age of 1 month. There were 3 courses of treatment, each included 2-week administration and 2-week break. All parameters were measured in 4-month aged rats.

Results: Introduction of MSG during the neonatal period leads to the NAFLD development in the 4-months old rats. For steatosis degree there was no significant difference between MSG-obesity group and lyophilized monocomponent probiotics groups (III–V). The highest manifestation of steatosis was observed for *B. animalis VKL* group (2.0 ± 0.25) as compared to *B. animalis VKB* (1.70 ± 0.21) and *L. casei IMVB-7280* (1.80 ± 0.20). The steatosis score changes between all monoprobiotics groups (III–V) were insignificant. Administration from birth of both alive (VII) and lyophilized (VI) probiotic mixture lead to a significant decrease by 69.5 % ($p < 0.001$) and 43.5 % ($p < 0.025$) of steatosis score respectively as compared to the MSG-obesity group (2.3 ± 0.21 %). For both alive and lyophilized probiotic mixtures, reduction of lobular inflammation was observed. These histological data were confirmed by the significant decrease of total lipids and triglycerides content in the liver approximately by 22–25 % in groups treated with probiotic mixtures (VI, VII) compared to the MSG-obesity group.

(Continued on next page)

* Correspondence: nazariikobyliak@gmail.com
[1]Bogomolets National Medical University, T. Shevchenko boulevard, 13, Kyiv 01601, Ukraine
Full list of author information is available at the end of the article

(Continued from previous page)

Conclusion: We established failure of NAFLD prevention with lyophilized monoprobiotic strains and the efficacy of probiotic mixture with the preference of alive probiotic strains.

Keywords: NAFLD, Prevention, Obesity, Lyophilized and alive probiotic strains, Monoprobiotic, Multistrain probiotics

Background

Non-alcoholic fatty liver disease (NAFLD) ranges from simple steatosis to non-alcoholic steatohepatitis (NASH) that can have different degrees of fibrosis and progress to liver cirrhosis and hepatocellular carcinoma [1]. NAFLD that is associated with obesity and type 2 diabetes has a prevalence of 15–20 % in the general population and 76–90 % in the obese [2]. NAFLD is currently a leading cause of chronic liver disease [3, 4], which has resulted in significant health concerns such as morbidity, mortality, and liver transplants [5].

According to Day's two-hit model of NAFLD pathogenesis insulin resistance as the first hit, causes lipid accumulation in hepatocytes and leads to the development of fatty liver. The second hit includes cellular insults such as oxidative stress and lipid oxidation, which damages the liver cells and triggers an inflammatory process that leads to pathological changes in hepatocytes that result in NASH [6]. Recent studies present a clear evidence that gut microbiota are strongly implicated in NAFLD pathogenesis and progression through several mechanisms [7].

The underlying mechanisms, which link altered gut microbiota composition to NAFLD are modulation of dietary choline metabolism [8] and production of endogenous ethanol [9], increased gut permeability [10] with subsequent endotoxemia and metabolic low-grade inflammation [11], increased energy harvest from the diet [12] and impaired short-chain fatty acids synthesis [13], decreased absorbtion of vitamins and biologically active compounds [12], altered bile acids metabolism, and FXR/TGR5 signaling [14]. Prebiotics and probiotics have physiologic functions that contribute to the health of gut microbiota and/or restoration of microflora, maintenance of a healthy body weight and control of factors associated with NAFLD through the various above mentioned pathways [15].

In our previous work, we have shown that periodic treatment with multiprobiotic containing biomass of 14 alive strains (*Lactobacillus, Lactococcus, Bifidobacterium, Propionibacterium, Acetobacter*) prevents, at least partially, the MSG-induced obesity [16] and NAFLD development [17]. However the question regarding the efficacy of different probiotic strains, their combination and form (alive or lyophilized) in the management of NAFLD remains open, which formed the current study aims.

Methods
Animals

This study was carried out in strict accordance with the recommendations in the Guide for the Care and Use of Laboratory Animals of the National Institutes of Health and the general ethical principles of animal experiments, approved by the First National Congress on Bioethics Ukraine (September 2001). The protocol was approved by the Committee on the Ethics of Animal Experiments of the Taras Shevchenko National University of Kyiv (Protocol number: 10/2014). The rats were kept in collective cages under controlled conditions of temperature (22 ± 3 °C), light (12 h light/dark cycle) and relative humidity (60 ± 5 %). The animals were fed laboratory chow (PurinaW) and tap water ad libitum.

Experiment design

The study included 70 male Wistar rats divided into 7 groups, of 10 animals in each (Fig. 1). Newborns rats of the control group (I) were administered with saline subcutaneously (s.c.) in the volume of 8 μl/g at 2nd, 4th, 6th, 8th and 10th postnatal days. Newborns rats of groups II–VII were injected with monosodium glutamate solution (MSG) (4.0 mg/g of body weight) s.c. at 2nd, 4th, 6th, 8th and 10th postnatal days [18]. Neonatal administration of MSG causes the significant accumulation of fat in the abdomen of the adult rats. This happens because of the neurotoxicity effects on the arcuate and ventromedial nuclei of the hypothalamus [19]. In our previous work, we have shown the development of NAFLD under conditions of the severe visceral obesity induced by MSG [17]. Thus, the obtained results confirmed the validity of the usage of MSG for NAFLD development.

The groups III–VII were treated with probiotics. The groups III–V received lyophilized monoprobiotics *B. animalis VKL*, *B. animalis VKB*, *L. casei IMVB-7280* respectively. The group VI received the mix of these three probiotic strains. The group VII was treated with multiprobiotic "Symbiter" which was supplied by Scientific and Production Company "O.D. Prolisok". It contains of 14 alive probiotic strains of *Lactobacillus* + *Lactococcus* (6×10^{10} CFU/g), *Bifidobacterium* (1×10^{10}/g), *Propionibacterium* (3×10^{10}/g), *Acetobacter* (1×10^{6}/g) genera.

Administration was started at the end of the 4th week after birth and continued intermittently by alternating a 2-week course and 2 weeks intervals of nontreatment.

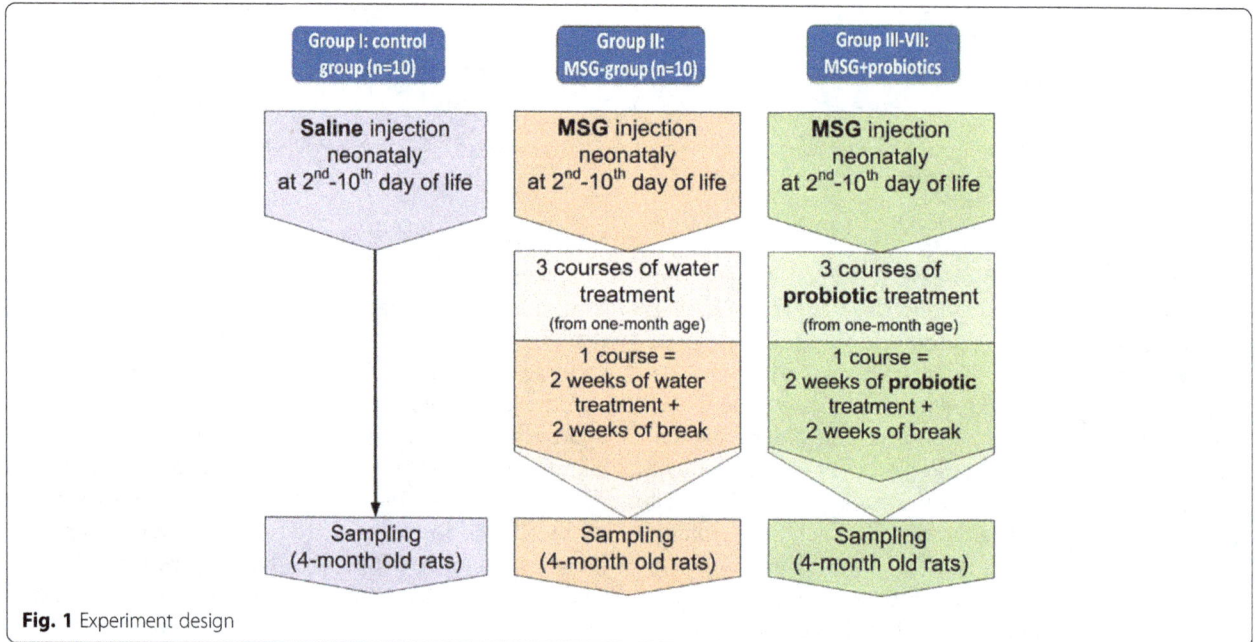

Fig. 1 Experiment design

Within 4 months after birth rats were on a normal diet. All parameters were measured in 4-months old rats.

Sample collection and blood biochemistry analysis

Rats of all groups were fasted for approximately 12 h prior sacrifice. Rats were sacrificed by cervical dislocation under urethane anesthesia. Blood was drawn from the apex of the cardiac ventricle and few blood drops were collected into a microcentrifuge tube containing a mixture of NaF and EDTA at a 2:1 (w/w) ratio. Blood sample was collected into a sterile tube and centrifuged at 3500 rpm (2260 g) for 15 min. After centrifugation serum supernatant for further analysis was aliquoted into microcentrifuge tubes and stored at −80 °C. Bilirubin, activity of alanine and aspartate aminotransferase in serum were determined by the standard biochemical methods.

Liver histology assessment

For histological analysis liver tissue samples from both the right and left hepatic lobes were taken (sample size 0.5 × 0.5 cm). After fixation for 24 h in a liquid Buena, liver fragments were dehydrated in alcohol of increasing concentrations (from 70 to 96 °), embedded in paraffin and then cut with a thickness of 5–6 microns and stained with hematoxylin-eosin. A pathologist blinded to group distributions performed the histological analyses of slides using light microscopy («Olympus», Japan). To assess morphological changes in the liver we used NAS (NAFLD activity score), which includes histological features and has been defined as unweighted sum of scores for steatosis (0–3), lobular inflammation (0–3) and ballooning (0–2). According to NAS scores ≥5 are diagnosed as non-alcoholic steatohepatitis (NASH), and cases with a NAS <3 are mentioned as not NASH [20]. Lipid extraction from the liver was performed according to Folch et al. [21].

Statistical analysis

Statistical analysis was performed with the SPSS-20 software. All data in this study were expressed as means ± standard error of the mean (M ± SEM) or %.

Table 1 Liver function tests of rats under MSG-induced obesity and probiotic correction

Parameters	Control rats (n = 10)	MSG-induced obesity (n = 10)	B. animalis VKL (n = 10)	B. animalis VKB (n = 10)	L. casei IMVB-7280 (n = 10)	Poliprobiotics (n = 10)	Symbiter (n = 10)
Total bilirubin, umol/l	12.9 ± 0.73	12.6 ± 0.58	13.6 ± 0.68	12.5 ± 0.3	13.3 ± 0.63	12.4 ± 0.47	13.4 ± 0.63
Indirect bilirubin, umol/l	8.3 ± 0.55	8.2 ± 0.35	8.6 ± 0.47	8.2 ± 0.29	8.5 ± 0.5	8.3 ± 0.33	8.3 ± 0.53
Direct bilirubin, mmol/l	4.6 ± 0.33	4.4 ± 0.3	5.0 ± 0.29	4.3 ± 0.26	4.8 ± 0.29	4.1 ± 0.27	5.1 ± 0.23
ALT, mkkat/l	0.231 ± 0.011	0.243 ± 0.015	0.230 ± 0.013	0.209 ± 0.010	0.221 ± 0.008	0.211 ± 0.014	0.212 ± 0.007
AST, mkkat/l	0.386 ± 0.007	0.397 ± 0.011	0.396 ± 0.015	0.382 ± 0.011	0.389 ± 0.014	0.373 ± 0.016	0.381 ± 0.018

Data are presented as the M ± SEM. One-way ANOVA or Kruskall-Wallis test were performed for data analysis. All differences were not significant ($p > 0.05$)

Table 2 Morphological changes in the rat liver assessed by NAFLD activity score (NAS)

Parameters	Intact rats (n = 10)	MSG-induced obesity (n = 10)	B. animalis VKL (n = 10)	B. animalis VKB (n = 10)	L. casei IMVB-7280 (n = 10)	Poliprobiotics (n = 10)	Symbiter (n = 10)
Steatosis (0–3)	0.10 ± 0.1^a	2.30 ± 0.21^d	2.0 ± 0.25^{cd}	1.70 ± 0.21^{cd}	1.80 ± 0.20^{cd}	1.30 ± 0.3^{bc}	0.70 ± 0.15^{ab}
Lobular inflammation (0–2)	0.0 ± 0.0^a	1.0 ± 0.21^b	0.60 ± 0.16^{ab}	0.40 ± 0.16^{ab}	0.40 ± 0.16^{ab}	0.30 ± 0.15^a	0.10 ± 0.1^a
Ballooning degeneration (0–2)	0.0 ± 0.0^a	0.20 ± 0.13^a	0.10 ± 0.1^a	0.10 ± 0.1^a	0.10 ± 0.1^a	0.0 ± 0.0^a	0.0 ± 0.0^a
Total NAS (0–8)	0.0 ± 0.0^a	3.60 ± 0.4^d	2.70 ± 0.36^{cd}	2.2 ± 0.25^c	2.30 ± 0.21^c	1.60 ± 0.3^{bc}	0.80 ± 0.2^{ab}
Prevalence of NASH, %	–	30	10	–	–	–	–

Data are presented as the M ± SEM. One-way ANOVA with post hoc Tukeys test for multiple comparisons were performed for data analysis. [a, b, c, d] Values at the same row with different superscript letters show significant differences at $p < 0.05$

Data distribution was analyzed using the Kolmogorov-Smirnov normality test. Continuous variables with parametric distribution were analyzed using Analysis of Variance (ANOVA) and if the results were significant, a post-hoc Tukeys test was performed. For data with non-parametric distribution Kruskall-Wallis and post-hoc Dunn's test were conducted for multiple comparisons. For comparisons of categorical variables we conducted χ^2 test. The difference between groups was defined to be statistically significant when a p-value was less than 0.05.

Results

We didn't find any significant difference in biochemical indicators (alanine transaminase (ALT), aspartate transaminase (AST), bilirubin) of liver in blood serum between intact, MSG-obesity and MSG-probiotics group (Table 1).

Liver histology changes, as assessed by the NAS score, associated with the administration of different types of probiotics are represented in Table 2. For steatosis degree there was no significant difference between the MSG-obesity group and lyophilized monocomponent probiotics groups (III–V) (Fig. 2a-d). The highest manifestation of steatosis was observed for B. animalis VKL group (2.0 ± 0.25) as compared to B. animalis VKB (1.70 ± 0.21) and L. casei IMVB-7280 (1.80 ± 0.20). The steatosis score changes between all monoprobiotics groups (III–V) were insignificant. Administration from birth of both alive (VII) and lyophilized (VI) probiotic mixture lead to a significant decrease by 69.5 % ($p < 0.001$) and 43.5 % ($p = 0.025$) of steatosis score respectively as compared to the MSG-obesity group (2.3 ± 0.21) (Fig. 3a and b).

Similar to steatosis score changes we found that administration of both alive and lyophilized probiotic

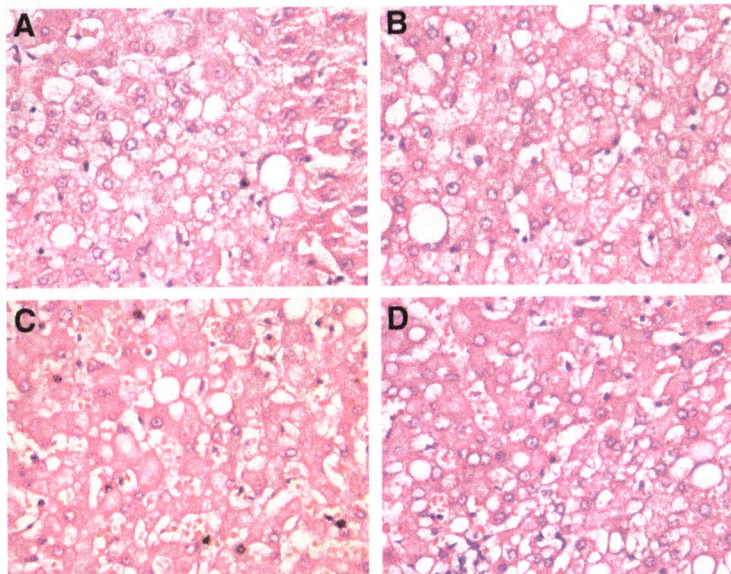

Fig. 2 Light microscopic micrographs of the rat liver tissue stained with hematoxylin and eosin, ×400. In micrographs predominantly microvesicular pronounced total steatosis were mainly observed. **a** - MSG-induced obesity group; **b** - B. animalis VKL group; **c** - B. animalis VKB group; **d** - L. casei IMVB-7280 group

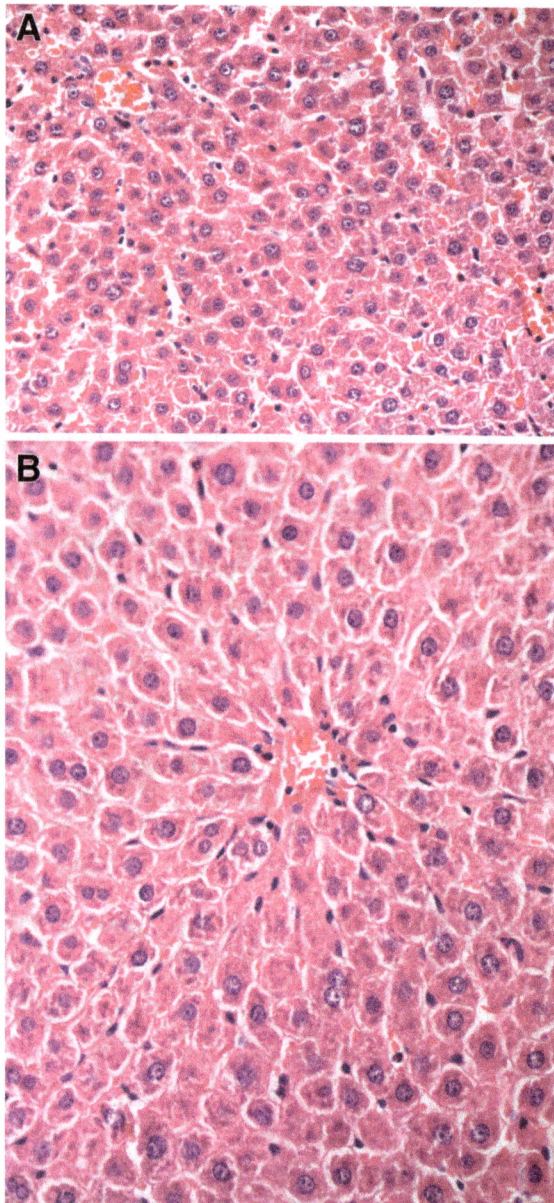

Fig. 3 Light microscopic micrographs of the rat liver tissue stained with hematoxylin and eosin, ×400. In micrographs focal mild microvesicular steatosis were mainly observed. **a** - Poliprobiotics group; **b** - Symbiter group

NAS score between MSG-induced obesity group and lyophilized monocomponent probiotics groups (III–V) were not found. The most prominent changes from all lyophilized groups were described for *B. animalis VKL*. Only in this group we diagnosed NASH in 10 % of animals that was significant ($p = 0.026$) as compared to MSG-obesity group with 30 % of animals with NASH. All groups were typically relative in histological presentation of ballooning degeneration due to the absence of any significant difference ($p > 0.05$) (Table 2).

The lowest total NAS score was observed after administration of alive multiprobiotic group (0.8 ± 0.2) that were insignificant in control rats and statistically lower as compared to all monoprobiotics groups (III–V). When used lyophilized (VI) probiotic mixture changes in total NAS score between other treated were insignificant.

In parallel with improving of total NAS score for both policomponent probiotic mixture, we observed a significant decrease of total lipids and triglycerides content in liver approximately by 22–25 % respectively as compared to the MSG-obesity group (Fig. 5a and b). After administration of lyophilized monocomponents probiotics (groups III–V) the changes in the amount of liver lipids were insignificant.

Discussion

Our study conclusively showed that short-term courses of probiotic mixtures from birth have a preventive effect on fatty liver disease development under condition of the MSG-induced obesity. Nevertheless therapeutic potential are more pronounced for alive probiotic multistrain mixture (VII) because only for Symbiter group significantly lower degree of steatosis and total NAS score were detected as compared to monocomponent probiotics groups (III–V) and any significant changes in liver histology assessment parameters were not found compared with intact rats.

In particular, different *Lactobacillus* та *Bifidobacterium* strains have specific effects on the markers of obesity in rodent models. The analysis of from the literature data published from January 2013 to July 2014 by Cani et al. showed that at least 15 different strains of *Lactobacillus* and 3 strains of *Bifidobacterium* do not equally influence hepatic lipids and NAFLD development in different animal models. Remarkably, 12 strains decreased hepatic tissue inflammation and 11 reduced the hepatic triglyceride content when given as a single treatment [22].

In contrast to our study, where we did not notice any significant single-strain specific changes in lipid metabolism and NAFLD development, a recent study compared the effects of four *Bifidobacteria* strains (*Bifidobacteria* L66-5, L75-4, M13-4 and FS31-12) on lipid metabolism in an high-fat diet obese mice. All

mixtures from 4th week after birth lead to a significant reduction of liver inflammation manifestation in the adulthood period in rats when compared with littermates with MSG-induced obesity. In the liver histology sections NASH specific lesions were observed. Specifically, the inflammation was mild and predominantly lobular rather than portal, with typically mixed infiltrates, which included chronic inflammatory cell phenotypes, such as lymphocytes, monocytes (Fig. 4a-d). Any significant changes in lobular inflammation as assessed by

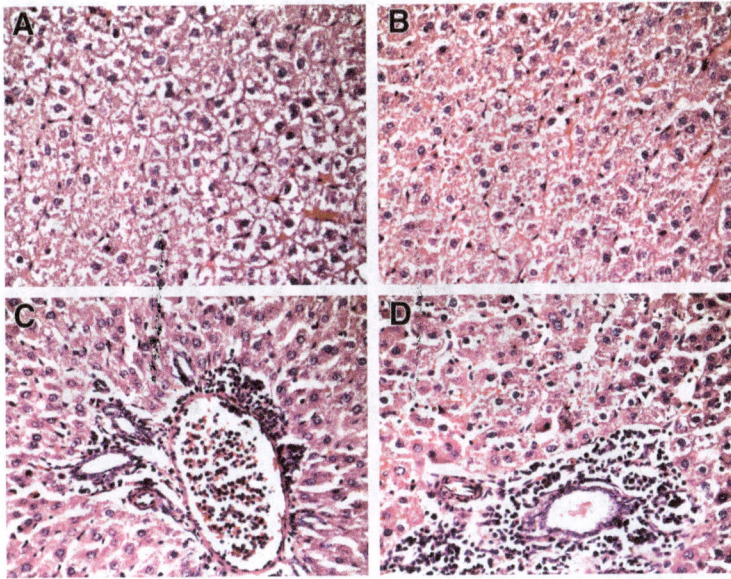

Fig. 4 Light microscopic micrographs of the rat liver tissue stained with hematoxylin and eosin, ×400. In micrographs microvesicular steatosis with perivascular leukocyte infiltration at zone 3 (mild lobular inflammation) (**c, d**) and focal necrosis as a result of hepatocytes ballooning degeneration – lack of nuclei (in center) (**a, b**) was observed. **a** - MSG-induced obesity group; **b** - B. *animalis* VKL group; **c** - B. *animalis* VKB group; **d** - L. *casei* IMVB-7280 group

the four strains could reduce serum and liver triglyceride and significantly alleviate the lipid deposition in the liver. As for total cholesterol only *Bifidobacteria* L66-5 and *Bifidobacteria* FS31-12 significantly decreased its amount in the liver [23].

Administration of single-strain probiotic of *Lactobacillus rhamnosus GG* protects mice from NAFLD development induced by a high-fructose diet through an increase of beneficial bacteria, restoration of the gut barrier function and subsequent attenuation of liver inflammation and steatosis [24]. Another study demonstrated that treatment with *Lactobacillus rhamnosus GG* for 13 weeks under condition of high fat diet improved insulin sensitivity and reduced lipid accumulation by stimulating adiponectin secretion and consequent activation of AMPK [25].

In addition, it was reported that an oral supplementation of *Bifidobacterium adolescentis* $(5 \times 10(7)$ CFU/ml) ad libitum for 12 weeks protected against a diet-induced NASH in C57BL/6 mice. Furthermore, mice treated with probiotic had significantly decreased liver damage, which was associated with prevention from lipid peroxidation, NFκB activation and finally inflammation in the liver [26].

On the other hand, our data find support in another recent study that established that single-strain probiotics of *Lactobacillus curvatus HY7601* significantly reduced liver fat accumulation as compared to *Lactobacillus plantarum KY1032* in diet-induced obesity. Combination of this probiotic was more effective for inhibiting gene expressions of various enzymes responsible for fatty acid synthesis in the liver, concomitant with decreases in fatty acid oxidation-related enzyme activities and their gene expressions [27].

Plaza-Diaz in Zucker rats with genetic determined obesity evaluated the effects of *Lactobacillus paracasei CNCM I-4034*, *Bifidobacterium breve CNCM I-4035* and *Lactobacillus rhamnosus CNCM I-4036* probiotic strains and their mixture on the hepatic steatosis development as compared to placebo. In this study only single-strain probiotic of *Lactobacillus rhamnosus or Bifidobacterium breve* and the mixture of *Bifidobacterium breve* and *Lactobacillus paracasei* decreased triacylglycerol content in the rat liver and reduced manifestation of hepatic steatosis in part by lowering serum LPS [28].

The improvement of NAFLD by probiotics strains can be achieved by various pathways. Mei et al. (2015) have shown that decrease in triglycerides level, total cholesterol, free fatty acids, and cholesterol low-density lipoproteins is associated with an increased uptake of cholesterol from the blood, its excretion with bile by the liver, and reduction of cholesterol synthesis under conditions of probiotic treatment of NAFLD [29]. Contrary to our findings, the scientists established the effectiveness of monostrains of *Lactobacillus* species. The influence of probiotics on lipid metabolism was associated with up- and downregulation of certain genes. The team has found an overexpression of low-density lipoproteins receptor that enhances the absorption of low-density lipoproteins by the liver. Besides, cholesterol 7α-hydroxylase

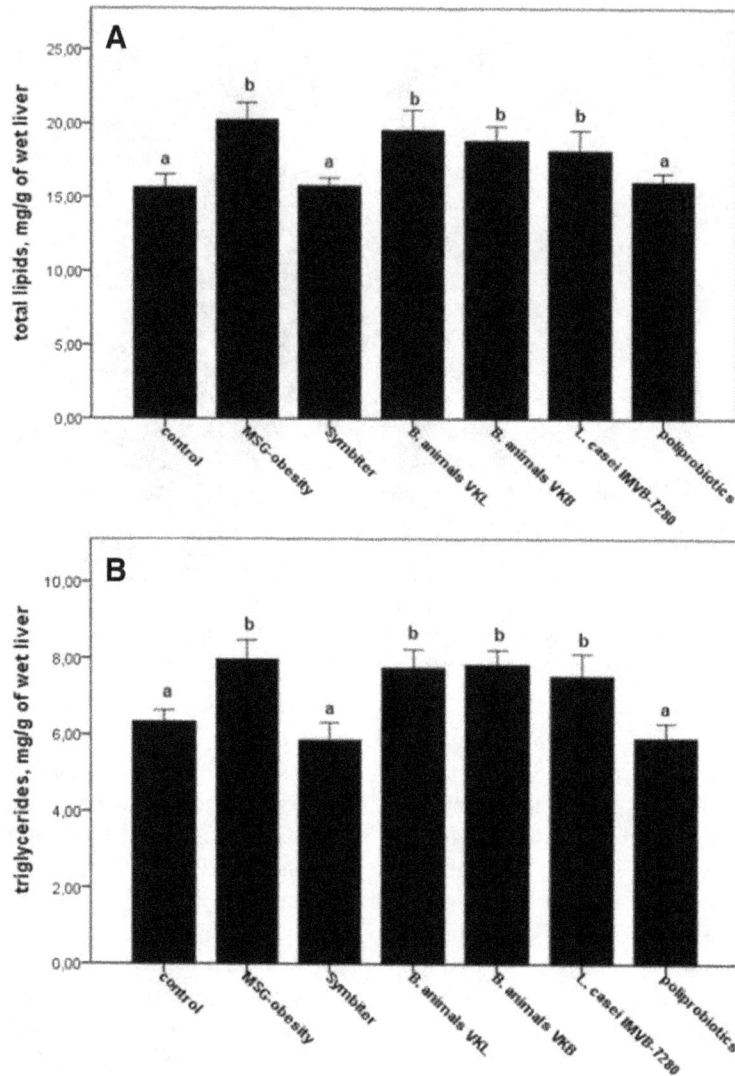

Fig. 5 Liver total lipids (**a**) and triglycerides (**b**) content of rats with the MSG-induced obesity and probiotic correction. Data are presented as the M ± SEM. One-way ANOVA with post hoc Tukeys test for multiple comparisons were performed for data analysis. [a, b] Values at the same row with different superscript letters show significant differences at $p < 0.05$

activity was elevated that proves the enhanced excretion of cholesterol with bile. Moreover, the farnesoid X receptor was up-regulated indicating the increased bile acid production. The reduction of cholesterol synthesis by probiotics was confirmed by the downregulation of 3-hydroxy-3-methyl glutaryl coenzyme A reductase and sterol regulatory element binding protein-1c. In addition, PPAR-α expression was high and PPAR-γ was low in rats with NAFLD and treated with probiotic strains that diverts lipid metabolism from fat deposition to β-oxidation of fatty acids [29].

Some light on the underlying mechanisms of probiotic impact was shed. It is known that symbiotic bacteria can produce short chain fatty acids, e.g. butyrate. This substance inhibits the activation of toll-like receptor (TLR)-dependent signalling cascades in the liver through strengthening gut tight junction, and reduction of bacterial endotoxin translocation to the liver that was shown on the model of western-style diet-induced NAFLD [30]. It was established that butyrate prevented lipid peroxidation through the reduction of 4-hydroxynonenal protein adducts level and downregulates inducible nitric oxide synthase that is critical for regulation not only NF-κB-depending signalling cascades in the development of NAFLD but also for expression of the TLR-4 adaptor protein myeloid differentiation primary response gene 88. Thus, production of butyrate results in attenuation of inflammation and TLR-dependent signalling in the liver under conditions of experimental NAFLD [30].

Conclusions

Postnatal administration of both alive (VII) and lyophilized (VI) probiotic mixture lead to significant decrease of hepatic steatosis, total lipids and triglycerides content in the liver as compared to MSG-obesity and may be more beneficial than single-strain probiotics. Thus, multicomponent probiotics have a preventive effect on fatty liver disease development. It may be related to more pronounced viability of the alive strains and their prevention of bacterial translocation. Multistrain or multispecies formed mutualistic interactions in mixtures and therefore were able to share with different metabolites, affect different receptors and produced various biologically active compounds. So, their synergistic overall effect is greater than the sum of their individual effects. On the other hand, most likely due to different putative mechanisms of action, strain-specific probiotics must be considered for novel investigation in different metabolic diseases.

Abbreviations

ANOVA: Analysis of Variance; NAFLD: non-alcoholic fatty liver disease; NASH: non-alcoholic steatohepatitis; TLR: toll-like receptor.

Competing interests

The authors declare that they have no competing interests.

Authors' contributions

PB, MS, DY, TB and LO designed the research. OV collected data and did sample analyses. NK, TF and GM analyzed data. NK, OV and TF wrote the manuscript. All authors have read and approved the final version to be published.

Authors' information

NK - PhD, assistant of Endocrinology Department, Bogomolets National Medical University.
OV - PhD, SRL 'Pharmacology and Experimental Pathology', Department of Biological and Biomedical Technology, ESC 'Institute of Biology', Taras Shevchenko National University of Kyiv.
FT - Ph.D., D.Sci., researcher of RL "Pharmacology and Experimental Pathology" Department of Biological and Biomedical Technology ESC «Institute of Biology» Taras Shevchenko National University of Kyiv.
GM, Ph.D., Assosiate Professor of Endocrinology Department, Bogomolets National Medical University.
PB, Ph.D., D.Sci., is a Professor, head of Endocrinology Department, Bogomolets National Medical University.
MYS Ph.D., D.Sci., is a Professor, a corresponding member of the National Academy of Sciences of Ukraine and the director of the Inteferon Department of Zabolotny Institute of Microbiology and Virology, NAS of Ukraine.
TB - Professor, Ph.D., D.Sci., SRL 'Pharmacology and Experimental Pathology', Department of Biological and Biomedical Technology, ESC 'Institute of Biology', Taras Shevchenko National University of Kyiv.
LO - Professor, Ph.D., D.Sci., SRL 'Pharmacology and Experimental Pathology', Head of Department of Biological and Biomedical Technology, ESC 'Institute of Biology', Taras Shevchenko National University of Kyiv.

Acknowledgment

We acknowledge the BMC Gastroenterology journal editorial team and BioMed Central team for the opportunity to publish this work.

Funding

The study was funded from the departmental resources.

Author details

[1]Bogomolets National Medical University, T. Shevchenko boulevard, 13, Kyiv 01601, Ukraine. [2]Taras Shevchenko National University of Kyiv, Volodymyrska Str., 64/13, Kyiv 01601, Ukraine. [3]Zabolotny Institute of Microbiology and Virology, National Academy of Sciences of Ukraine, Zabolotny Str., 154, Kyiv 03680, Ukraine. [4]Scientific and Production Company "O.D. Prolisok", Kyiv, Ukraine.

References

1. Kobyliak N, Abenavoli L. The role of liver biopsy to assess non-alcoholic fatty liver disease. Rev Recent Clin Trials. 2014;9:159–69.
2. Angulo P. Medical progress: nonalcoholic fatty liver disease. N Engl J Med. 2002;346:1221–31.
3. Farrell GC, Larter CZ. Nonalcoholic fatty liver disease: from steatosis to cirrhosis. Hepatology. 2006;43:99–112.
4. Weston SR, Leyden W, Murphy R, Bass NM, Bell BP, Manos MM. Racial and ethnic distribution of nonalcoholic fatty liver in persons with newly diagnosed chronic liver disease. Hepatology. 2005;41:372–9.
5. Musso G, Gambino R, Cassader M, Pagano G. Meta-analysis: natural history of nonalcoholic fatty liver disease (NAFLD) and diagnostic accuracy of non-invasive tests for liver disease severity. Ann Med. 2011;43:617–49.
6. Day CP, James OF. Steatohepatitis: a tale of two "hits"? Gastroenterology. 1998;114:842–5.
7. Arslan N. Obesity, fatty liver disease and intestinal microbiota. World J Gastroenterol. 2014;20:16452–63.
8. Buchman AL, Dubin MD, Moukarzel AA, Jenden DJ, Roch M, Rice M, et al. Choline deficiency: a cause of hepatic steatosis during parenteral nutrition that can be reversed with intravenous choline supplementation. Hepatology. 1995;22:1399–403.
9. Volynets V, Küper MA, Strahl S, Maier IB, Spruss A, Wagnerberger S, et al. Nutrition, intestinal permeability, and blood ethanol levels are altered in patients with nonalcoholic fatty liver disease (NAFLD). Dig Dis Sci. 2012;57:1932–41.
10. Kashyap PC, Marcobal A, Ursell LK, Smits SA, Sonnenburg ED, Costello EK, et al. Genetically dictated change in host mucus carbohydrate landscape exerts a diet-dependent effect on the gut microbiota. Proc Natl Acad Sci U S A. 2013;110:17059–64.
11. Cani PD, Bibiloni R, Knauf C, Waget A, Neyrinck AM, Delzenne NM, et al. Changes in gut microbiota control metabolic endotoxemia-induced inflammation in high-fat diet-induced obesity and diabetes in mice. Diabetes. 2008;57:1470–81.
12. Turnbaugh PJ, Ley RE, Mahowald MA, Magrini V, Mardis ER, Gordon JI. An obesity-associated gut microbiome with increased capacity for energy harvest. Nature. 2006;444:1027–31.
13. Le Poul E, Loison C, Struyf S, Springael JY, Lannoy V, Decobecq ME, et al. Functional characterization of human receptors for short chain fatty acids and their role in polymorphonuclear cell activation. J Biol Chem. 2003;278:25481–9.
14. Jiang C, Xie C, Li F, Zhang L, Nichols RG, Krausz KW, et al. Intestinal farnesoid X receptor signaling promotes nonalcoholic fatty liver disease. J Clin Invest. 2014;125:386–402.
15. Kobyliak N, Conte C, Cammarota G, Haley AP, Styriak I, et al. Probiotics in prevention and treatment of obesity: a critical view. Nutr Metab. 2016;13:14.
16. Savcheniuk O, Kobyliak N, Kondro M, Virchenko O, Falalyeyeva T, Beregova T. Short-term periodic consumption of multiprobiotic from childhood improves insulin sensitivity, prevents development of non-alcoholic fatty liver disease and adiposity in adult rats with glutamate-induced obesity. BMC Complement Altern Med. 2014;14:247.
17. Kondro M, Kobyliak N, Virchenko O, Falalyeyeva T, Beregova T, Bodnar P. Multiprobiotic therapy from childhood prevents the development of nonalcoholic fatty liver disease in adult monosodium glutamate-induced obese rats. Curr Issues Pharm Med Sci. 2014;27:243–5.
18. Kondro M, Mykhalchyshyn G, Bodnar P, Kobyliak N, Falalyeyeva T. Metabolic profile and morpho-functional state of the liver in rats with glutamate-induced obesity. Curr Issues Pharm Med Sci. 2013;26:379–81.
19. Nakagawa T, Ukai K, Ohyama T, Gomita Y, Okamura H. Effects of chronic administration of sibutramine on body weight, food intake and motor

activity in neonatally monosodium glutamate-treated obese female rats: relationship of antiobesity effect with monoamines. Exp Anim. 2000;49:239–49.

20. Kleiner DE, Brunt EM, Van Natta M, Behling C, Contos MJ, Cummings OW, et al. Design and validation of a histological scoring system for nonalcoholic fatty liver disease. Hepatology. 2005;41:1313–21.

21. Folch J, Lees M, Stanley GHS. A simple method for the isolation and purification of total lipids from animal tissues. J Biol Chem. 1957;226:497–509.

22. Cani PD, Van Hul M. Novel opportunities for next-generation probiotics targeting metabolic syndrome. Curr Opin Biotechnol. 2014;32:21–7.

23. Yin YN, Yu QF, Fu N, Liu XW, Lu FG. Effects of four Bifidobacteria on obesity in high-fat diet induced rats. World J Gastroenterol. 2010;16:3394–401.

24. Ritze Y, Bárdos G, Claus A, Ehrmann V, Bergheim I, Schwiertz A, et al. Lactobacillus rhamnosus GG protects against non-alcoholic fatty liver disease in mice. PLoS One. 2014;9, e80169.

25. Kim SW, Park KY, Kim B, Kim E, Hyun CK. Lactobacillus rhamnosus GG improves insulin sensitivity and reduces adiposity in high-fat diet-fed mice through enhancement of adiponectin production. Biochem Biophys Res Commun. 2013;431:258–63.

26. Reichold A, Brenner SA, Spruss A, Förster-Fromme K, Bergheim I, Bischoff SC. Bifidobacterium adolescentis protects from the development of nonalcoholic steatohepatitis in a mouse model. J Nutr Biochem. 2014;25:118–25.

27. Yoo SR, Kim YJ, Park DY, Jung UJ, Jeon SM, Ahn YT, et al. Probiotics L. plantarum and L. curvatus in combination alter hepatic lipid metabolism and suppress diet-induced obesity. Obesity (Silver Spring). 2013;21:2571–8.

28. Plaza-Diaz J, Gomez-Llorente C, Abadia-Molina F, Saez-Lara MJ, Campaña-Martin L, Muñoz-Quezada S, et al. Effects of Lactobacillus paracasei CNCM I-4034, Bifidobacterium breve CNCM I-4035 and Lactobacillus rhamnosus CNCM I-4036 on hepatic steatosis in Zucker rats. PLoS One. 2014;9, e98401.

29. Mei L, Tang Y, Li M, Yang P, Liu Z, Yuan J, Zheng P. Co-administration of cholesterol-lowering probiotics and anthraquinone from Cassia obtusifolia L. ameliorate non-alcoholic fatty liver. PLoS One. 2015;10, e0138078.

30. Jin C, Sellmann C, Engstler AJ, Ziegenhardt D, Bergheim I. Supplementation of sodium butyrate protects mice from the development of non-alcoholic steatohepatitis (NASH). Br J Nutr. 2015;114:1745–55.

21

Niclosamide induced cell apoptosis via upregulation of ATF3 and activation of PERK in Hepatocellular carcinoma cells

Shunyan Weng[1,2,3†], Liang Zhou[2†], Qing Deng[2], Jiaxian Wang[1], Yan Yu[2], Jianwei Zhu[1] and Yunsheng Yuan[1,2*]

Abstract

Background: Hepatocellular carcinoma (HCC) is one of most common and aggressive human malignancies in the world, especially, in eastern Asia, and its mortality is very high at any phase. We want to investigate mechanism of niclosamide inducing cell apoptosis in HCC.

Methods: Two hepatoma cell lines were used to evaluate activity of niclosamide inducing cell apoptosis and study its mechanism. Quantitative real-time PCR and western blotting were used in analysis of genes expression or protein active regulated by niclosamide.

Results: Niclosamide remarkably induced cell apoptosis in hepatoma cells. Furthermore, our study revealed that RNA-dependent protein kinase-like kinase (PERK) is activated and its expression is up-regulated in HCC cells which are exposed to niclosamide. niclosamide also significantly increase activating transcription factor 3 (ATF3), activating transcription factor 4 (ATF4) and CCAAT/enhancer-binding protein-homologous protein (CHOP) expression in HCC cells. It's suggested that the function of niclosamide was abrogated by PERK inhibitor or absent ATF3. Expression of PERK and CHOP is correlated with ATF3 level in the cells.

Conclusion: Taken together, our results indicate that ATF3 plays an integral role in ER stress activated and cell apoptosis induced by niclosamide in HCC cells. In this study, the new mechanism of niclosamide as anti-cancer we investigated, too.

Keywords: Activating transcription factor 3, Endoplasmic reticulum stress, Reactive oxygen species, Liver cancer

Background

Hepatocellular carcinoma (HCC) is one of the most common and aggressive human malignancies in the world [1]. It is a major public health issue worldwide according to epidemiological data, and the incidence is high in East Asia.

HCC often develops caused by chronic tissue damage due to liver cirrhosis which could be induced by HBV, HCV, alcohol intake, hemochromatosis, nonalcoholic steatohepatits and so on [2].

Surgical resection is the primary treatment option for patients with early stage of HCC [2]. After surgical treatment, patients should accept chemotherapy. However the rate of total 5-years survival is very low due to side effects of chemotherapeutic drugs and the chemo-resistance of tumor cells. Therefore it is very important to develop new drugs for HCC treatment [3]. It is well known that Endoplasmic Reticulum (ER) stress could induce cell apoptosis or cell death in many tumor categories, including breast cancer [4], neuroectodermal tumor [5], HCC [6], etc. ER stress could activate un-folded protein response (UPR) whose signaling network consists of three stress sensors, namely protein kinase RNA like ER kinase (PERK) or RNA-dependent kinase-like kinase, inositol-requiring enzyme 1α (IRE1α),

* Correspondence: yunsheng@sjtu.edu.cn
†Equal contributors
[1]Engineering Research Center of Cell and Therapeutic Antibody, Ministry of Education, School of Pharmacy, Shanghai Jiao Tong University, 800 Dongchuan Rd, Biology and Pharmacy Building, suite 6-208, Shanghai 200240, People's Republic of China
[2]The Shanghai Municipality Key Laboratory of Veterinary Biotechnology, School of Agriculture and Biology, Shanghai Jiao Tong University, 800 Dongchuan Rd, Shanghai 200240, People's Republic of China
Full list of author information is available at the end of the article

and activating transcription factor 6 (ATF6) [7]. In cancer cells, UPR could be activated by exposure to hypoxia, oxidative stress and nutrient starvation. The tumor microenvironment usually features hypoxia and high content of reactive oxygen species (ROS) because of the highly active proliferation and metabolism status of cancer cells. Hypoxia and ROS could direct PERK activation, which in turn activates eukaryotic translation initiation factor 2α (eIF2α) which would induce the expression of activating transcription factor 4 (ATF4) for regulating redox homeostasis and metabolic homeostasis [8]. However CCAAT/enhancer-binding protein-homologous protein (CHOP, also known as GADD153), a downstream element to ATF4 in the PERK pathway, induces apoptosis or cell death under intensive or prolonged ER stress conditions [9, 10]. Interestingly, activating transcription factor 3 (ATF3), a bZIP DNA-binding protein, is associated with CHOP and thus integrated into the PERK/eIF2α pathway under ER stress backgrounds [11]. Expression of ATF3 could be induced by ER stress and involved in regulation of cell apoptosis [12]. In the tumors, ATF3 might induce cell apoptosis or improve cell survival depending on tumor types. Currently, several studies have shown that ATF3 plays tumor suppressing roles in different cancer types, including colon cancer [11] and esophageal squamous cell carcinomas (ESCC) [13]. It's also reported that the overexpression of ATF3 suppresses growth of HeLa cells [14]. Other data showed that niclosamide, an antihelminthic drug for treatment of tapeworm infections approved by FDA, has exhibited anticancer function in different tumor types, including leukemia, colon cancer, glioma, etc [15]. We hypothesized that niclosamide also has effective function in anti-HCC. In this study, We demonstrated a new mechanism of niclosamide as anticancer with HCC cells.

Methods

Cell culture and drug treatment

HepG2 and QGY7701 cell lines were obtained from the Cell Bank of Shanghai Institute of Cell Biology (Chinese Academy of Sciences, Shanghai) and maintained in DMED (Hyclone, Logan, UT,) high glucose medium, supplemented with 10 % FBS (Gibco, NY). All cells were cultured in humidified 37 °C incubator supplied with 5 % CO2. Niclosamide (Sigma-Aldrich, St. Louis, MO) was dissolved in DMSO (Sigma-Aldrich, St. Louis, MO). To explore the regulation of niclosamide upon signal pathways, cells were seeded in 6-well plate and incubated for 24 h. Then cells were fed with fresh medium containing different concentrations of niclosamide or DMSO only as control. After 24 h of niclosamide treatment, cells was lysed with 1 % SDS lysis buffer (1%SDS,25 mM EDTA, 45 mM Tris-HCl, ph6.5) for western analysis, and total RNA was isolated directly with Trizol reagent

(Life technologies, CA). In order to block ER stress, GSK2606414 (Selleck Chemicals, Houston, TX) was used to pretreat cells for 1 h before cells treated with niclosamide.

DNA constructs and lenti-virus packaging

Oligo of ATF3 shRNA was synthesized and inserted in pGV298 lentiviral vector (GeneChem, Shanghai). The ATF3 target sequence was 5'-GCAAAGTGCCGAAAC AAGA-3' according to as described in publication [16]. The control GFP shRNA plasmid was purchased from GeneChem inc (GeneChem, Shanghai). The lentiviral vector is cotransfected with pVSV-G, pRev, pTat and pGag-pol (Gifts from Dr. Cheng, UMCM, Baltimore) in order to produce lentivirus particles in HEK293T cells with lipfectimin2000 (life technologies, CA) and supernatant were collected and were used to transduce HepG2 cells.

Stable ATF3 knockout HepG2 cell line

HepG2 cells were planted to 6-well plate and incubated overnight. Cells were fed with medium contained ATF3 shRNA lentivirus particles and 10 μg.ml^{-1} polybrene(Santa Cruz, CA) which could improve the efficiency of lentivirus transduction. The medium was changed after 24 h of lentivirus transduction. Positive cells were selected with 10 μM puromycin (Santa Cruz, CA) and efficiency of ATF3 knockout was analyzed with western blotting.

Cell viability assay

HepG2 and QGY7701 cells were seeded to 96-well plates and incubated overnight. Cells were fed with fresh complete medium containing different concentrations of niclosamide every 24 h and maintained for 3 days. Then cell viability was analyzed with CCK8 kit (Dojindo, Japan). Data were normalized with control group and presented as average ± SD. For the analysis of cell viability in ATF3 knock-down HepG2 and control cell lines, HepG2-ATF3^{KD} and HepG2-control cells were planted in 96-well plates. Cells were treated with niclosamide or DMSO and cell number was counted every day for three days. Data was presented as average ± SD. Student t-test was used in statist analysis.

Terminal deoxynucleotidyl transferase-mediated dUTP nick end labeling (TUNEL) assay

TUNEL assay was performed to analyze cells apoptosis induced by niclosamide. HepG2 and QGY7701 cells grown on polylysine-coated cover slides were fixed with 4 % Paraformalclehyde after 24 h of 10 μM niclosamide treatment. TUNEL APO-GREEN detect kit (biotool, Shanghai, China) was used in DNA labeling according to manufacturer's instruction. Images were taken by NIKON fluorescence microscope (Nikon, Japan).

Flow cytometry
HepG2 and QGY7701 cells were treated with niclosamide, niclosamide/GSK2606414 or DMSO as control. Cells were harvested at 24 h of drug treatment and washed twice with cold PBS on ice. Cell pellets were resuspended with PBS and FITC-Annexin V Apoptosis Detection Kit (Wanlei Bio, Shenyang, China) was used to stain cells according to manufacturer's manual book. Cells apoptosis were analyzed with flow cytometer (BD Bioscience, US).

RNA preparation and quantitative real-time PCR
Total RNA was extracted with Trizol reagents (Life technologies, CA) according to manufacturer's instruction. Reverse transcription and quantitative Real-time PCR (qRT-PCR) were performed as previously described [17]. For detecting gene expression induced by niclosamide, ATF3 and ER stress associated genes were selected for qRT-PCR and GAPDH was used as control. All primers were synthesized by Life technologies company (Shanghai, China) and the sequences were listed in Table 1. 2 μg total RNA was used as template to synthesize the first strand of cDNA with M-MLV reverse transcriptase (Takara, Dalian, China) in a 20 μl reaction system. PCR reactions were carried out with 200x diluted cDNAs, 100 nmol of each primer, and SYB Premix Ex Taq II (TaKaRa, Dalian, China) in a 20 μl reaction system. qRT-PCR reactions were performed with ABI (life technologies, CA) and PCR parameters involved the following steps: 95 °C for 5 min, 1 cycle; 94 °C for 5 s and 60 °C for

30 s, 40 cycles. Final data were normalized with GAPDH and presented as ratio to control.

Western immunoblotting
Western immunoblotting was performed as previously described [15]. The primary antibodies used in this study were anti-cleaved caspase 3 and anti- phospho-eIF2α (Ser51) (Cell signaling tech, Danvers), anti-GAPDH (Proteintech, Chicago), anti-ATF4 (Wanlei Bio, Shenyang, China), anti-GADD153/CHOP (Wanlei Bio, Shenyang,China), anti-ATF3, anti-eIF2α, anti-pPERK and anti-PERK (Santa Cruz biotech, Santa Cruz). HRP conjunct secondary Antibodies were purchased from Jackson immune Research-laboratories (Western Grove, PA). The PVDF membrane was purchased from Millipore (Millipore, Billerica) and ECL substrate was purchased from Thermo Fisher (Thermo Fisher, Waltham).

Immunofluorescence staining and confocal microscopy
HepG2 and QGY7701 cells were grown on polylysine-coated cover slides and were fixed with cold methanol after 24 h of 2 μM niclosamide treatment. The cells were incubated in block buffer (3%BSA in TBST) at room temperature (RT) for 30 min. Then, anti-ATF3 or anti-GADD153/CHOP antibodies was diluted to 1:100 in blotting buffer (1 % BSA in TBST with 0.3 % TritonX-100) and were used to blot cells overnight at 4 °C. After the cells were washed three times with TBST, Alex®488-goat anti-rabbit IgG (Life technologies, CA) were used to incubate cells at RT for 1 h. Cell nucleus was stained with Hoechst 33342 (Sigma-Aldrich, St. Louis, MO). Confocal images were taken with Leica SP8 confocal microscope (Leica, Wetzlar, Germany).

Table 1 Primers for qRT-PCR

Gene Accession	Gene ID	Primer	Sequence
NM_001030287	ATF3	Forward(5'-3')	CGAAGACTGGAGCAAAATG ATG
		Reverse(5'-3')	CATCCAGGCCAGGTCTCTGCCTCAG
NM_001675	ATF4	Forward(5'-3')	TGGACTTCGAGCAAGAGATG
		Reverse(5'-3')	AGGAAGGAAGGCTGGAAGAG
NM_001195053	DDIT3(CHOP)	Forward(5'-3')	TGCTTTCAGGTGTGGTGATG TATG
		Reverse(5'-3')	AATCAGAGCTGGAACCTGAGGA
NM_004836	EIF2AK3(PERK)	Forward(5'-3')	CTTATGCCAGACACACAGGA CAA
		Reverse(5'-3')	TCCATCTGAGTGCTGAATGGAATAC
NM_007348	ATF6A	Forward(5'-3')	GCCGCCGTCCCAGATATTA
		Reverse(5'-3')	GCAAAGAGAGCAGAATCCCA
NM_001433	ERN1(IRE1A)	Forward(5'-3')	ATTGTGTACCGGGGCATGTT
		Reverse(5'-3')	TTCTCCGTGCAGAAGTAGCG
NM_001256799	GAPDH	Forward(5'-3')	CTCAGACACCATGGGGAAG GTGA
		Reverse(5'-3')	ATGATCTTGAGGCTGTTGTCATA

Statistical analysis

All calculations and statistical analyses were performed with Excel software (Microsoft, WA). Student t test was used in comparing two groups in experiments. All data were presented as average ± SD. All tests were two-sided, and P values less than 0.05 were considered to be statistically significant.

Results

Niclosamide suppressed cells growth by inducing ER-stress in HCC cells

Niclosamide significantly suppressed HCC growth in vitro as indicated by results of cell viability assay (Fig. 1a, b). The results of western blotting showed that niclosamide remarkably activated caspase-3 active and level of the poly ADP-ribose polymerase (PARP), a substrate of activated caspase-3, in niclosamide treatment cells was significantly less than in control cells (Fig. 1c, d, e). These data demonstrated activity of inducing apoptosis in hepatoma cells. To investigate the role of in ER-stress, the transcription levels of PERK, ATF6 and IRE1α, which are expressed specifically under the background of ER-stress, were analyzed using qRT-PCR. Interestingly, mRNA level of PERK but not ATF6 or IRE1α was significantly upregulated by niclosamide in both of HepG2 and QGY7701 cells (Fig. 2a).

ATF4 and CHOP are the most important downstream genes in the PERK-eIF2α pathway and modulate cell

apoptosis [9]. Therefore, the expression of ATF3, ATF4 and CHOP were analyzed with RT-PCR and results showed that all of their mRNA levels were remarkably increased after niclosamide treatment (Fig. 2b, c, d). It's also shown in our study that CHOP mRNA level was increased by over 20 times. To identify whether PERK pathway is activated by niclosamide, different doses of niclosamide was used to treat hepatoma cells and certain protein levels were analyzed with western blotting. We found protein levels of ATF4, ATF3 and CHOP, which are important transcription factors of the PERK pathway, were significantly increased in a dose dependent manner in accordance with the elevation of PERK protein level (Fig. 3a, b). In turn, phosphorylation of eIF2α was enhanced by active PERK (Fig. 3a, c). Interestingly, under normal conditions ATF3 level was low in HCC cells, but its elevation was more significant than ATF4 or CHOP (Fig. 3b). Our data suggested that niclosamide also activated caspase3 in both HepG2 and QGY7701 cells (Fig. 3a).

Niclosamide increased nuclear accumulation of ATF3 and CHOP in HCC

ATF3 and CHOP are critical transcription factors in the PERK pathway and they should bind to DNA to regulate gene transcription. To investigate whether ATF3 and CHOP upregulated by niclosamide localized in nucleus of hepatoma cells, Anti-ATF3 and Anti-CHOP primary

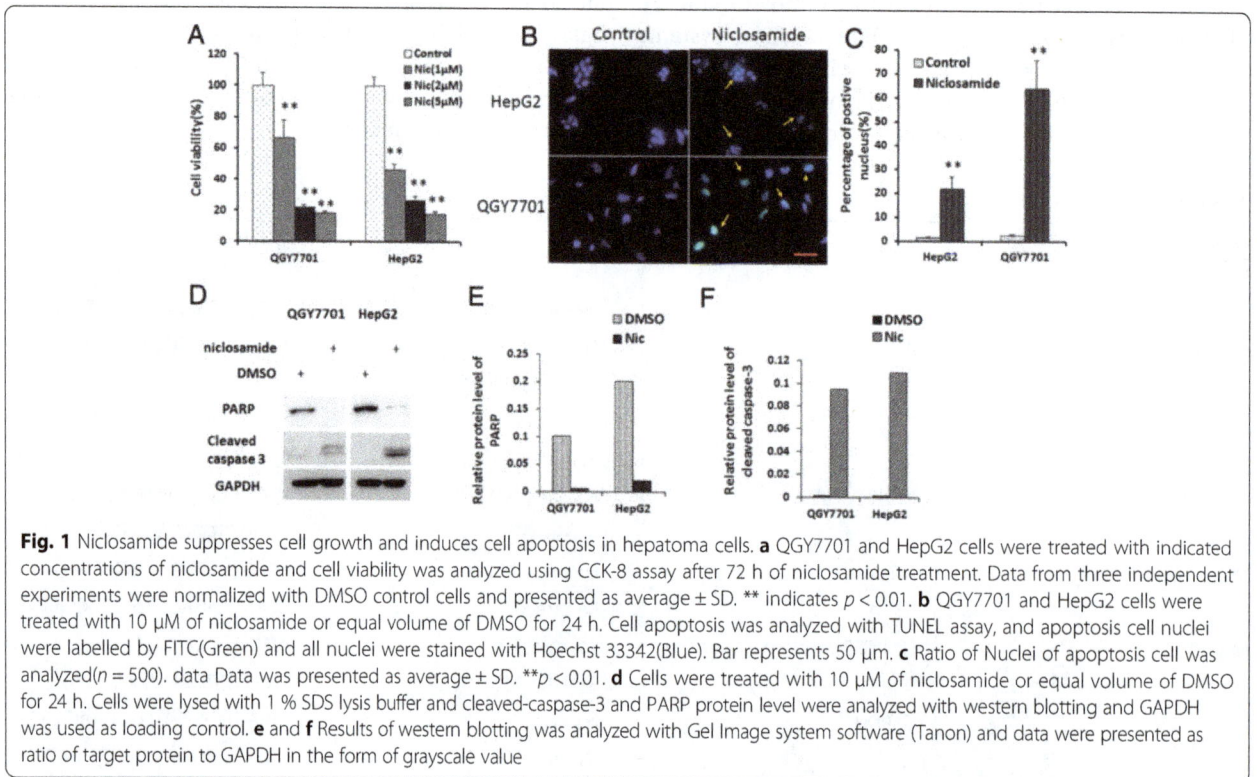

Fig. 1 Niclosamide suppresses cell growth and induces cell apoptosis in hepatoma cells. **a** QGY7701 and HepG2 cells were treated with indicated concentrations of niclosamide and cell viability was analyzed using CCK-8 assay after 72 h of niclosamide treatment. Data from three independent experiments were normalized with DMSO control cells and presented as average ± SD. ** indicates $p < 0.01$. **b** QGY7701 and HepG2 cells were treated with 10 μM of niclosamide or equal volume of DMSO for 24 h. Cell apoptosis was analyzed with TUNEL assay, and apoptosis cell nuclei were labelled by FITC(Green) and all nuclei were stained with Hoechst 33342(Blue). Bar represents 50 μm. **c** Ratio of Nuclei of apoptosis cell was analyzed(n = 500). data Data was presented as average ± SD. **$p < 0.01$. **d** Cells were treated with 10 μM of niclosamide or equal volume of DMSO for 24 h. Cells were lysed with 1 % SDS lysis buffer and cleaved-caspase-3 and PARP protein level were analyzed with western blotting and GAPDH was used as loading control. **e** and **f** Results of western blotting was analyzed with Gel Image system software (Tanon) and data were presented as ratio of target protein to GAPDH in the form of grayscale value

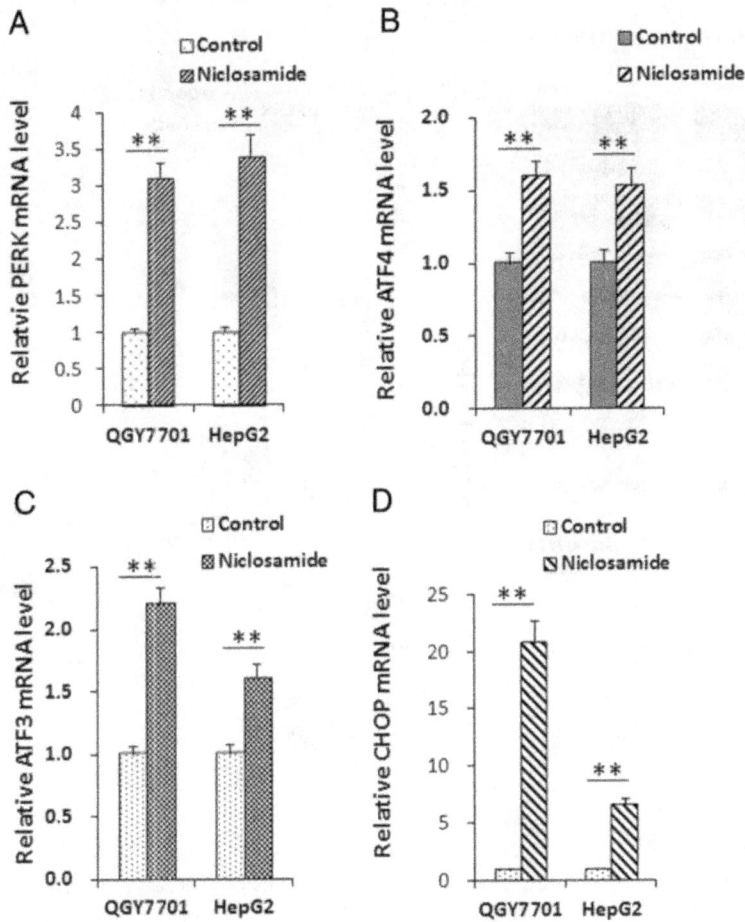

Fig. 2 Expression of PERK signal pathway related genes was induced by niclosamide in hepatoma cells. QGY7701 and HepG2 cells were harvested and total RNA was extracted post treatment with 10 μM niclosamide in the medium for 24 h. **a** Expression level of PERK and its downstream genes, **b** ATF4, **c** ATF3 and **d** CHOP, were analyzed with qRT-PCR. Data were normalized with control group and presented as change-fold. All experiments were repeated for at least three times. ** indicates $p < 0.01$

antibodies was used in immunofluorescence assays. The results showed that niclosamide increase both ATF3 and CHOP levels and increase their accumulation in the nucleus of HepG2 and QGY7701 cells (Fig. 4a, b). These results demonstrated that niclosamide might upregulate ATF3 and CHOP expression, and such expression products would localize in nucleus to exert their roles.

Niclosamide induced apoptosis in the HCC suppressed by PERK inhibition

Since PERK pathway was activated by niclosamide, we tried to investigate whether PERK pathway had its roles in the apoptosis induced by niclosamide. Our data showed that GSK2606414, an inhibitor of PERK pathway, could improve cell survival under niclosamide treatment (Fig. 5a). The results of western blot showed that GSK2606414 significantly suppress activation of caspase3 in HepG2 and QGY7701 cells (Fig. 5b). According to the cell flow cytometry assay data for cell

apoptosis, GSK2606414 decrease percentage of apoptotic cells after niclosamide treatment (Fig. 5c). These evidences confirmed that PERK pathway contributes to cells apoptosis induced by niclosamide.

ATF3 upregulation during cell apoptosis induced by niclosamide

To verify the role of ATF3 in ER stress activated by niclosamide in HCC, we tried to down-regulate ATF3 in hepatoma cell lines with small hair RNA (ATF3-shRNA) targeting ATF3 gene and GFP gene (GFP-shRNA) as control. Our data showed there is no difference in cell proliferation between control cells and ATF3 knockdown (ATF3KD) cells in normal cell culture medium. However, ATF3KD cells had higher cell viability than control cells post niclosamide treatment (Fig. 6a). ATF3 knock-down might abrogate PERK and CHOP expression induced by niclosamide (Fig. 6b, c, d). In turn, ATF3 knock-down also reduced caspase3 activity

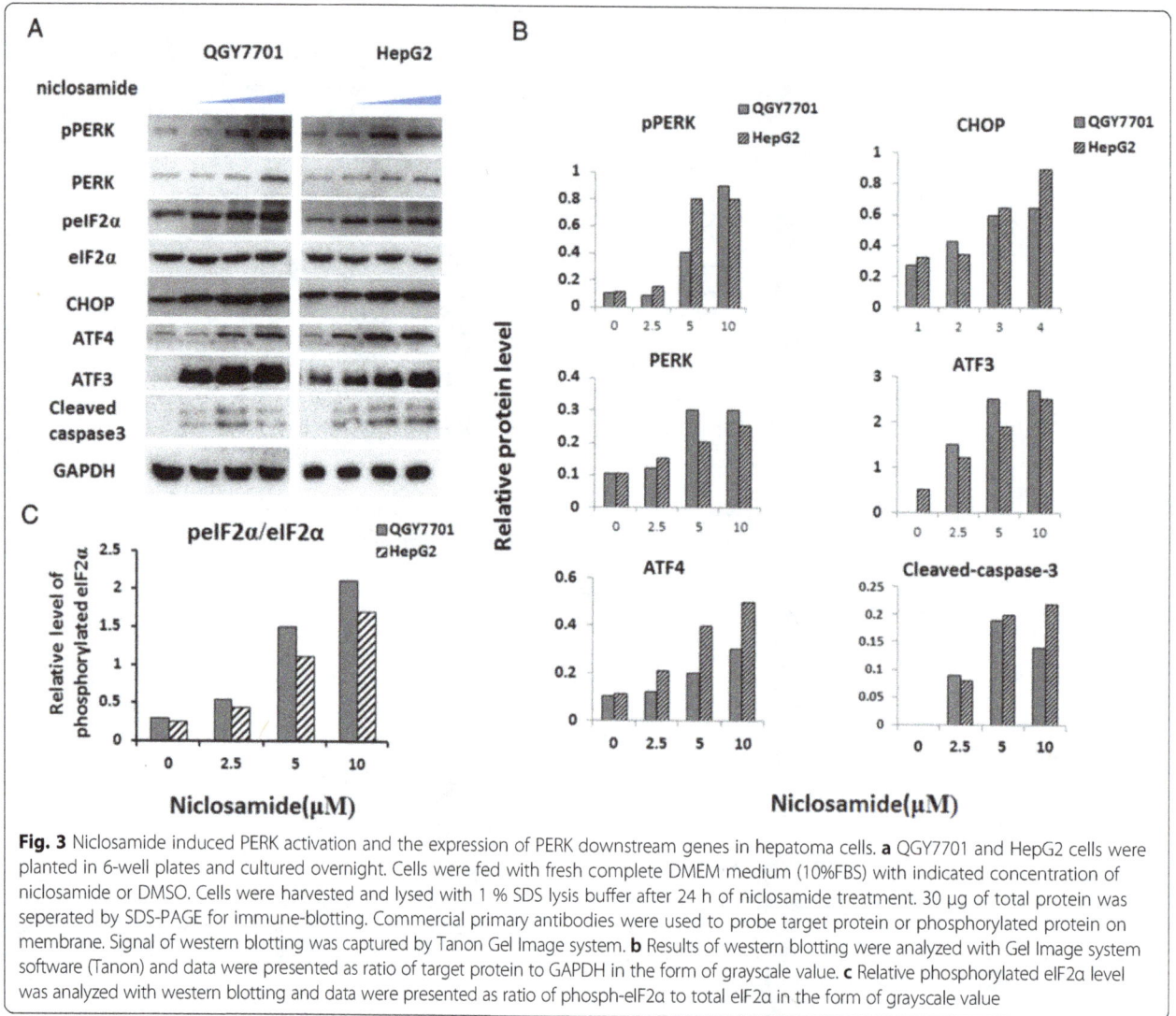

Fig. 3 Niclosamide induced PERK activation and the expression of PERK downstream genes in hepatoma cells. **a** QGY7701 and HepG2 cells were planted in 6-well plates and cultured overnight. Cells were fed with fresh complete DMEM medium (10%FBS) with indicated concentration of niclosamide or DMSO. Cells were harvested and lysed with 1 % SDS lysis buffer after 24 h of niclosamide treatment. 30 μg of total protein was seperated by SDS-PAGE for immune-blotting. Commercial primary antibodies were used to probe target protein or phosphorylated protein on membrane. Signal of western blotting was captured by Tanon Gel Image system. **b** Results of western blotting were analyzed with Gel Image system software (Tanon) and data were presented as ratio of target protein to GAPDH in the form of grayscale value. **c** Relative phosphorylated eIF2α level was analyzed with western blotting and data were presented as ratio of phosph-eIF2α to total eIF2α in the form of grayscale value

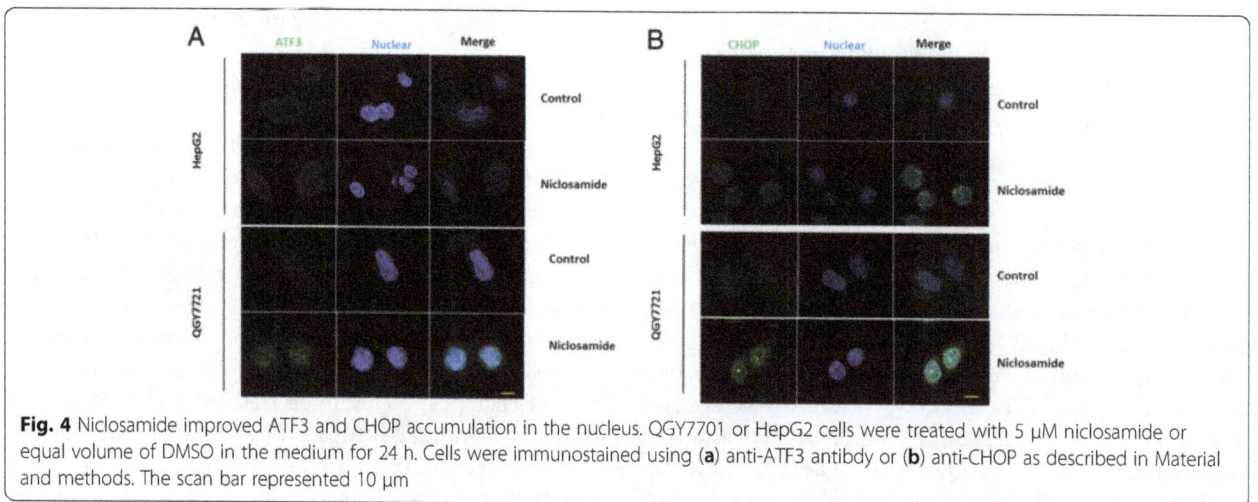

Fig. 4 Niclosamide improved ATF3 and CHOP accumulation in the nucleus. QGY7701 or HepG2 cells were treated with 5 μM niclosamide or equal volume of DMSO in the medium for 24 h. Cells were immunostained using (**a**) anti-ATF3 antibdy or (**b**) anti-CHOP as described in Material and methods. The scan bar represented 10 μm

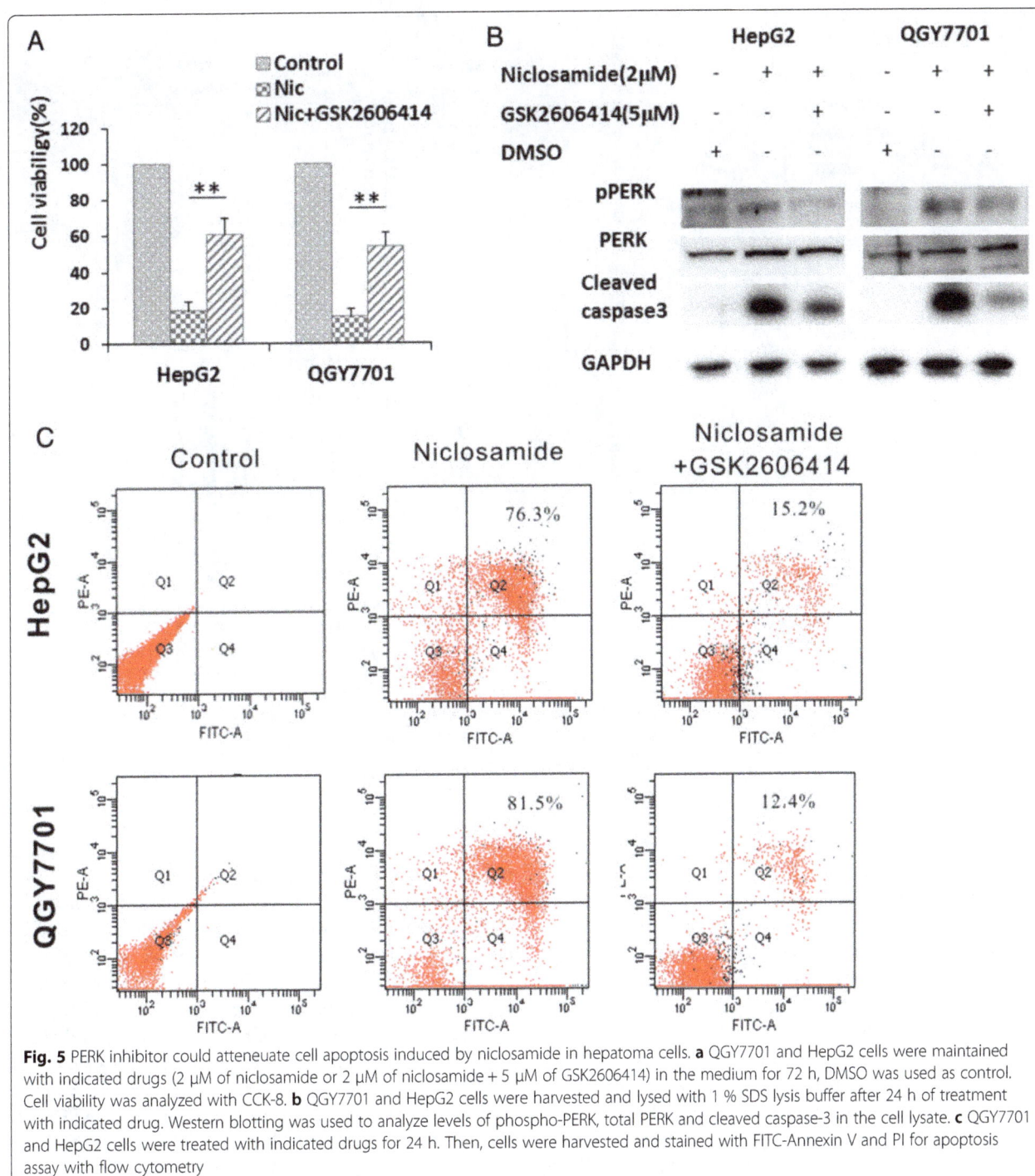

Fig. 5 PERK inhibitor could atteneuate cell apoptosis induced by niclosamide in hepatoma cells. **a** QGY7701 and HepG2 cells were maintained with indicated drugs (2 μM of niclosamide or 2 μM of niclosamide + 5 μM of GSK2606414) in the medium for 72 h, DMSO was used as control. Cell viability was analyzed with CCK-8. **b** QGY7701 and HepG2 cells were harvested and lysed with 1 % SDS lysis buffer after 24 h of treatment with indicated drug. Western blotting was used to analyze levels of phospho-PERK, total PERK and cleaved caspase-3 in the cell lysate. **c** QGY7701 and HepG2 cells were treated with indicated drugs for 24 h. Then, cells were harvested and stained with FITC-Annexin V and PI for apoptosis assay with flow cytometry

induced by niclosamide (Fig. 6b). So our data suggested that ATF3 plays a central role in ER-stress activated and apoptosis induced by niclosamide in HepG2 cells.

Discussion

In this study, our data suggested that niclosamide remarkably induced cell apoptosis (Fig. 1b) and increase

expression level of PERK and its down-stream genes in HCCs (Fig. 2). It's known that sustaining ER stress could sequentially activate IRE1α, ATF6 and PERK pathways [4, 8]. PERK/ATF4/CHOP pathway is one of most important pathways to induce cancer cell apoptosis in the UPR [18]. ATF3 is an important factor for stress response in cells and it interact with ATF4 and CHOP,

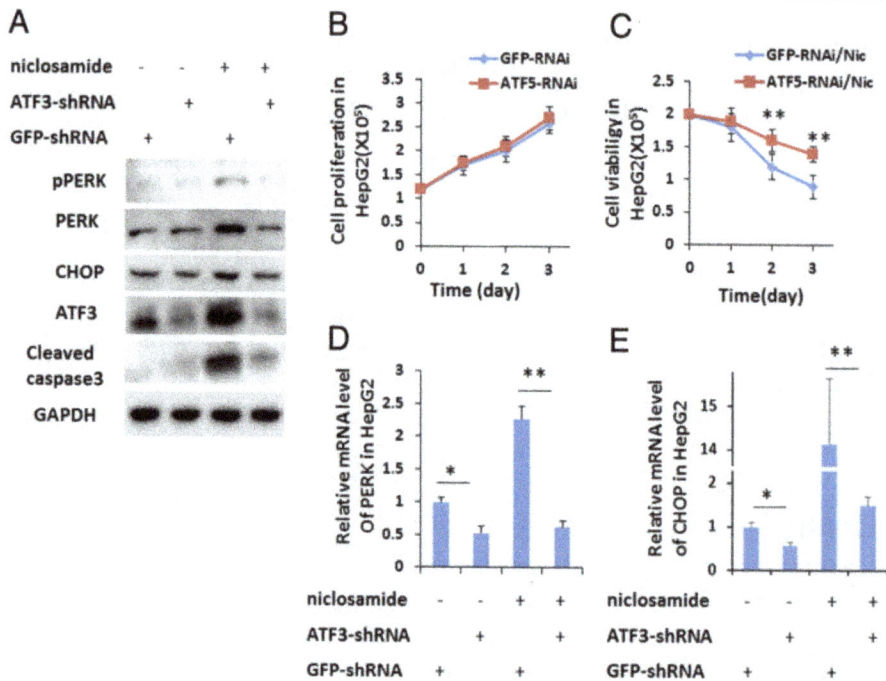

Fig. 6 ATF3 was involved in modulation of cell apoptosis induced by niclosamide. **a** ATF3 knockdown HepG2 cell line (HepG2-ATF3^{KD}) and control cell lines (GFP knockdown, HepG2-Control) was treated with indicated chemicals for 24 h and cells were harvested and lysed with 1 % SDS lysis buffer. 30 μg of total protein was seperated by SDS-PAGE for western blotting assay. Indicated primary antibodies were used for immunoblotting. HepG2-ATF3^{KD} and HepG2-control cells were planted in 96-well plates and maintained (**b**) without or with (**c**) 10 μM of niclosamide for 3 days. Cell number was countered every day. Data from three independent experiments were analyzed and presented as average ± SD. ** indicates $p < 0.01$. D and E, HepG2-ATF3^{KD} and HepG2-Control cells were treated with or without 10 μM of niclosamide for 24 h. Then, total RNA was extracted and cDNA was synthesized. Relative mRNA level of (**d**) PERK and (**e**) CHOP were analyzed with qRT-PCR. Data was presented as average ± SD. *$p < 0.05$,**$p < 0.01$

these two transcription factors being PERK targeting genes under ER stress conditions [5, 9]. Current study demonstrated that ATF3 was involved in regulation of PERK function [19]. We further tried to reveal whether their protein levels are related with dose of niclosamide or not. Data of western blotting indicated that niclosamide upregulates PERK, ATF4, ATF3 and CHOP depending on the niclosamide concentration (Fig. 3). The results also demonstrated that caspase-3 is activated under niclosamide treatment (Fig. 3). Many studies had shown that niclosamide blocked cancer cells proliferation in a number of tumors types by suppressing the activities of several oncogenic pathways, including NF-kB, STAT3, notch and Wnt [20-22]. It also increases the level of reactive oxygen species (ROS) in acute myelogenous leukemia cells and enhances sensitivity to ROS in lung cancer cells [23]. Recently, it was identified that niclosamide could suppress HCC proliferation by blocking Wnt pathway [24]. Interestingly, we found that PERK pathway should play a critical role in HCC apoptosis induced by niclosamide. The apoptosis-inducing role of niclosamide in HCC could be abrogated by PERK inhibitor, GSK2606414 (Fig. 5). Several studies have

suggested PERK/ATF4/CHOP pathway being involved in regulation of cells apoptosis and death in HCC [6, 25, 26].

Current studies have demonstrated that ATF3 plays an integral role in the PERK-eIF2α pathway in regulation of downstream gene expression when ER-stress is activated [27]. ATF3 is integrated in the PERK pathway, and its expression is regulated by PERK [19]. In the PERK pathway, ATF3 also modulates CHOP expression and regulates eIF2α activation by negative feedback [27]. In clinical HCC samples, the expression level of ATF3 is significantly low [28]. It's also reported that ATF3 expression was low in HepG2 and QGY7701 cells. Niclosamide not only increases ATF3 mRNA and protein levels in HCCs, but also stimulates ATF3 accumulation in nucleus of HepG2 or QGY7701 cells (Fig. 4a). Because ATF3 functions in regulation of cancer cell survival and apoptosis depending on tumor types, its function in HCC was still unclear. Our data showed that downregulation of ATF3 expression level in HepG2 could remarkably abrogate effects of niclosamide on cell viability and activate caspase-3 level (Fig. 6a, b, c). Especially, PERK and CHOP expression levels were lower in ATF3 knock down cells than wild type cells either with or without

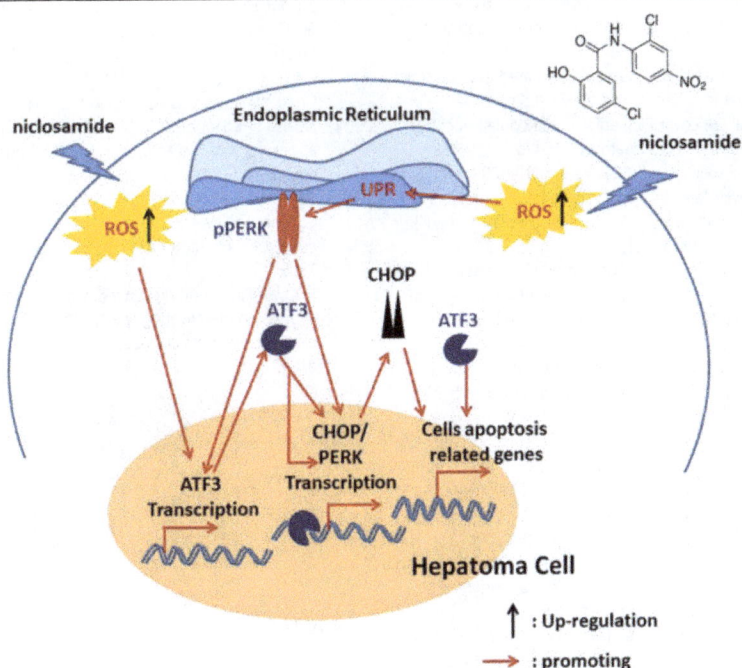

Fig. 7 A model of niclosamide inducing cell apoptosis through ATF3-dependent PERK activation in hepatoma cells. In hepatoma cells, niclosamide could induce ROS which in turn activates the PERK pathway. Both activated PERK pathway and ROS could enhance ATF3 expression. PERK pathway and ATF3 directly regulate CHOP expression. ATF3 and CHOP would induce cells apoptosis. In addition, ATF3 also regulates PERK pathway through modulating PERK expression

niclosamide treatment (Fig. 6d, e). Several observations suggested that ATF3, an integrated player coordinating the expression of ER stress response related genes, directly regulates target gene expression which induce cell death or apoptosis in p53-dependent or independent ways in cancer cells under ER stress [16, 19]. It represses cancer-related chemokine expression and regulates cancer cells micro-environment under ER stress [11]. In our study, expression of ER stress target genes was repressed in an ATF3-absent condition in HepG2 and QGY7701 cells. Our study demonstrates a series of crucial roles of ATF3 in PERK/CHOP pathway activation and cells apoptosis induction resulting from niclosamide treatment in HCC (Fig. 7).

Conclusion

Our study reveals that niclosamide activates PERK and up-regulates both of ATF3 and CHOP expression in HCCs. The function of niclosamide could be abrogated by PERK inhibitor and suppression of ATF3 expression. Especially, ATF3 upregulates PERK and CHOP level in HCCs being exposed to niclosamide. Our data indicates that ATF3 plays a central role in the induction of cell apoptosis by niclosamide in HCC.

Competing interest
All authors declared that they have no conflict of interest in this work.

Authors' contributions
SW, LZ and YY performed most of experiments. QD and JW did cells apoptosis analysis by FACS. YY, JZ and YY designed and guided experiments. YY wrote manuscript and all of authors discussed this manuscript. All authors read and approved the final manuscript.

Acknowledgment
We would like to thank Weifeng Ma and Hao Xu from Shanghai Jiao Tong University(SJTU) help us to prepare some solutions and Evhy He from SJTU help us to review the manuscript. This work was supported by the National Natural and Science Foundation of China (Yunsheng Yuan, 81302825) and the Shanghai Key Laboratory of Veterinary Biotechnology (Yunsheng Yuan, klab201501).

Author details
[1]Engineering Research Center of Cell and Therapeutic Antibody, Ministry of Education, School of Pharmacy, Shanghai Jiao Tong University, 800 Dongchuan Rd, Biology and Pharmacy Building, suite 6-208, Shanghai 200240, People's Republic of China. [2]The Shanghai Municipality Key Laboratory of Veterinary Biotechnology, School of Agriculture and Biology, Shanghai Jiao Tong University, 800 Dongchuan Rd, Shanghai 200240, People's Republic of China. [3]School of Life Sciences and Biotechnology, Shanghai Jiao Tong University, 800 Dongchuan Rd, Shanghai 200240, People's Republic of China.

References
1. Worns MA, Galle PR. HCC therapies–lessons learned. Nat Rev Gastroenterol Hepatol. 2014;11(7):447–52.
2. Tejeda-Maldonado J, Garcia-Juarez I, Aguirre-Valadez J, Gonzalez-Aguirre A, Vilatoba-Chapa M, Armengol-Alonso A, Escobar-Penagos F, Torre A, Sanchez-Avila JF, Carrillo-Perez DL. Diagnosis and treatment of hepatocellular carcinoma: an update. World J Hepatol. 2015;7(3):362–76.

3. Greten TF, Wang XW, Korangy F. Current concepts of immune based treatments for patients with HCC: from basic science to novel treatment approaches. Gut. 2015;64(5):842–8.

4. Moenner M, Pluquet O, Bouchecareilh M, Chevet E. Integrated endoplasmic reticulum stress responses in cancer. Cancer Res. 2007;67(22):10631–4.

5. Armstrong JL, Flockhart R, Veal GJ, Lovat PE, Redfern CP. Regulation of endoplasmic reticulum stress-induced cell death by ATF4 in neuroectodermal tumor cells. J Biol Chem. 2009;285(9):6091–100.

6. Koh IU, Lim JH, Joe MK, Kim WH, Jung MH, Yoon JB, Song J. AdipoR2 is transcriptionally regulated by ER stress-inducible ATF3 in HepG2 human hepatocyte cells. FEBS J. 2010;277(10):2304–17.

7. Wang WA, Groenendyk J, Michalak M. Endoplasmic reticulum stress associated responses in cancer. Biochim Biophys Acta. 2014;1843(10):2143–9.

8. Kato H, Nishitoh H. Stress responses from the endoplasmic reticulum in cancer. Front Oncol. 2015;5:93.

9. Xu L, Su L, Liu X. PKCdelta regulates death receptor 5 expression induced by PS-341 through ATF4-ATF3/CHOP axis in human lung cancer cells. Mol Cancer Ther. 2012;11(10):2174–82.

10. Liao Y, Fung TS, Huang M, Fang SG, Zhong Y, Liu DX. Upregulation of CHOP/GADD153 during coronavirus infectious bronchitis virus infection modulates apoptosis by restricting activation of the extracellular signal-regulated kinase pathway. J Virol. 2013;87(14):8124–34.

11. Park SH, Kim J, Do KH, Park J, Oh CG, Choi HJ, Song BG, Lee SJ, Kim YS, Moon Y. Activating transcription factor 3-mediated chemo-intervention with cancer chemokines in a noncanonical pathway under endoplasmic reticulum stress. J Biol Chem. 2014;289(39):27118–33.

12. Spohn D, Rossler OG, Philipp SE, Raubuch M, Kitajima S, Griesemer D, Hoth M, Thiel G. Thapsigargin induces expression of activating transcription factor 3 in human keratinocytes involving Ca2+ ions and c-Jun N-terminal protein kinase. Mol Pharmacol. 2010;78(5):865–76.

13. Xie JJ, Xie YM, Chen B, Pan F, Guo JC, Zhao Q, Shen JH, Wu ZY, Wu JY, Xu LY, et al. ATF3 functions as a novel tumor suppressor with prognostic significance in esophageal squamous cell carcinoma. Oncotarget. 2014;5(18):8569–82.

14. Lu D, Chen J, Hai T. The regulation of ATF3 gene expression by mitogen-activated protein kinases. Biochem J. 2007;401(2):559–67.

15. Xiang D, Yuan Y, Chen L, Liu X, Belani C, Cheng H. Niclosamide, an anti-helminthic molecule, downregulates the retroviral oncoprotein Tax and pro-survival Bcl-2 proteins in HTLV-1-transformed T lymphocytes. Biochem Biophys Res Commun. 2015;464(1):221–8.

16. Wang H, Mo P, Ren S, Yan C. Activating transcription factor 3 activates p53 by preventing E6-associated protein from binding to E6. J Biol Chem. 2010; 285(17):13201–10.

17. Yuan Y, Wu X, Ou Q, Gao J, Tennant BC, Han W, Yu Y. Differential expression of the genes involved in amino acids and nitrogen metabolisms during liver regeneration of mice. Hepatol Res. 2009; 39(3):301–312.

18. Dicks N, Gutierrez K, Michalak M, Bordignon V, Agellon LB. Endoplasmic reticulum stress, genome damage, and cancer. Front Oncol. 2015;5:11.

19. Edagawa M, Kawauchi J, Hirata M, Goshima H, Inoue M, Okamoto T, Murakami A, Maehara Y, Kitajima S. Role of activating transcription factor 3 (ATF3) in endoplasmic reticulum (ER) stress-induced sensitization of p53-deficient human colon cancer cells to tumor necrosis factor (TNF)-related apoptosis-inducing ligand (TRAIL)-mediated apoptosis through up-regulation of death receptor 5 (DR5) by zerumbone and celecoxib. J Biol Chem. 2014;289(31):21544–61.

20. Jin Y, Lu Z, Ding K, Li J, Du X, Chen C, Sun X, Wu Y, Zhou J, Pan J. Antineoplastic mechanisms of niclosamide in acute myelogenous leukemia stem cells: inactivation of the NF-kappaB pathway and generation of reactive oxygen species. Cancer Res. 2010;70(6):2516–27.

21. Li R, Hu Z, Sun SY, Chen ZG, Owonikoko TK, Sica GL, Ramalingam SS, Curran WJ, Khuri FR, Deng X. Niclosamide overcomes acquired resistance to erlotinib through suppression of STAT3 in non-small cell lung cancer. Mol Cancer Ther. 2013;12(10):2200–12.

22. Osada T, Chen M, Yang XY, Spasojevic I, Vandeusen JB, Hsu D, Clary BM, Clay TM, Chen W, Morse MA, et al. Antihelminth compound niclosamide downregulates Wnt signaling and elicits antitumor responses in tumors with activating APC mutations. Cancer Res. 2011;71(12):4172–82.

23. Lee SL, Son AR, Ahn J, Song JY. Niclosamide enhances ROS-mediated cell death through c-Jun activation. Biomed Pharmacother. 2014;68(5):619–24.

24. Tomizawa M, Shinozaki F, Motoyoshi Y, Sugiyama T, Yamamoto S, Sueishi M, Yoshida T. Niclosamide suppresses Hepatoma cell proliferation via the Wnt pathway. Onco Targets Ther. 2013;6:1685–93.

25. Shi YH, Ding ZB, Zhou J, Hui B, Shi GM, Ke AW, Wang XY, Dai Z, Peng YF, Gu CY, et al. Targeting autophagy enhances sorafenib lethality for hepatocellular carcinoma via ER stress-related apoptosis. Autophagy. 2011; 7(10):1159–72.

26. Chen YJ, Su JH, Tsao CY, Hung CT, Chao HH, Lin JJ, Liao MH, Yang ZY, Huang HH, Tsai FJ, et al. Sinulariolide induced hepatocellular carcinoma apoptosis through activation of mitochondrial-related apoptotic and PERK/eIF2alpha/ATF4/CHOP pathway. Molecules. 2013;18(9):10146–61.

27. Jiang HY, Wek SA, McGrath BC, Lu D, Hai T, Harding HP, Wang X, Ron D, Cavener DR, Wek RC. Activating transcription factor 3 is integral to the eukaryotic initiation factor 2 kinase stress response. Mol Cell Biol. 2004;24(3): 1365–77.

28. Xiaoyan L, Shengbing Z, Yu Z, Lin Z, Chengjie L, Jingfeng L, Aimin H. Low expression of activating transcription factor 3 in human hepatocellular carcinoma and its clinicopathological significance. Pathol Res Pract. 2014; 210(8):477–81.

22

Influence of light alcohol consumption on lifestyle-related diseases: a predictor of fatty liver with liver enzyme elevation in Japanese females with metabolic syndrome

Masahiro Sogabe[1,2,3*], Toshiya Okahisa[1,2], Tadahiko Nakagawa[2], Hiroshi Fukuno[4], Masahiko Nakasono[5], Tetsu Tomonari[2], Takahiro Tanaka[2], Hironori Tanaka[2], Tatsuya Taniguchi[2], Naoki Muguruma[2] and Tetsuji Takayama[2]

Abstract

Background: Although heavy drinking is known to lead to liver injury, some recent studies have reported that light alcohol consumption (LAC) may play a protective role against fatty liver in the general population, and may even play a protective role against non-alcoholic fatty liver disease (NAFLD) in males with metabolic syndrome (MS). However, the association between LAC and fatty liver with liver enzyme elevation in females with MS is unclear.

Methods: Participants of this study were 20,853 females who underwent a regular health check-up between April 2008 and March 2012 at our hospital. Enrolled subjects were 1141 females with MS, who underwent all necessary tests and drank less than 20 g/day of alcohol. We investigated the presence of fatty liver with liver enzyme elevation, defined in this study as alanine aminotransferase (ALT) levels $\geqq 31$ IU/l, and the association between LAC and fatty liver with ALT elevation.

Results: There was no significant difference in the prevalence of fatty liver and ALT between light drinkers and non-drinkers. The prevalence of individuals receiving a treatment for dyslipidemia and impaired glucose tolerance (IGT) was significantly lower in light drinkers than in non-drinkers. Body mass index (BMI), waist circumference (WC), diastolic blood pressure (DBP), triglyceride (TG), uric acid (UA), IGT, and visceral fat type MS (V-type MS) were significant predictors of the prevalence of fatty liver with ALT elevation in logistic regression analysis. The odds ratio [OR] (95 % confidence interval [CI], p value) for fatty liver with ALT elevation were as follows: BMI, 2.181 (1.445–3.293, $p < 0.001$); WC, 1.853 (1.280–2.684, $p < 0.01$); DBP, 1.604 (1.120–2.298, $p < 0.05$); TG, 2.202 (1.562–3.105, $p < 0.001$); UA, 2.959 (1.537–5.698, $p < 0.01$); IGT, 1.692 (1.143–2.506, $p < 0.01$); and V-type MS, 3.708 (2.529–5.437, $p < 0.001$).

Conclusions: There was no significant difference in the prevalence of fatty liver with ALT elevation in females with MS between light drinkers and non-drinkers, suggesting that other factors such as BMI, WC, V-type MS, and lifestyle-related disease may be more important than LAC for the prevalence of fatty liver with ALT elevation.

Keywords: Light alcohol consumption, Fatty liver with ALT elevation, Females, Metabolic syndrome

* Correspondence: tokushimakenananshi@yahoo.co.jp
[1]Department of General Medicine and Community Health Science, Institute of Biomedical Sciences, Tokushima University Graduate School, 3-18-15 Kuramoto-cho, Tokushima City, Tokushima 770-8503, Japan
[2]Department of Gastroenterology and Oncology, Institute of Biomedical Sciences, Tokushima University Graduate School, Tokushima, Japan
Full list of author information is available at the end of the article

Background

The prevalence of MS defined as obese individuals with abnormalities in hypertension, glucose metabolism, and dyslipidemia, has been increasing in countries of both advanced and emerging economies. This increase in prevalence is problematic due to the association of MS and various other diseases, as well as an increase medical expenses. Additionally, in Asian and western countries, the prevalence of non-alcoholic fatty liver disease (NAFLD), which is strongly associated with MS, has also been increasing [1, 2]. Although heavy drinking is believed to lead to liver injury [3], several recent studies have reported that moderate or light drinking plays a protective role against fatty liver [4–8]. Drinking may be problematic for persons with MS due to the differences in clinical background between persons with and without MS and the increase in total caloric intake due to drinking. Although light alcohol consumption (LAC) was shown to play a protective role against NAFLD in males with MS in a recent study [9], the prevalence of MS and NAFLD, and the influence of alcohol consumption are known to differ markedly between males and females. The present study investigated the association between LAC and fatty liver with alanine aminotransferase (ALT) elevation in females with MS.

Methods

Subjects and study design

Subjects were 20,853 females (mean age ± standard deviation 49.2 ± 11.5 years range 17–88), residing around Takamatsu city, who underwent a regular health check-up at our hospital between April 2008 and March 2012. We excluded subjects who did not fulfill the diagnostic criteria for MS, who were positive for hepatitis B surface antigen (HBsAg) and/or hepatitis C antibody (HCVAb), who did not hope to undergo ultrasound examination, or who consumed 20 g/day or more of alcohol. All subjects were informed that their clinical data may be retrospectively analyzed for an epidemiological study, and informed consent was obtained. This study was a cross-sectional study elucidating the association between LAC and fatty liver with ALT elevation in females with MS. The study design was approved by the Ethics Committees of Kagawa Prefectural Cancer Detection Center, and the study was performed in conformity with the Declaration of Helsinki.

Physical examination and serum biochemistry

Height and body weight were obtained from the participants. Height was measured to the nearest 0.1 cm and body weight was measured to the nearest 0.1 kg. Body mass index (BMI) was calculated as the weight (in kilograms) divided by the square of the height (in meters). Waist circumference (WC) was measured at the umbilical

level. Venous blood samples were taken from all subjects following a 12-h overnight fast. Aspartate aminotransferase (AST), ALT, gamma-glutamyl transpeptidase (GGT), total cholesterol (T-CHO), high-density lipoprotein (HDL) cholesterol, triglycerides (TG), low-density lipoprotein (LDL) cholesterol, uric acid (UA), fasting plasma glucose (FPG), and hemoglobin A1c (HbA1c) (National Glycohemoglobin Standardization Program [NGSP]) were analyzed immediately by common enzymatic methods using an auto analyzer (TBA-80FR; Toshiba Medical System Tokyo, Japan).

Evaluation of alcohol consumption

Lifestyle-related information such as medical history, smoking status, and alcohol consumption were obtained by a common standardized self-response questionnaire. The amount of alcohol consumed per drinking day was calculated in grams using representative percent alcohol by volume for each type of alcoholic beverages: 5 % for beer, 10 % for wine, 16 % for Japanese sake, 25 % for shochu, and 34 % for whiskey. Subjects were divided into two categories by the drinking information: nondrinkers, those drinking 12 drinks (one drink means less 10 g) or less per year of less than one drink/drinking day; and light drinkers those drinking, from more than zero to less than 20 g/drinking day. In addition, light drinkers were divided into two subcategories: minimal drinkers, those drinking from more than zero to less than 10 g/drinking day; and very light drinkers, those drinking from 10 g to less than 20 g/drinking day.

Diagnosis of MS

There are several diagnostic criteria for MS. We used the diagnostic criteria for MS proposed by the International Diabetes Federation (IDF) because this criteria has been used worldwide [10]. The MS criteria used in this study were as follows: WC must exceed 80 cm, and two or more of the following components must be present: (1) hypertension: blood pressure ≥130/85 mmHg or medicated for hypertension (2) dyslipidemia: HDL-C <50 mg/dl and/or TG ≥150 mg/dl, or medicated for dyslipidemia (3) impaired glucose tolerance: FPG ≥100 mg/dl or medicated for diabetes.

Ultrasonography

Standard ultrasonography was performed with the subjects to assess the abdomen including the liver, gallbladder, pancreas, kidney, and spleen, in a morning fasting state by trained technicians. A Xario SSA-660A instrument was used with a 3.5 MHz convex-array probe (Toshiba Medical System, Tokyo, Japan) for ultrasonography. During ultrasound examination, more than 20 abdominal images were saved in the database and reviewed by gastroenterologists, who had more than 10 years of experience in ultrasonography, without knowledge of the results of the subject's data, such as blood-test screening. We defined fatty liver by ultrasonography by the presence of liver-kidney echo contrast and liver brightness, as well as having deep attenuation and/or liver vessel blurring [11]. A liver biopsy is known to be the gold standard for the diagnosis of NAFLD. However, liver biopsy is not realistic to perform in a medical check-up because this method has a risk of bleeding. Thus, we investigated fatty liver with ALT elevation in the present study. Alanine aminotransferase elevation was defined as an ALT level of ≥ 31 IU/l in this study. Also, visceral fat was assessed by the abdominal wall fat index (AFI), defined by the ratio of preperitoneal and subcutaneous fat thicknesses [12]. This procedure has been widely employed in medical check-ups for the assessment of visceral fat due to the significant correlation between the ratio of visceral and subcutaneous fat area by computed tomography (CT) and AFI by ultrasonography [12]. Although CT is the best method for assessment of the visceral fat, radiation exposure by CT is a risk for young females. Therefore, we selected the use of ultrasonography to assess visceral fat in the present study.

Statistical analysis

This study was a cross-sectional study investigating the association between LAC and fatty liver with ALT elevation in females with MS. Baseline data are expressed as means ± standard deviation (SD) for all continuous variables and as subject number (%) for categorical variables. All statistical differences were considered significant at a P value of less than 0.05. The $\chi 2$-test or Student's t-test was used to compare and determine differences between two groups for independent samples and the P value was adjusted for confounding variables using analysis of covariance. Factors with a significant influence on the prevalence of fatty liver with ALT elevation were then determined by univariate analysis. Age, BMI, WC, SBP, DBP, TG, HDL-C, UA, IGT, MS type, smoking status, and drinking status were then subjected to a multivariate logistic regression analysis. Results are presented as odds ratios (ORs) with 95 % confidence interval (CI) for each variable. All statistical analyses were performed using Med Calc Software (Broekstraat, Mariakerke, Belgium).

Results

Enrollment

Enrolled subjects are shown in Fig. 1. Initial participants were 20,853 females who underwent a regular health check-up between April 2008 and March 2012 at our hospital. Subjects were enrolled after application of the inclusion and exclusion criteria described in the Methods section (Subjects and study design). Of the 20,853 subjects, 2606 (12.5 %) females fulfilled the diagnostic criteria for MS. Of the 2606 subjects, 1306 subjects answered the self-

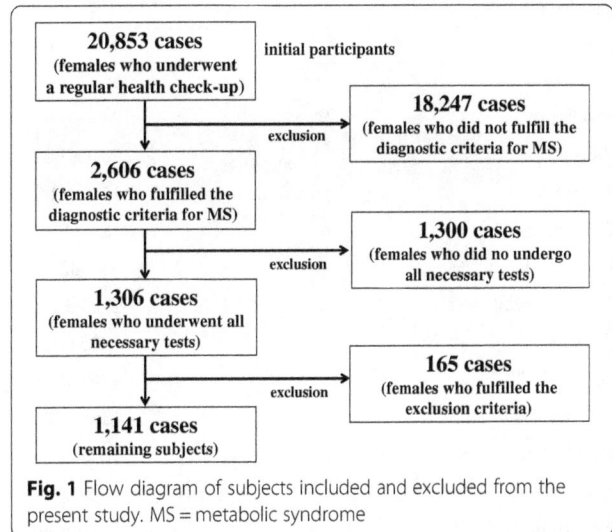

Fig. 1 Flow diagram of subjects included and excluded from the present study. MS = metabolic syndrome

response questionnaire, underwent physical examinations, blood-test screening, and abdominal ultrasonography. Of the 1306 subjects, we excluded 165 subjects who fulfilled the exclusion criteria, and the remaining 1141 subjects were enrolled in this study.

Subject characteristics

The characteristics of enrolled subjects are shown in Table 1. Mean age BMI, and WC was 56.6 ± 8.3 years (range, 29–85), 26.3 ± 3.6 kg/m^2 (range, 18.5–50.8), and 90.0 ± 7.2 cm (range, 80–117.5), respectively. Prevalence of hypertension, dyslipidemia, and impaired glucose tolerance (IGT) was 82.1, 93.4, and 74.7 %, respectively. The prevalence of fatty liver in all subjects was 56.3 %. Of the 1141 subjects with MS, the number of subjects with visceral type MS (V-type MS) and subcutaneous type MS (S-type MS) was 170 (14.9 %) and 971 (85.1 %), respectively. The proportion of light drinkers was 30.1 % in all subjects.

Clinical characteristics in light drinkers and non-drinkers

The comparison of clinical characteristics in females with MS between light drinkers and non-drinkers is shown in Table 2. The P^a value was adjusted for confounding variables including age, BMI, WC, smoking history, dyslipidemia, hypertension, and IGT. Age, BMI, and WC were significantly lower in light drinkers than in non-drinkers. There was no significant difference in the prevalence of hypertension, dyslipidemia, and IGT between light drinkers and non-drinkers. HbA1c were significantly lower in light drinkers than in non-drinkers. Regarding liver enzyme, there was no significant difference in ALT or AST between light drinkers and non-drinkers. In addition, there was no significant difference in the prevalence of fatty liver or fatty liver with ALT elevation between light drinkers and non-drinkers.

Table 1 Subject characteristics

Number	1141
Age (years)	56.6 ± 8.3
BMI (kg/m²)	26.3 ± 3.6
WC (cm)	90.0 ± 7.2
SBP (mmHg)	131.1 ± 14.1
DBP (mmHg)	78.0 ± 9.4
Hypertension, n (%)	937 (82.1 %)
T-CHO (mg/dl)	212.2 ± 33.3
TG (mg/dl)	122.5 ± 62.8
HDL (mg/dl)	59.8 ± 13.8
LDL (mg/dl)	135.9 ± 30.1
Dyslipidemia, n (%)	1066 (93.4 %)
UA (mg/dl)	4.9 ± 1.1
FPG (mg/dl)	107.9 ± 19.0
HbA1c (NGSP) (%)	6.0 ± 0.7
IGT, n (%)	852 (74.7 %)
ALT (IU/l)	27.2 ± 19.4
AST (IU/l)	23.7 ± 10.8
GGT (IU/l)	34.1 ± 31.2
FIB-4 index	2.7 ± 0.7
Fatty liver, n (%)	642 (56.3 %)
V-type MS, n (%)	170 (14.9 %)
Light drinker, n (%)	344 (30.1 %)
Past history of smoking, n (%)	103 (9.0 %)

Data are given as means ± standard deviation (SD), and as number (%) for categorical variables

ALT alanine aminotransferase, *AST* aspartate aminotransferase, *BMI* body mass index, *DBP* diastolic blood pressure, *FPG* fasting plasma glucose, *GGT* gamma-glutamyl transpeptidase, *HbA1c* hemoglobin A1c, *HDL* high density lipoprotein, *IGT* impaired glucose tolerance, *LDL* low density lipoprotein, *MS* metabolic syndrome, *NGSP* National Glycohemoglobin Standardization Program, *SBP* systolic blood pressure, *T-CHO* total cholesterol, *TG* triglyceride, *UA* uric acid, *V-type* visceral type, *WC* waist circumference. Light drinkers were subjects who drank from more than zero to less than 20 g/day of alcohol

Clinical characteristics in minimal drinkers and very light drinkers

The comparison of clinical characteristics in females with MS between minimal drinkers and very light drinkers is shown in Table 3. The P^a value was adjusted for confounding variables including age, BMI, WC, smoking history, dyslipidemia, hypertension, and IGT. There was no significant difference in age, BMI, and WC between minimal drinkers and very light drinkers. SBP, DBP, and the prevalence of hypertension were significantly lower in minimal drinkers than in very light drinkers. HDL was significantly higher in very light drinkers than in minimal drinkers. HbA1c was significantly lower in very light drinkers than in minimal drinkers. The prevalence of fatty liver and ALT was significantly lower in very light drinkers than in minimal drinkers.

Treatment for lifestyle-related diseases in light drinkers and non-drinkers

The comparison of those receiving treatment for lifestyle-related diseases between light drinkers and non-drinkers in females with MS is shown in Table 4. The P^a value was adjusted for confounding variables including age, BMI, WC, smoking history, dyslipidemia, hypertension, and IGT. There was no significant difference in the prevalence of those receiving treatment for hypertension, SBP, or DBP between light drinkers and non-drinkers. The prevalence of those receiving treatment for dyslipidemia was significantly lower in light drinkers than in non-drinkers. The prevalence of those receiving treatment for IGT or FBS in those receiving treatment for IGT was significantly lower in light drinkers than in non-drinkers.

Predictors of fatty liver with ALT elevation

Univariate and multivariate independent predictors of fatty liver with ALT elevation in females with MS are shown in Table 5. Of the 20 items related to the clinical background of subjects with or without fatty liver with ALT elevation, 14 items were identified as significant factors by univariate analysis. Multiple logistic regression analysis was performed with 12 items, with age, BMI, WC, SBP, DBP, TG, HDL, UA, IGT, MS type, drinking status, and smoking status as covariates. BMI, WC, DBP, TG, UA, IGT, and V-type MS were significant and independent predictors of an increased prevalence of fatty liver with ALT elevation. The odds ratio [OR] (95 % confidence interval [CI], p value) for fatty liver with ALT elevation were as follows: BMI, 2.181 (1.445–3.293, $p < 0.001$); WC 1.853 (1.280–2.684, $p < 0.01$); DBP 1.604 (1.120–2.298, $p < 0.05$); TG 2.202 (1.562–3.105, $p < 0.001$); UA 2.959 (1.537–5.698, $p < 0.01$); IGT 1.692 (1.143–2.506, $p < 0.01$); and V-type MS 3.708 (2.529–5.437, $p < 0.001$).

Discussion

This cross-sectional study explored the association between LAC and fatty liver with ALT elevation in females with MS. The association between MS and NAFLD has been shown to be mutually very strong [13, 14], and NAFLD is thought to be a manifestation of MS in the liver [13, 15, 16]. Light or moderate drinking has been reported to play a protective role against fatty liver in several studies [4–8]. Moreover, a recent study showed that the prevalence of NAFLD was significantly lower in light drinkers than in non-drinkers, and LAC was one of the significant factors of decreased prevalence of NAFLD, including males with MS [9]. However, the prevalence of MS, NAFLD including fatty liver, and the influence of alcohol consumption has been known to differ markedly between males and females. Additionally, females have been known to be more sensitive to the hepatic effects of alcohol than males in clinical and

Table 2 Comparison of clinical characteristics in females with MS between light drinkers and non-drinkers

	Light drinkers (n = 344)	Non-drinkers (n = 797)	P-value (P^a-value)
Age (years)	54.6 ± 7.9	57.5 ± 8.3	<0.001
BMI (kg/m²)	25.9 ± 3.5	26.4 ± 3.6	<0.05
WC (cm)	89.1 ± 7.1	90.3 ± 7.2	<0.05
SBP (mmHg)	129.7 ± 13.3	131.7 ± 14.4	(NS)
DBP (mmHg)	77.9 ± 9.3	78.0 ± 9.4	(NS)
Hypertension, n (%)	282 (82.0 %)	655 (82.2 %)	(NS)
T-CHO (mg/dl)	214.6 ± 34.8	211.1 ± 32.6	(NS)
TG (mg/dl)	121.5 ± 64.8	122.9 ± 62.0	(NS)
HDL (mg/dl)	60.2 ± 13.8	59.7 ± 13.8	(NS)
LDL (mg/dl)	138.0 ± 31.1	135.0 ± 29.6	(NS)
Dyslipidemia, n (%)	324 (99.4 %)	742 (93.1 %)	(NS)
UA (mg/dl)	4.9 ± 1.1	4.9 ± 1.1	(NS)
FPG (mg/dl)	106.5 ± 14.4	108.5 ± 20.6	(NS)
HbA1c (NGSP) (%)	5.9 ± 0.6	6.1 ± 0.8	(<0.05)
IGT, n (%)	261 (75.9 %)	591 (74.2 %)	(NS)
ALT (IU/l)	27.2 ± 21.4	27.2 ± 18.5	(NS)
AST (IU/l)	23.0 ± 9.9	24.0 ± 11.2	(NS)
GGT (IU/l)	32.3 ± 27.4	34.8 ± 32.6	(NS)
FIB-4 index	2.5 ± 0.6	2.7 ± 0.7	(NS)
Fatty liver, n (%)	188 (54.7 %)	454 (57.0 %)	(NS)
FL with ALT elevation, n (%)	76 (22.1 %)	177 (22.2 %)	(NS)
V-type MS, n (%)	55 (16.0 %)	115 (14.4 %)	(NS)
Past history of smoking, n (%)	49 (14.2 %)	54 (6.8 %)	<0.001

Data are given as means ± standard deviation (SD), and as number (%) for categorical variables. P-value is based on the X2 test or Student's t-test. Significant is at the 5 % level

ALT alanine aminotransferase, *AST* aspartate aminotransferase, *BMI* body mass index, *DBP* diastolic blood pressure, *FL* fatty liver, *FPG* fasting plasma glucose, *GGT* gamma-glutamyl transpeptidase, *HbA1c* hemoglobin A1c, *HDL* high density lipoprotein, *IGT* impaired glucose tolerance, *LDL* low density lipoprotein, *MS* metabolic syndrome, *NGSP* National Glycohemoglobin Standardization Program, *NS* not significant, *SBP* systolic blood pressure, *T- CHO* total cholesterol, *TG* triglyceride, *UA* uric acid, *V-type* visceral type, *WC* waist circumference. ALT elevation was defined as ALT level of >31 IU/l in this study. Light drinkers were subjects who drank from more than zero to less than 20 g/day of alcohol. Non-drinkers were subjects who drank 12 drinks (one drink means less 10 g) or less per year of less than 10 g/drinking day

[a]Adjusted for age, BMI, WC, smoking history, dyslipidemia, hypertension, and IGT

experimental studies [17–19]. However, the association between LAC and fatty liver with ALT elevation in females with MS is unclear. Results from this study demonstrated that there was no significant difference in the prevalence of fatty liver with ALT elevation between light drinkers and non-drinkers; however, the prevalence of those undergoing treatment for dyslipidemia and IGT was significantly lower in light drinkers than in non-drinkers in females with MS. BMI, WC, V-type MS, and lifestyle-related disease were important factors for the prevalence of fatty liver with ALT elevation in females with MS.

Ethanol induces hepatic lipid synthesis and may reduce hepatic fatty acid oxidation [20]. However alcohol consumption is known to cause fatty liver in some cases [20, 21]. Light or moderate drinking was associated with a lower incidence of hypertransaminasemia [5, 6] and a

decreased risk of fatty liver [4, 7, 8] in recent clinical studies. The prevalence of fatty liver was reported to be significantly decreased by light or moderate drinking in a study with asymptomatic Japanese male subjects [7]. However, the influence of alcohol intake is known to differ between males and females [17–19, 22], and the association between liver enzyme, NAFLD including fatty liver, and LAC in females has been controversial. It was reported that the odds ratio for MS was decreased to less than 1 in females with LAC [23], and the prevalence of fatty liver in females was reported to be significantly lower in drinkers than in non-drinkers [8]. On the other hand, it was reported in a recent study that there was no association between the prevalence of elevated liver enzyme levels and alcohol consumption in females [24]. Additionally, in a recent prospective study from the UK, excess body weight was reported to contribute to almost

Table 3 Comparison of clinical characteristics in females with MS between minimal drinkers and very light drinkers

	Minimal drinkers ($n = 250$)	Very light drinkers ($n = 94$)	P-value (P^a-value)
Age (years)	54.6 ± 7.9	54.5 ± 7.8	NS
BMI (kg/m^2)	25.8 ± 3.3	26.0 ± 4.0	NS
WC (cm)	89.0 ± 6.8	89.5 ± 8.0	NS
SBP (mmHg)	128.9 ± 13.4	131.8 ± 12.8	(<0.01)
DBP (mmHg)	77.3 ± 9.9	79.6 ± 7.5	(<0.01)
Hypertension, n (%)	197 (78.8 %)	85 (90.4 %)	(<0.001)
T-CHO (mg/dl)	213.2 ± 34.8	218.5 ± 34.5	(NS)
TG (mg/dl)	123.3 ± 67.7	116.6 ± 56.3	(NS)
HDL (mg/dl)	59.3 ± 13.9	62.8 ± 13.2	(<0.05)
LDL (mg/dl)	137.1 ± 31.0	140.3 ± 31.5	(NS)
Dyslipidemia, n (%)	235 (94.0 %)	89 (94.7 %)	(NS)
UA (mg/dl)	4.9 ± 1.1	5.1 ± 1.1	(NS)
FPG (mg/dl)	106.7 ± 14.7	105.9 ± 13.6	(NS)
HbA1c (NGSP) (%)	6.0 ± 0.6	5.8 ± 0.4	(<0.05)
IGT, n (%)	186 (74.4 %)	75 (79.8 %)	(NS)
ALT (IU/l)	28.5 ± 23.2	23.9 ± 15.2	(<0.05)
AST (IU/l)	23.0 ± 10.4	22.0 ± 8.0	(NS)
GGT (IU/l)	30.5 ± 22.9	36.9 ± 36.6	(NS)
FIB-4 index	2.5 ± 0.6	2.5 ± 0.6	(NS)
Fatty liver, n (%)	148 (59.2 %)	40 (42.6 %)	(<0.01)
FL with ALT elevation, n (%)	60 (24.0 %)	16 (17.0 %)	(NS)
V-type MS, n (%)	39 (15.6 %)	16 (17.0 %)	(NS)
Past history of smoking, n (%)	28 (11.2 %)	21 (22.3 %)	<0.05

Data are given as means ± standard deviation (SD), and as number (%) for categorical variables. P-value is based on the X2 test or Student's t-test. Significant is at the 5 % level

ALT alanine aminotransferase, AST aspartate aminotransferase, BMI body mass index, DBP diastolic blood pressure, FL fatty liver, FPG fasting plasma glucose, GGT gamma-glutamyl transpeptidase, HbA1c hemoglobin A1c, HDL high density lipoprotein, IGT impaired glucose tolerance, LDL low density lipoprotein, MS metabolic syndrome, NGSP National Glycohemoglobin Standardization Program, NS not significant, SBP systolic blood pressure, T-CHO total cholesterol, TG triglyceride, UA uric acid, V-type visceral type, WC waist circumference. ALT elevation was defined as ALT level of >31 IU/l in this study. Minimal drinkers were subjects who drank from more than zero to less than 10 g/day of alcohol. Very light drinkers were subjects who drank from 10 to less than 20 g/day of alcohol
[a]Adjusted for age, BMI, WC, smoking history, dyslipidemia, hypertension, and IGT

20 % of liver cirrhosis-related hospital admission and deaths in middle-aged female subjects, and alcohol consumption contributed to almost 50 % [25]. However, in the majority of reports on the effect of alcohol consumption on MS, subjects were almost always from a general population and were not divided into those with and without MS, or those with fatty liver were not divided with respect to liver enzyme elevation. To address this, the present study was limited to only female subjects with MS, and showed that there was no significant difference in the prevalence of fatty liver with ALT elevation between light drinkers and non-drinkers.

The mechanism of this inverse association between drinking and NAFLD including fatty liver remains unclear. Light to moderate drinking may enhance insulin sensitivity [21, 26] and reduce the risk of non-alcoholic steatohepatitis, possibly due to reduced insulin resistance [4]. Although the present study showed that there

was no significant difference in the prevalence of fatty liver with ALT elevation or IGT between light drinkers and non-drinkers, the prevalence of those undergoing treatment for IGT was significantly lower in light drinkers than in non-drinkers in females with MS. It is known that obesity increases fat deposition in hepatocytes and the progression of fatty liver, which may lead to inflammation, liver fibrosis, and liver cirrhosis [27]. The improvement of insulin sensitivity by light drinking may have been weak because subjects in the present study were obese with MS. The beneficial effects of reducing a risk of fatty liver may be weak in light female drinkers with MS, due to the lack of significant difference in insulin sensitivity between light drinkers and non-drinkers in females with MS.

Although it was reported that drinking had a positive effect on HDL-C levels [28], there was no significant difference in HDL levels between light drinkers and non-

Table 4 Comparison of those receiving treatment for lifestyle-related diseases between light drinkers and non-drinkers in females with MS

Lifestyle-related disease	Presence of treatment	Light drinkers (n = 344)	Non-drinkers (n = 797)	P-value (Pª-value)
Hypertension	Treatment (+), n (%)	128 (37.2 %)	330 (41.4 %)	NS
	SBP (mmHg)	130.5 ± 13.7	133.2 ± 15.7	(NS)
	DBP (mmHg)	77.3 ± 8.6	78.6 ± 9.2	(NS)
	Treatment (−), n (%)	216 (62.8 %)	467 (58.6 %)	
	SBP (mmHg)	129.2 ± 13.0	130.6 ± 13.4	(NS)
	DBP (mmHg)	78.3 ± 9.7	77.6 ± 9.6	(NS)
Dyslipidemia	Treatment (+), n (%)	85 (24.7 %)	320 (40.2 %)	<0.01
	T-CHO (mg/dl)	197.8 ± 32.4	201.0 ± 26.5	(NS)
	TG (mg/dl)	116.3 ± 49.4	113.4 ± 52.6	(NS)
	HDL (mg/dl)	63.8 ± 13.8	63.0 ± 14.0	(NS)
	LDL (mg/dl)	119.2 ± 26.3	122.7 ± 23.4	(NS)
	Treatment (−), n (%)	259 (75.3 %)	477 (59.8 %)	
	T-CHO (mg/dl)	220.2 ± 33.8	218.0 ± 34.5	(NS)
	TG (mg/dl)	123.2 ± 69.1	129.3 ± 66.9	(NS)
	HDL (mg/dl)	59.1 ± 13.6	57.4 ± 13.1	(NS)
	LDL (mg/dl)	144.2 ± 30.1	143.3 ± 30.5	(NS)
IGT	Treatment (+), n (%)	17 (4.9 %)	72 (9.0 %)	<0.05
	FBS (mg/dl)	124.1 ± 25.4	138.1 ± 33.4	(<0.05)
	HbA1c (NGSP) (%)	6.9 ± 0.9	7.2 ± 1.1	(NS)
	Treatment (−), n (%)	327 (95.1 %)	725 (91.0 %)	
	FBS (mg/dl)	105.6 ± 13.0	105.5 ± 16.2	(NS)
	HbA1c (NGSP) (%)	5.9 ± 0.5	6.0 ± 0.7	(NS)

Data are given as means ± standard deviation (SD), and as number (%) for categorical variables. P-value is based on the $x2$ test or Student's t-test. Significant is at the 5 % level

DBP diastolic blood pressure, FPG fasting plasma glucose, HbA1c hemoglobin A1c, HDL high density lipoprotein, IGT impaired glucose tolerance, LDL low density lipoprotein, NGSP National Glycohemoglobin Standardization Program, NS not significant, SBP systolic blood pressure, T-CHO total cholesterol, TG triglyceride, Light drinkers were subjects who drank from more than zero to less than 20 g/day of alcohol. Non-drinkers were subjects who drank 12 drinks (one drink means less 10 g) or less per year ofless than 10 g/drinking day

ªAdjusted for age, BMI, WC, smoking history, dyslipidemia, hypertension, and IGT

drinkers in females with MS in the present study. Interestingly, HDL was significantly higher in very light drinkers than in minimal drinkers. The effect of alcohol consumption on MS in the general population remains controversial. Although several reports have shown that the prevalence of MS is associated with alcohol consumption, irrespective of the amount consumed [29, 30], some another studies have reported beneficial effects of alcohol consumption on MS [31, 32]. It was recently reported that the prevalence of fatty liver was decreased along with the level of alcohol consumption in males subjects with MS, and alcohol consumption was associated with higher blood pressure, higher fasting plasma glucose, and a lower level of HDL-C in the male subjects who drank from more than zero to an excess of 280 g/week [23]. Although the present study showed that there was no significant difference in the prevalence of fatty liver with ALT elevation, hypertension, dyslipidemia, or IGT between light drinkers and non-drinkers, the prevalence

of those undergoing treatment for dyslipidemia or IGT was significantly higher in non-drinkers than light drinkers. These results suggest that females may differ from males in sensitivity to the hepatic effects of alcohol due to some factors, such as pharmacokinetics or metabolism of alcohol [18]. Additionally, the present results may also be influenced by the difference in adipose tissue distribution [33, 34], estrogen-related sex hormones [35, 36], treatment for lifestyle-related disease, and other social lifestyle factors, such as physical activity, exercise, diet, and drinking patterns between males and females. Further investigation is warranted, due to the lack of more detailed investigation on social lifestyle factors.

We do not suggest that drinking is recommended for non-drinkers because LAC was not a significant factor of a decreased prevalence of fatty liver with ALT elevation in the present study, and the effects of drinking differ among individuals. Increased drinking is also not recommended for minimal drinkers. Although ALT and

Table 5 Results of univariate and multivariate: independent predictors of fatty liver with ALT elevation in females with MS

	Univariate analysis			Multivariate analysis		
	FL with ALT elevation (+) (n = 253)	FL with ALT elevation (−) (n = 888)	P-value	OR	95 % CI	P-value
Age (≧50/< 50 years)	187/66	739/149	<0.01	1.003	0.677–1.484	NS
BMI (≧25/< 25 kg/m²)	199/54	469/419	<0.001	2.181	1.445–3.293	<0.001
WC (≧90/< 90 cm)	166/87	348/540	<0.001	1.853	1.280–2.684	<0.01
SBP (≧130/< 130 mmHg)	138/115	557/331	<0.05	0.756	0.543–1.053	NS
DBP (≧85/< 85 mmHg)	76/177	197/691	<0.05	1.604	1.120–2.298	<0.05
Hypertension (+/−)	209/44	728/160	NS			
T-CHO (≧220/< 220 mg/dl)	103/150	340/548	NS			
TG (≧150/< 150 mg/dl)	105/148	206/682	<0.001	2.202	1.562–3.105	<0.001
HDL (<50/≧ 50 mg/dl)	96/157	217/671	<0.001	1.362	0.955–1.942	NS
LDL (≧140/< 140 mg/dl)	118/135	365/523	NS			
Dyslipidemia (+/−)	236/17	58/830	NS			
UA (≧7.0/< 7.0 mg/dl)	24/229	23/865	<0.001	2.959	1.537–5.698	<0.01
FPG (≧100/< 100 mg/dl)	202/51	641/247	<0.05			
HbA1c (≧6.5/< 6.5 % NGSP)	70/183	110/778	<0.001			
IGT (+/−)	204/49	648/240	<0.05	1.692	1.143–2.506	<0.01
AST (≧31/< 31 IU/l)	140/113	21/867	<0.001			
GGT (≧51/< 51 IU/l)	90/163	94/794	<0.001			
V-type MS/S-type MS	82/171	88/800	<0.001	3.708	2.529–5.437	<0.001
Light drinker/Non-drinker	76/177	268/620	NS	0.988	0.699–1.396	NS
Past history of smoking (+/−)	31/222	72/816	NS	1.182	0.705–1.981	NS

Significant is at the 5 % level

ALT alanine aminotransferase, AST aspartate aminotransferase, BMI body mass index, CI confidence interval, DBP diastolic blood pressure, FL fatty liver, FPG fasting plasma glucose, GGT gamma-glutamyl transpeptidase, HbA1c hemoglobin A1c, HDL high density lipoprotein, IGT impaired glucose tolerance, LDL low density lipoprotein, MS metabolic syndrome, NGSP National Glycohemoglobin Standardization Program, NS not significant, OR odds ratio, SBP systolic blood pressure, S-type subcutaneous-type, T-CHO total cholesterol, TG triglyceride, UA uric acid, V-type visceral type, WC waist circumference. Light drinkers were subjects who drank from more than zero to less than 20 g/day of alcohol. Non-drinkers were subjects who drank 12 drinks (one drink means less 10 g) or less per year of less than 10 g/drinking day. ALT elevation was defined as ALT level of >31 IU/l in this study

the prevalence of fatty liver were significantly lower in very light drinkers than in minimal drinkers, the prevalence of hypertension was significantly higher in very light drinkers than in minimal drinkers. Alanine aminotransferase and lifestyle-related diseases, such as hypertension, dyslipidemia, and IGT, may be more affected in non-drinkers and minimal drinkers with MS by the increased eating duration due to alcohol consumption. Interestingly, the prevalence of hypertension in light daily drinkers (from more than zero to less than 10 g/ every day) was shown to be significantly higher than in non-drinkers in the present study (data not shown). In addition, individuals with MS and patients with risk of drinking abuse should not be advised to drink heavily. In particular, heavy drinking should not be recommended for individuals with MS because excess alcohol consumption is known to be a risk for mortality and death from noncardiovascular causes [37, 38], and MS is known to be a risk factor for arteriosclerotic diseases and ischemic heart disease [39]. Despite the possibility that heavy drinking may have a beneficial effect against

fatty liver and on liver enzyme, we emphasize that heavy drinking should not be recommended for individuals with MS.

There are some limitations that should be noted in the present study. First the present study did not investigate the underlying mechanism between the association of LAC and fatty liver with ALT elevation in females with MS, due to the nature of the cross-sectional design. Second, detailed data, such as contents of subjects' diets, eating duration, total caloric intake, and physical activity were not investigated. Third, although the subjects in the present study were females, the state of menses was not investigated, and the levels of estrogen-related sex hormones were not measured. Fourth, there was a possibility that the proportion of those with mild steatosis undetectable by ultrasound may have been higher in light drinking subjects than in non-drinkers, because the sensitivity of detecting steatosis by ultrasound is known to be below 20–30 %. Fifth, although ALT is known to be a simple marker of liver enzymes, ALT is unable to reflect the severity of NAFLD. Last, there was a possibility of selection bias subjects in the present study may have high interest in health because they hoped to undergo a medical check-up in Ningen Dock. Further studies will be required to resolve these limitations.

Conclusion

The present study showed that there was no significant difference in the prevalence of fatty liver with ALT elevation between light drinkers and non-drinkers in females with MS. Body mass index, WC, DBP, TG, UA, IGT, and V-type MS were significant factors of an increased prevalence of fatty liver with ALT elevation, and the prevalence of individuals undergoing treatment for dyslipidemia or IGT was significantly lower in light drinkers than in non-drinkers in females with MS. We believe that BMI, WC, V-type MS, and lifestyle-related disease may be more important factors for the prevalence of fatty liver with ALT elevation than LAC in Japanese females with MS.

Abbreviations
AFI: abdominal wall fat index; ALT: alanine aminotransferase; AST: aspartate aminotransferase; BMI: body mass index; CI: confidence interval; DBP: diastolic blood pressure; DM: diabetic mellitus; FPG: fasting plasma glucose; GGT: gamma-glutamyl transpeptidase; HbA1c: hemoglobin A1c; HBsAg: hepatitis B surface antigen; HCVAb: hepatitis C antibody; HDL: high-density lipoprotein; IDF: International Diabetes Federation; IGT: impaired glucose tolerance; LAC: light alcohol consumption; LDL: low-density lipoprotein; MS: metabolic syndrome; NAFLD: non-alcoholic fatty liver disease; NGSP: National Glycohemoglobin Standardization Program; NS: not significant; OR: odds ratio; SBP: systolic blood pressure; SD: standard deviation; S-type: subcutaneous type; T-CHO: total cholesterol; TG: triglyceride; UA: uric acid; V-type: visceral type; WC: waist circumference.

Competing interests
The authors declare that they have no conflict of interest to report present study.

Authors' contributions
MS designed the study, coordinated it, and wrote the manuscript. TO co-designed the study and helped to improve the manuscript. TN was responsible for the statistical analysis. HF was responsible for the assessment of ultrasonography, and performed laboratory data collection. MN contributed to the advice of study design and discussed the data. TT performed laboratory data collection and the statistical analysis. TT was responsible for the assessment of ultrasonography. HT performed laboratory data collection. TT performed the statistical analysis. NM co-designed the study. TT contributed to the advice of study design. All authors read and approved the final manuscript.

Acknowledgments
The authors would like to thank all subjects in our study.

Author details
[1]Department of General Medicine and Community Health Science, Institute of Biomedical Sciences, Tokushima University Graduate School, 3-18-15 Kuramoto-cho, Tokushima City, Tokushima 770-8503, Japan. [2]Department of Gastroenterology and Oncology, Institute of Biomedical Sciences, Tokushima University Graduate School, Tokushima, Japan. [3]Department of Gastroenterology, Kagawa Prefectural Cancer Detection Center, Takamatsu, Japan. [4]Department of Internal Medicine, Higashi Tokushima Medical Center, Tokushima, Japan. [5]Department of Internal Medicine, Tsurugi Municipal Handa Hospital, Tokushima, Japan.

References

1. Caballeria L, Auladell MA, Toran P, Miranda D, Aznar J, Pera G, Gil D, Munoz L, Planas J, Canut S, Bernad J, Auba J, Pizarro G, Aizpurua MM, Altaba A, Tibau A. Prevalence and factors associated with the presence of non alcoholic fatty liver disease in an apparently healthy adult population in primary care units. BMC Gastroenterol. 2007;7:41.
2. Amarapurkar DN, Hashimoto E, Lesmana LA, Sollano JD, Chen PJ, Goh KL. How common is non-alcoholic fatty liver disease in the Asia-Pacific region and are there local differences? J Gastroenterol Hepatol. 2007;22: 788–93.
3. Ruhl CE, Everhart JE. Joint effects of body weight and alcohol on elevated serum alanine aminotransferase in the United States population. Clin Gastroenterol Hepatol. 2005;3:1260–8.
4. Dixon JB, Bhathal PS, O'Brien PE. Nonalcoholic fatty liver disease: predictors of nonalcoholic steatohepatitis and liver fibrosis in the severely obese. Gastroenterology. 2001;121:91–100.
5. Suzuki A, Angulo P, St Sauver J, Muto A, Okada T, Lindor K. Light to moderate alcohol consumption is associated with lower frequency of hypertransaminasemia. Am J Gastroenterol. 2007;102:1912–9.
6. Dunn W, Xu R, Schwimmer JB. Modest wine drinking and decreased prevalence of suspected non-alcoholic fatty liver disease. Hepatology. 2008; 47:1947–54.
7. Gunji T, Matsuhashi N, Sato H, Fujibayashi K, Okumura M, Sasabe N, Urabe A. Light and moderate alcohol consumption significantly reduces the prevalence of fatty liver in the Japanese male population. Am J Gastroenterol. 2009;104:2189–95.
8. Moriya A, Iwasaki Y, Ohguchi S, Kayashima E, Mitsumune T, Taniguchi H, Ikeda F, Shiratori Y, Yamamoto K. Alcohol consumption appears to protect against non-alcoholic fatty liver disease. Aliment Pharmacol Ther. 2011;33: 378–88.
9. Sogabe M, Okahisa T, Taniguchi T, Tomonari T, Tanaka T, Tanaka H, Nakasono M, Takayama T. Light alcohol consumption plays a protective role against non-alcoholic fatty liver disease in Japanese men with metabolic syndrome. Liver Int. 2015;35:1707–14.
10. The IDF consensus worldwide definition of the metabolic syndrome [article online]. Available from http://www.idf.org/home.
11. Hamaguchi M, Kojima T, Itoh Y, Harano Y, Fujii K, Nakajima T, Kato T, Takeda N, Okuda J, Ida K, Kawahito Y, Yoshikawa T, Okanoue T. The severity of ultrasonographic findings in nonalcoholic fatty liver disease reflects the metabolic syndrome and visceral fat accumulation. Am J Gastroenterol. 2007;102:2708–15.
12. Suzuki R, Watanabe S, Hirai Y, Akiyama K, Nishide T, Matsushima Y, Murayama H, Ohshima H, Shinomiya M, Shirai K. Abdominal wall fat index, estimated by ultrasonography, for assessment of the ratio of visceral fat to subcutaneous fat in the abdomen. Am J Med. 1993;95:309–14.
13. Neuschwander-Tetri BA. Nonalcoholic steatohepatitis and the metabolic syndrome. Am J Med Sci. 2005;330:326–35.
14. Marchesini G, Bugianesi E, Forlani G, Cerrelli F, Lenzi M, Manini R, Natale S, Vanni E, Villanova N, Melchionda N, Rizzetto M. Nonalcoholic fatty liver, steatohepatitis, and the metabolic syndrome. Hepatology. 2003;37:917–23.
15. Marchesini G, Brizi M, Bianchi G, Tomassetti S, Bugianesi E, Lenzi M, McCullough AJ, Natale S, Forlani G, Melchionda N. Nonalcoholic fatty liver disease: a feature of the metabolic syndrome. Diabetes. 2001;50:1844–50.
16. Eckel RH, Grundy SM, Zimmet PZ. The metabolic syndrome. Lancet. 2005; 365:1415–28.
17. Becker U, Deis A, Sorensen TI, Gronbaek M, Borch-Johnsen K, Muller CF, Schnohr P, Jensen G. Prediction of risk of liver disease by alcohol intake, sex, and age: a prospective population study. Hepatology. 1996;23:1025–9.
18. Sato N, Lindros KO, Baraona E, Ikejima K, Mezey E, Jarvelainen HA, Ramchandani VA. Sex difference in alcohol-related organ injury. Alcohol Clin Exp Res. 2001;25(Suppl):40S–5.
19. Jarvelainen HA, Lukkari TA, Heinaro S, Sippel H, Lindros KO. The antiestrogen toremifene protects against alcoholic liver injury in female rats. J Hepatol. 2001;35:46–52.
20. You M, Crabb DW. Recent advances in alcoholic liver disease II. Minireview: molecular mechanisms of alcoholic fatty liver. Am J Physiol Gastrointest Liver Physiol. 2004;287:G1–6.
21. Donohue Jr TM. Alcohol-induced steatosis in liver cells. World J Gastroenterol. 2007;13:4974–8.
22. Taniai M, Hashimoto E, Tokushige K, Kodama K, Kogiso T, Torii N, Shiratori K. Roles of gender, obesity, and lifestyle-related diseases in alcoholic liver

disease: obesity does not influence the severity of alcoholic liver disease. Hepatology Research. 2012;42:359–67.

23. Hamaguchi M, Kojima T, Ohbora A, Takeda N, Fukui M, Kato T. Protective effect of alcohol consumption for fatty liver but not metabolic syndrome. World J Gastroenterol. 2012;18:156–67.

24. Park EY, Lim MK, Oh JK, Cho H, Bae MJ, Yun EH, Kim DI, Shin HR. Independent and Supra-Additive Effects of Alcohol Consumption, Cigarette Smoking, and Metabolic Syndrome on the Elevation of Serum Liver Enzyme Levels. PLoS One. 2013;8:e63439.

25. Liu B, Balkwill A, Reeves G, Beral V. Body mass index and risk of liver cirrhosis in middle aged UK women: prospective study. BMJ. 2010;340:c912.

26. Zhou YJ, Li YY, Nie YQ, Ma JX, Lu LG, Shi SL, Chen MH, Hu PJ. Prevalence of fatty liver disease and its risk factors in the population of South China. World J Gastroenterol. 2007;13:6419–24.

27. Farrell GC, Larter CZ. Nonalcoholic fatty liver disease: from steatosis to cirrhosis. Hepatology. 2006;43:S99–112.

28. Rimm EB, Williams P, Fosher K, Criqui M, Stampfer MJ. Moderate alcohol intake and lower risk of coronary heart disease: meta-analysis of effects on lipids and haemostatic factors. BMJ. 1999;319:1523–8.

29. Baik I, Shin C. Prospective study of alcohol consumption and metabolic syndrome. Am J Clin Nutr. 2008;87:1455–63.

30. Yokoyama H, Hiroshi H, Ohgo H, Hibi T, Saito I. Effects of excessive ethanol consumption on the diagnosis of the metabolic syndrome using its clinical diagnostic criteria. Intern Med. 2007;46:1345–52.

31. Gigleux I, Gagnon J, St-Pierre A, Cantin B, Dagenais GR, Meyer F, Despres JP, Lamarche B. Moderate alcohol consumption is more cardioprotective in men with the metabolic syndrome. J Nutr. 2006;136:3027–32.

32. Freiberg MS, Cabral HJ, Heeren TC, Vasan RS, Curtis Ellison R. Alcohol consumption and the prevalence of the Metabolic Syndrome in the US: a cross-sectional analysis of data from the Third National Health and Nutrition Examination Survey. Diabetes Care. 2004;27:2954–9.

33. Kvist H, Chowdhury B, Grangard U, Tylen U, Sjostrom L. Total and visceral adipose-tissue volumes derived from measurements with computed tomography in adult men and women: predicted equations. Am J Clin Nutr. 1988;48:1351–61.

34. Lemieux S, Prud'homme D, Bouchard C, Tremblay A, Despres JP. Sex differences in the relation of visceral adipose tissue accumulation to total body fatness. Am J Clin Nutr. 1993;58:463–7.

35. Suzuki A, Abdelmalek MF. Nonalcoholic fatty liver disease in women. Womens Health (Lond Engl). 2009;5:191–203.

36. Ayonrinde OT, Olynyk JK, Beilin LJ, Mori TA, Pennell CE, de Klerk N, Oddy WH, Shipman P, Adams LA. Gender-specific differences in adipose distribution and adipocytokines influence adolescent nonalcoholic fatty liver disease. Hepatology. 2011;53:800–9.

37. Fuchs CS, Stampfer MJ, Colditz GA, Giovannucci EL, Manson JE, Kawachi I, Hunter DJ, Hankinson SE, Hennekens CH, Rosner B. Alcohol consumption and mortality among women. N Engl J Med. 1995;332:1245–50.

38. Thun MJ, Peto R, Lopez AD, Monaco JH, Henley SJ, Heath Jr CW, Dorr R. Alcohol consumption and mortality among middle-aged and elderly U.S. adults. N Engl J Med. 1997;337:1705–14.

39. Lakka HM, Laaksonen DE, Lakka TA, Niskanen LK, Kumpusalo E, Tuomilehto J, Salonen JT. The metabolic syndrome and total and cardiovascular disease mortality in middle-aged men. JAMA. 2002;288:2709–16.

Permissions

The contributors of this book come from diverse backgrounds, making this book a truly international effort. This book will bring forth new frontiers with its revolutionizing research information and detailed analysis of the nascent developments around the world.

We would like to thank all the contributing authors for lending their expertise to make the book truly unique. They have played a crucial role in the development of this book. Without their invaluable contributions this book wouldn't have been possible. They have made vital efforts to compile up to date information on the varied aspects of this subject to make this book a valuable addition to the collection of many professionals and students.

This book was conceptualized with the vision of imparting up-to-date information and advanced data in this field. To ensure the same, a matchless editorial board was set up. Every individual on the board went through rigorous rounds of assessment to prove their worth. After which they invested a large part of their time researching and compiling the most relevant data for our readers.

The editorial board has been involved in producing this book since its inception. They have spent rigorous hours researching and exploring the diverse topics which have resulted in the successful publishing of this book. They have passed on their knowledge of decades through this book. To expedite this challenging task, the publisher supported the team at every step. A small team of assistant editors was also appointed to further simplify the editing procedure and attain best results for the readers.

Apart from the editorial board, the designing team has also invested a significant amount of their time in understanding the subject and creating the most relevant covers. They scrutinized every image to scout for the most suitable representation of the subject and create an appropriate cover for the book.

The publishing team has been an ardent support to the editorial, designing and production team. Their endless efforts to recruit the best for this project, has resulted in the accomplishment of this book. They are a veteran in the field of academics and their pool of knowledge is as vast as their experience in printing. Their expertise and guidance has proved useful at every step. Their uncompromising quality standards have made this book an exceptional effort. Their encouragement from time to time has been an inspiration for everyone.

The publisher and the editorial board hope that this book will prove to be a valuable piece of knowledge for researchers, students, practitioners and scholars across the globe.

List of Contributors

Dae Yeong Kim, Kyung Joo Cho and Hye-Lim Ju
Institute of Gastroenterology, Yonsei University College of Medicine, Seoul 120-752, South Korea

Sook In Chung and Hyuk Moon
Institute of Gastroenterology, Yonsei University College of Medicine, Seoul 120-752, South Korea
Brain Korea 21 Project for Medical Science College of Medicine, Yonsei University, Seoul 120-752, South Korea

Do Young Kim, Sang Hoon Ahn and Kwang-Hyub Han
Department of Internal Medicine, Yonsei University College of Medicine, Seoul 120-752, South Korea

Simon Weonsang Ro
Institute of Gastroenterology, Yonsei University College of Medicine, Seoul 120-752, South Korea
Room 407, ABMRC, Severance Hospital, Yonsei University College of Medicine, Yonsei-ro 50-1, Seoul 120-752, South Korea

Wei Li
Department of Interventional Radiology, the Affiliated Hospital of Qingdao University, Qingdao, Shandong 266003, China

Chengwei Dong
Department of Hepatobiliary Surgery, Weifang People's Hospital, Weifang, Shandong 261041, China

Renan Spode, Nicolas Glaser, Nico Buettner, Tobias Boettler, Christoph Neumann-Haefelin, Michael Schultheiss and Robert Thimme
Department of Medicine II, Medical Center University of Freiburg, Faculty of Medicine, University of Freiburg, Hugstetter Str. 55, D-79106 Freiburg, Germany

Dominik Bettinger
Department of Medicine II, Medical Center University of Freiburg, Faculty of Medicine, University of Freiburg, Hugstetter Str. 55, D-79106 Freiburg, Germany
Berta-Ottenstein-Programme, Faculty of Medicine, University of Freiburg, Freiburg, Germany

Thomas Baptist Brunner and Eleni Gkika
Department of Radiation Oncology, Medical Center University of Freiburg,Faculty of Medicine, University of Freiburg, Robert-Koch-Str. 3, D-79106 Freiburg, Germany

Lars Maruschke
Department of Radiology, Medical Center University of Freiburg, Faculty of Medicine, University of Freiburg, Hugstetter Str. 55, D-79106 Freiburg, Germany

Aleena Jain
Department of Pathology, Seth GSMC & KEMH, Parel, Mumbai, India

Rachana Chaturvedi, Amita Joshi and Mangesh Londhe
Department of Pathology, Seth GSMC & KEMH, Mumbai, India

Chetan Kantharia
G. I. Surgery, Seth GSMC & KEMH, Mumbai, India

Mayura Kekan
Department of Pathology, TNMC & Nair Ch hospital, Mumbai, India

Chun-Yi Tsai, Motoi Nojiri, Yukihiro Yokoyama, Tomoki Ebata, Takashi Mizuno and Masato Nagino
Division of Surgical Oncology, Department of Surgery, Nagoya University Graduate School of Medicine, 65 Tsurumai-cho, Showa-ku, Nagoya 466-8550, Japan

Rui Yu and Lidong Chen
Department of Gastroenterology, The First Affiliated Hospital of Zhengzhou University, Zhengzhou, China

Qiangwei Shi
Department of Cardiology, The First Affiliated Hospital of Zhengzhou University, Zhengzhou, China

Lei Liu
Department of Nasology, The First Affiliated Hospital of Zhengzhou University, Zhengzhou, China

Bingsong Huang, Yi Shi, Suxiong Deng, Maogen Chen, Jun Li, Yi Ma and Ronghai Deng
Organ Transplant Center, the First Affiliated Hospital, Sun Yat-sen University, No. 58 Zhongshan 2nd Road, Guangzhou 510080, China

Jun Liu
Department of Respiratory, the First People's Hospital affiliated to Guangzhou Medical University, Guangzhou 510080, China

Paul M. Schroder
Department of Surgery, Duke University Medical Center, 10 Duke Medicine Circle Durham, Durham, NC 27710, USA

Rolf Hultcrantz and Per Stål
Unit of Liver Diseases, Department of Upper GI, C1-77 Huddinge, Karolinska University Hospital, Karolinska Institutet, 141 86 Stockholm, Sweden

Joel Marmur
Unit of Liver Diseases, Department of Upper GI, C1-77 Huddinge, Karolinska University Hospital, Karolinska Institutet, 141 86 Stockholm, Sweden
Unit of Gastroenterology and Hepatology, Department of Medicine, Ersta Hospital, Karolinska Institutet, Stockholm, Sweden

Soheir Beshara, Gösta Eggertsen and Liselotte Onelöv
Unit of Clinical Chemistry, Department of Laboratory Medicine, Karolinska University Hospital, Karolinska Institutet, Stockholm, Sweden

Nils Albiin
Department of Radiology, Ersta Hospital, Karolinska Institutet, Stockholm, Sweden

Olof Danielsson
Unit of Pathology, Department of Laboratory Medicine, Karolinska University Hospital, Karolinska Institutet, Stockholm, Sweden

Zhimin Liu, Zhifeng Zhang, Mei Huang, Bojia Liu, Qiyang Guo and Zhijun Duan
Second department of Gastroenterology, First Affiliated Hospital of Dalian Medical University, Dalian 116011, China

Xiaoping Sun and Qingshan Chang
The Sixth People's Hospital of Dalian, Dalian 116021, China

Birgit Tsaknakis, Rawan Masri, Ahmad Amanzada, Golo Petzold, Volker Ellenrieder, Albrecht Neesse and Steffen Kunsch
Department Gastroenterology and Gastrointestinal Oncology, University Medical Centre Goettingen Georg-August-University, Robert-Koch-Str. 40, 37075 Goettingen, Germany

Shuzhen Wang, Xin Zhang and Hui-Guo Ding
Department of Gastroenterology and Hepatology, Beijing You'an Hospital, Affiliated with Capital Medical University, Fengtai District, Beijing 100069, China

Tao Han
Department of Gastroenterology, Tianjin Third Central Hospital
Tianjin, China

Wen Xie
Department of Hepatology, Beijing Ditan Hospital, Affiliated with Capital Medical University, Beijing, China

Yonggang Li
Department of Hepatology, PLA 302 Hospital, Beijing, China

Hong Ma
Liver Diseases Center, Beijing Friendship Hospital, Affiliated with Capital Medical University, Beijing, China

Roman Liebe and Honglei Weng
Department of Medicine II, Section Molecular Hepatology, Medical Faculty Mannheim, Heidelberg University, Mannheim, Germany

Manping Huang, Bin Huang and Guowen Li
Department of Intervention, Hunan Cancer Hospital & The Affiliated Cancer Hospital of Xiangya School of Medicine, Central SouthUniversity, No.283, Tongzipo Road, Changsha 410013, People's Republic of China

Sainan Zeng
Infection Controlling Center, The Third Xiangya Hospital of Central South University, Tongzipo Road, Yuelu District, Changsha 410013, People's Republic of China

Heng-Yuan Hsu, Yi-Ping Liu, Tsung-Han Wu and Wei-Chen Lee
Department of Surgery, Linkou Chang Gung Memorial Hospital, No.5, Fuxing St, Guishan Dist, Taoyuan City 33305, Taiwan, Republic of China

Miin-Fu Chen
Department of Surgery, Linkou Chang Gung Memorial Hospital, No.5, Fuxing St, Guishan Dist, Taoyuan City 33305, Taiwan, Republic of China
College of Medicine, Chang Gung University, Guishan, Taoyuan, Taiwan, Republic of China

Hao-Tsai Cheng
College of Medicine, Chang Gung University, Guishan, Taoyuan, Taiwan, Republic of China
Graduate Institute of Clinical Medical Sciences, Chang Gung University, Guishan, Taoyuan, Taiwan, Republic of China
Department of Gastroenterology and Hepatology, Linkou Chang Gung Memorial Hospital, No.5, Fuxing St, Guishan Dist, Taoyuan City 33305, Taiwan, Republic of China

Chao-Wei Lee
Department of Surgery, Linkou Chang Gung Memorial Hospital, No.5, Fuxing St, Guishan Dist, Taoyuan City 33305, Taiwan, Republic of China
College of Medicine, Chang Gung University, Guishan, Taoyuan, Taiwan, Republic of China
Graduate Institute of Clinical Medical Sciences, Chang Gung University, Guishan, Taoyuan, Taiwan, Republic of China

Hsin-I Tsai
Graduate Institute of Clinical Medical Sciences, Chang Gung University, Guishan, Taoyuan, Taiwan, Republic of China
Department of Anesthesiology, Linkou Chang Gung Memorial Hospital, No.5, Fuxing St, Guishan Dist, Taoyuan City 33305, Taiwan, Republic of China

Wei-Ting Chen
Department of Gastroenterology and Hepatology, Linkou Chang Gung Memorial Hospital, No.5, Fuxing St, Guishan Dist, Taoyuan City 33305, Taiwan, Republic of China

Chien-Chih Chiu
Department of Nursing, Linkou Chang Gung Memorial Hospital, No.5, Fuxing St, Guishan Dist, Taoyuan City 33305, Taiwan, Republic of China

Ming-Chin Yu
Department of Surgery, Linkou Chang Gung Memorial Hospital, No.5, Fuxing St, Guishan Dist, Taoyuan City 33305, Taiwan, Republic of China
College of Medicine, Chang Gung University, Guishan, Taoyuan, Taiwan, Republic of China
Department of Surgery, Xiamen Chang Gung Hospital, Xiamen, China

Chang Seok Bang
Department of Internal Medicine, Hallym University College of Medicine, Chuncheon, Republic of Korea

Il Han Song
Division of Hepatology, Department of Internal Medicine, Dankook University College of Medicine, Cheonan, Korea, Republic of Korea

Sanae Haga and Michitaka Ozaki
Department of Biological Response and Regulation, Faculty of Health Sciences, Hokkaido University, N-12, W-5, Kita-ku, Sapporo, Hokkaido 060-0812, Japan.

Yimin
Department of Advanced Medicine, Graduate School of Medicine, Hokkaido University, N-15, W-7, Kita-ku, Sapporo, Hokkaido 060-8638, Japan

Jihyun An, Young-Suk Lim, Wonhee Jeong, Danbi Lee, Ju Hyun Shim, Hanu Lee and Yung Sang Lee
Department of Gastroenterology, Liver Center, Asan Medical Center, University of Ulsan College of Medicine, 88, Olympic-ro 43-gil, Songpa-gu, Seoul 05505, Korea

Gi-Ae Kim
Health Screening and Promotion Center, Asan Medical Center, Seoul, Republic of Korea

Seong-bong Han
Department of Applied Statistics, Gachon University, Seongnam-si, Gyeonggi-do, Republic of Korea

Bin Li
Department of Hepatobiliary & Pancreatovascular Surgery, First affiliated Hospital of Xiamen University, Xiamen, China

Yan-Ming Zhou
Department of Hepatobiliary & Pancreatovascular Surgery, First affiliated Hospital of Xiamen University, Xiamen, China
Department of Special Treatment, Eastern Hepatobiliary Surgery Hospital, Second Military Medical University, Shanghai, China

Xiao-Feng Zhang, Jia-Mei Yang and Cheng-Jun Sui
Department of Special Treatment, Eastern Hepatobiliary Surgery Hospital, Second Military Medical University, Shanghai, China

Marcello Persico, Mario Masarone and Tommaso Bucci
Internal Medicine and Hepatology Unit, PO G. Da Procida – AOU- San Giovanni e Ruggi D'Aragona, University of Salerno, Via Salvatore Calenda 162, CAP: 84126 Salerno, Italy

Antonio Damato, Mariateresa Ambrosio and Albino Carrizzo
Vascular Physiopathology Unit IRCCS, INM Neuromed, Pozzilli, IS, Italy

Alessandro Federico
Hepato-Gastroenterology Division, University of Campania "L. Vanvitelli", Naples, Italy

Valerio Rosato
Internal Medicine and Hepatology Department, University of Campania "L. Vanvitelli", Naples, Italy

Carmine Vecchione
Department of Medicine and Surgery, University of Salerno, Salerno, Italy

Norihiro Kishida, Osamu Itano, Masahiro Shinoda, Minoru Kitago, Hiroshi Yagi, Yuta Abe, Taizo Hibi and Yuko Kitagawa
Department of Surgery, School of Medicine, Keio University, 35 Shinanomachi, Shinjuku-ku, Tokyo 160-8582, Japan

Sachiko Matsuda
Department of Surgery, School of Medicine, Keio University, 35 Shinanomachi, Shinjuku-ku, Tokyo 160-8582, Japan
Chugai Pharmaceutical Endowed Research Chair in Molecular Targeted Therapy of Gastrointestinal Cancer, School of Medicine, Keio University, Tokyo, Japan

Yohei Masugi and Michiie Sakamoto
Department of Pathology, School of Medicine, Keio University, Tokyo, Japan

Koichi Aiura
Department of Surgery, Kawasaki Municipal Hospital, Kawasaki-ku, Japan

Nazarii Kobyliak, Galyna Mykhalchyshyn and Petro Bodnar
Bogomolets National Medical University, T. Shevchenko boulevard, 13, Kyiv 01601, Ukraine

Tetyana Falalyeyeva, Oleksandr Virchenko, Tetyana Beregova and Lyudmyla Ostapchenko
Taras Shevchenko National University of Kyiv, Volodymyrska Str., 64/13, Kyiv 01601, Ukraine

Mykola Spivak
Zabolotny Institute of Microbiology and Virology, National Academy of Sciences of Ukraine, Zabolotny Str., 154, Kyiv 03680, Ukraine

Dmytro Yankovsky
Scientific and Production Company "O.D. Prolisok", Kyiv, Ukraine

Jiaxian Wang and Jianwei Zhu
Engineering Research Center of Cell and Therapeutic Antibody, Ministry of Education, School of Pharmacy, Shanghai Jiao Tong University, 800 Dongchuan Rd, Biology and Pharmacy Building, suite 6-208, Shanghai 200240, People's Republic of China

Yunsheng Yuan
Engineering Research Center of Cell and Therapeutic Antibody, Ministry of Education, School of Pharmacy, Shanghai Jiao Tong University, 800 Dongchuan Rd, Biology and Pharmacy Building, suite 6-208, Shanghai 200240, People's Republic of China
The Shanghai Municipality Key Laboratory of Veterinary Biotechnology, School of Agriculture and Biology, Shanghai Jiao Tong University, 800 Dongchuan Rd, Shanghai 200240, People's Republic of China

Liang Zhou, Qing Deng and Yan Yu
The Shanghai Municipality Key Laboratory of Veterinary Biotechnology, School of Agriculture and Biology, Shanghai Jiao Tong University, 800 Dongchuan Rd, Shanghai 200240, People's Republic of China

Shunyan Weng
Engineering Research Center of Cell and Therapeutic Antibody, Ministry of Education, School of Pharmacy, Shanghai Jiao Tong University, 800 Dongchuan Rd, Biology and Pharmacy Building, suite 6-208, Shanghai 200240, People's Republic of China
The Shanghai Municipality Key Laboratory of Veterinary Biotechnology, School of Agriculture and Biology, Shanghai Jiao Tong University, 800 Dongchuan Rd, Shanghai 200240, People's Republic of China
School of Life Sciences and Biotechnology, Shanghai Jiao Tong University, 800 Dongchuan Rd, Shanghai 200240, People's Republic of China

Toshiya Okahisa
Department of General Medicine and Community Health Science, Institute of Biomedical Sciences, Tokushima University Graduate School, 3-18-15 Kuramoto-cho, Tokushima City, Tokushima 770-8503, Japan
Department of Gastroenterology and Oncology, Institute of Biomedical Sciences, Tokushima University Graduate School, Tokushima, Japan

Tadahiko Nakagawa, Tetsu Tomonari, Takahiro Tanaka, Hironori Tanaka, Tatsuya Taniguchi, Naoki Muguruma and Tetsuji Takayama
Department of Gastroenterology and Oncology, Institute of Biomedical Sciences, Tokushima University Graduate School, Tokushima, Japan

Masahiro Sogabe
Department of General Medicine and Community Health Science, Institute of Biomedical Sciences, Tokushima University Graduate School, 3-18-15 Kuramoto-cho, Tokushima City, Tokushima 770-8503, Japan
Department of Gastroenterology and Oncology, Institute of Biomedical Sciences, Tokushima University Graduate School, Tokushima, Japan
Department of Gastroenterology, Kagawa Prefectural Cancer Detection Center, Takamatsu, Japan

Hiroshi Fukuno
Department of Internal Medicine, Higashi Tokushima Medical Center, Tokushima, Japan

Masahiko Nakasono
Department of Internal Medicine, Tsurugi Municipal Handa Hospital, Tokushima, Japan

Index